The Public/Private Sector Mix in Healthcare Delivery

International Policy Exchange Series

Published in collaboration with the
Center for International Policy Exchanges
University of Maryland

Series Editors
Douglas J. Besharov
Neil Gilbert

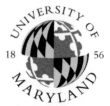

SCHOOL of
PUBLIC POLICY

The Public/Private Sector Mix in Healthcare Delivery

A Comparative Study

Edited by

HOWARD A. PALLEY, PHD

Professor Emeritus of Social Policy
School of Social Work
University of Maryland Baltimore
Baltimore, MD, USA

and

Distinguished Fellow
Institute for Human Services Policy
University of Maryland Baltimore
Baltimore, MD, USA

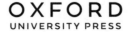

OXFORD
UNIVERSITY PRESS

OXFORD
UNIVERSITY PRESS

Oxford University Press is a department of the University of Oxford. It furthers
the University's objective of excellence in research, scholarship, and education
by publishing worldwide. Oxford is a registered trade mark of Oxford University
Press in the UK and certain other countries.

Published in the United States of America by Oxford University Press
198 Madison Avenue, New York, NY 10016, United States of America.

Library of Congress Cataloging-in-Publication Data
Names: Palley, Howard A., editor.
Title: The public/private sector mix in healthcare delivery : a comparative study /
[edited by] Howard A. Palley.
Other titles: International policy exchange series.
Description: New York, NY : Oxford University Press, [2023] |
Series: International policy exchange series |
Includes bibliographical references and index. |
Identifiers: LCCN 2022027430 (print) | LCCN 2022027431 (ebook) |
ISBN 9780197571101 (hardback) | ISBN 9780197571125 (epub) |
ISBN 9780197571132 (online)
Subjects: MESH: Delivery of Health Care | Public-Private Sector
Partnerships | Quality of Health Care | Health Equity | Health
Inequities | Comparative Study
Classification: LCC RA418 (print) | LCC RA418 (ebook) | NLM W 84.1 |
DDC 362.1—dc23/eng/20220727
LC record available at https://lccn.loc.gov/2022027430
LC ebook record available at https://lccn.loc.gov/2022027431

DOI: 10.1093/oso/9780197571101.001.0001

1 3 5 7 9 8 6 4 2

Printed by Sheridan Books, Inc., United States of America

To: the Future
My grandchildren:
Amelia and Charlotte Vitale
Emma, Harry, and Thomas Palley

Contents

Acknowledgments

I would like to acknowledge the encouragement, advice, and support of Douglas J. Besharov, Brody Professor of Public Policy, University of Maryland, and Neil Gilbert, Chernin Professor of Social Welfare and Social Services, University of California (Berkeley), in this endeavor. They serve as the co-editors-in-chief in the Oxford University Press Library on International Social Policy. Their support provided the incentive to go forward with this project. I would also be remiss if I did not thank Dana Bliss, Executive Editor at Oxford University Press, for his helpfulness and graciousness in responding to my numerous questions "along the way." Also, I would like to thank Janice C. Hicks, MSM, School of Social Work, University of Maryland, for her competence and graciousness in "putting things together" for the submission of the manuscript.

Contributors

Sara Allin, Associate Professor, Institute for Health Policy, Management, and Evaluation, and Director, North American Observatory on Health Systems and Policies, University of Toronto, Ontario, Canada

Xavier Ballart, Professor, Department of Political Science and Public Administration, Autonomous University of Barcelona, Barcelona, Spain

Pamela Bernales-Baksai, Research Associate, Facultad Latinoamericana de Ciencias Sociales (FLASCO Chile), Santiago, Chile

Luciene Burlandy, Professor, Faculty of Nutrition, Graduate Program in Nutritional Science and Graduate Program in Social Policy, Fluminense Federal University, Niteroi, Brazil

Tatiana Chubarova, Head, Center for Economic Theory of Social Sector, Institute of Economics, Russian Academy of Sciences, Moscow, Russian Federation

Stephen Duckett, Honorary Enterprise Professor, School of Population and Global Health, University of Melbourne, Melbourne, Victoria, Australia

Guillermo Fuentes, Professor, Institute of Political Science, University of the Republic, Montevideo, Uruguay

Anna Häger Glenngård, Associate Professor and Senior Lecturer, School of Economics and Management, Lund University, Lund, Sweden

Natalya Grigorieva, Professor, Department of Political Analysis, School of Public Administration, Lomonosov Moscow State University, Moscow, Russian Federation

Colleen M. Grogan, Professor, Crown Family School of Social Work, Policy, and Practice; Director, Center of Health Policy and Administration, University of Chicago, IL, USA

Michael K. Gusmano, Professor of Health Policy and Associate Dean of Academic Programs, College of Health, Lehigh University, Bethlehem, PA, USA; Research Scholar, The Hastings Center, Garrison, NY, USA

Patrick Jeurissen, Professor of Sustainable Health Care Systems, IQ Healthcare Scientific Institute for Quality of Healthcare, Radboud Institute for Health Sciences, Radboud University Medical Center, Nijmegen, the Netherlands

Florien M. Kruse, Postdoctoral Researcher, IQ Healthcare Scientific Institute for Quality of Healthcare, Radboud Institute for Health Sciences, Radboud University Medical Center, Nijmegen, the Netherlands

Ricardo Velázquez Leyer, Professor, Department of Social and Political Sciences, Universidad Iberoamericana, Cuidad de México, México

Lenaura de Vasconcelos Costa Lobato, Professor, School of Social Work and Post Graduate Program in Social Policy, Fluminense Federal University, Neteroi, Brazil

Gregory P. Marchildon, Professor and Ontario Research Chair of Health Policy and System Design, Institute of Health Policy, Management, and Evaluation, University of Toronto, Toronto, Ontario, Canada, and Founding Director, North American Observatory on Health Systems and Policies

Zeynep Or, Research Director, Institute for Research and Information on Health Economics (IRDES), Paris, France

Howard A. Palley, Professor Emeritus of Social Policy, School of Social Work, and Distinguished Fellow, Institute of Human Services Policy, University of Maryland, Baltimore, MD, USA

Aurélie Pierre, Health Economist, Institute for Research and Information on Health Economics (IRDES), Paris, France

Monica de Castro Maia Senna, Professor, School of Social Work and Post Graduate Program in Social Policy, Federal Fluminense University, Niteroi, Brazil

Federico Toth, Professor, Department of Political and Social Sciences, University of Bologna, Bologna, Italy

1

Introduction

Comments on the Public/Private Sector Mix in Healthcare Delivery

Howard A. Palley

This volume examines the public/private sector mix in a number of national healthcare systems and their interface with the goals of health equity and quality of healthcare. Moreover, there is a consideration of public accountability. The unique significance of this collection of national studies involving the public/private sector mix of healthcare services and/or finances is that it provides insights into the factors that enhance the public/private sector mix in fulfilling the goals of health equity and the quality of healthcare services as well as an understanding of the circumstances in which elements of the public/private sector mix may be harmful for the achievement of such goals in a variety of national settings. The contributions to this volume provide a variety of perspectives in dealing with these objectives.

Addressing Health Equity and Quality of Healthcare

Broadly, the term *social equity* refers to whether comparable services are provided to consumers of healthcare and social welfare services with similar needs regardless of income or the mix of public and private insurance coverage (Cohen, Grogan, and Horwitt 2017; Palley and Oktay 1983; Stone 2012). Moreover, the achievement of health equity (social equity limited to healthcare delivery) includes a dimension that involves a standard of quality of care. Braverman (2014, 6) defined health equity as the pursuit of "the highest possible standard of health for all people and giving special attention to the needs of those at greatest risk of poor health, based on social conditions." The term *health equity* refers to outputs that would serve equally persons with similar needs at a level that best meets those needs. Contributors in this

Howard A. Palley, *Introduction* In: *The Public/Private Sector Mix in Healthcare Delivery*. Edited by: Howard A. Palley, Oxford University Press. © Oxford University Press 2023. DOI: 10.1093/oso/9780197571101.003.0001 volume also direct their attention to the achievement of "quality of care." The Institute of Medicine of the US National Academy of Medicine defined high quality of healthcare as that which the attributes of being effective and safe, timely, patient centered, efficient and equitable (2001). Herein, a definition that also tries to "tackle" this matter was discussed by Campbell, Rolland, and Buetow (2000), who noted: "There are two principle dimensions to quality of care for . . . patients: access and effectiveness. . . . [Do] users get the care they need, and is the care effective when they get it" (1611). They further noted that two key components are "effectiveness of clinical care and effectiveness of interpersonal care" and how this effectiveness relates to the context of "the structure of the health care system, the process of care, and the outcomes relating from such care" (1611).

Contributors address concerns relating to quality of healthcare in a variety of ways within various national contexts. In so doing, these studies involve examination of the degree of achievement of public accountability for healthcare delivery in various national contexts (Björkman and Venkat Raman 2020; Dutton 2007; Fox and Jordan 2011; Grogan 2015; Pérez Durán 2020).

The Complexity of National Contexts

An important factor in understanding national healthcare policies is the complexity of each national context. In his discussion of reforms initiated in particular national healthcare systems, Björkman noted that to comprehend why nations take a variety of paths "not only external and internal pressures for change must be investigated but also structural features of social policy making that enable politicians and policy entrepreneurs to change the system despite the fact that institutional legacies and popular support for existing arrangements create barriers to change" (Björkman 2011 1066). Thus, there are prismatic differences in varied refracted national and subnational healthcare polices (Costa-Font and Greer 2013; Fierlbeck and Palley 2020; Maioni and Marmor 2005; Nathanson 2015; Okma and Crevelli 2010; Okma 2018b; Riggs 1964; Tuohy 2009). As Costa-Font and Greer concluded in their study of European health and social care: "Few generalizations hold well because of the complexity of politics, institutions, powers, and finances in each country . . . . An observer who expects German federalism to make the Lander powerful actors in health policy or French decentralization to produce territorial divergence, is inattentive to politics and institutional details and will be accordingly surprised" (2013, 276). Also, the studies included in this volume involve some attention to examination of vertical and horizontal linkages necessary "to integrate government responses to complex policy issues" (Björkman 2017, 71). Furthermore, organizational matters that are included in contributed articles involve examining the process with which public accountability is (or is not) reached at national and local levels (Chubarova and Gregorieva 2020; Grogan 2015; Kohli 2004; Pérez Durán 2020).

Comparative Analysis and Delivery of Healthcare

Comparative analysis of healthcare policies and programs, an area of comparative public policy analysis, includes a number of approaches; sorting out significant factors shaping national healthcare policies is a key concern. Such factors may include elements that are situational, cultural, political, and historical (Adolino and Blake 2010; Dodds 2018; Fischer, Miller, and Sidney 2007; Ingram, Schneider, and deLeon 2007; Marmor, Freeman, and Okma 2005; Tikkanen et al. 2020; Wilensky 1997). Our authors approach such dimensions in a variety of ways. In this volume, various chapters examine aspects of governmental structure, including the degree of centralization or decentralization and the ways in which healthcare policy is implemented in various national contexts.

In reality, different healthcare system analyses must be viewed in terms of the framework presented. Different analyses have different emphases. Some analyses primarily examine the question of what factors lead to the development of particular healthcare policies or programs. Others focus on the differences in the architecture of different healthcare programs with regard to funding, administration, and benefits. Still others focus on the need to assess comparative healthcare programs with regard to such dimensions of adequacy, equity, and the efficiency of policy outcomes. Often comparative healthcare studies focus as much on "how policies workout as on their genesis" (Klein 2010, lx).

The contributors to this volume examine how different variations of public/private sector financing and organization affect the delivery of healthcare services in a variety of nations. In the studies that follow, the public/private sector mix varies dependent on financial arrangements, the mix of ownership in the organization of healthcare, and the extent of private insurance arrangements, the nature of the regulatory process, as well as purchase of care arrangements within the public healthcare systems.

In this volume, the various national studies presented are indicative of the diversity of such arrangements. Also, the articles in this volume broadly address whether public/private sector arrangements in the provision of healthcare services and/or the financing of such services benefit or erode health equity and quality of healthcare in the various nations. The main focus of this volume examines an institutional arrangement, the public/private sector mix of financing and services, and how it affects public policy outcomes in national healthcare delivery systems. A number of the studies in this volume indicate that the achievement of a level of health equity requires adequate financing as low-income groups and low-income regions lack "market leverage" and also that the use of public funds to enhance health equity requires a viable system of national public accountability.

Some Further Comments

It is useful to review some of the literature examining the various elements that affect the dynamics resulting in national policies regarding healthcare delivery. As we have previously observed, a comprehensive comparative method of examining national healthcare policies and programs may address certain policy areas, which could include the following: organization, which is the extent to which the state directly provides healthcare services or extends this function to other private providers; the extent and nature of the regulatory process and the degree of private sector oversight by a public accountability process; as well as the nature of financial incentives and sanctions with respect to the behavior of insurers, healthcare providers, and the users of healthcare services (Bevan, Connolly, and Mays 2020; Dutton 2007; Okma 2018a; Maioni and Marmor 2015; Toth 2020, 2021). These criteria encompass what Tuohy referred to as the institutional mix of hierarchy, market, and peer control (collegiality) factors and the structural balance that includes the categories of state actors, healthcare providers, and private financial interests (Björkman and Nemec 2017; Bevan et al. 2020; Duckett 2020; Glover 2020; Tuohy 2009). While these factors can be discerned and are influential, there is always a dynamic process that may result in incremental or major reforms dependent on the nature of the structural constraints, including the nature of the cultural values, the political process, the initiative of political actors, and the structure of political institutions (Tuohy 2018; Sances and Clinton 2019). Nevertheless, these factors offer a basis for examining and comparing diverse national healthcare organizations and policies (Bjorkman and Nemec 2017; Dutton 2007; Maioni and Marmor 2015; Nathanson 2007; Okma and Crevelli 2010; Segatto, Béland, and Marchildon 2020).

In their discussion of comparative approaches to the examination of national healthcare systems, Marmor, Freeman, and Okma (2005, 342) noted that an approach to comparative study may involve examining "a number of individual countries that employ a common framework of analysis . . . addressing a particular theme of health policy, for example competition or privatization. . . . This approach allows comparative generalizations" (also see Fierlbeck and Palley 2020; Okma and Crevelli 2010). Further, Blank and Burau noted that the use of comparative healthcare studies allow us to obtain cross-cultural insights that indicate what works and what doesn't work with respect to a wide variety of institutional and cultural contexts (Blank, Burau, and Kuhlmann 2018). They went on to note that given the complexity of healthcare delivery and the plentitude of healthcare systems, only a comparative approach can generate the evidence that allows us to consider the choices adopted.

Examining the Public/Private Sector Mix Organizationally In National Health Settings

In a discussion of the public/private sector interface in healthcare delivery, Venkat Raman and Björkman provided a definition regarding an idealized notion of a successful "public/private partnership." They stated:

> Partnerships are collaborative efforts with mutually agreed obligations, clear accountability, and a willingness to share risks within well-defined management structures in order to produce or deliver public goods, with specified performance outcomes, within a stipulated period of time by harmonizing public and private interests. (Venkat Raman and Björkman 2015, 378)

The problem with the application of this definition is that, while optimal, this situation is infrequently reached. More often, there is a "falling short" of the ideal (Flood and Gross 2014). For instance in the United States, many nursing homes fail to meet the federal statutory requirement of adequate nursing home care structures or quality of care by "gaming the system" (Olson 2016). As Olson noted:

> The . . . public/private "partnerships" for LTSS [long-term supports and services] extract extreme value from our nation's resources for the for-profit sector to the detriment of our seniors and disabled young adults. . . . Complicated legal arrangements for nursing homes and home health agencies have allowed several layers of companies and related entities to pocket large portions of the Medicare and Medicaid pie while sheltering the businesses from consumer lawsuits and government sanctions for deficient and sometimes harmful care. (172–173)

Some other observations related to the difficulty in achieving health equity and quality in nursing home care and "chronic care" policy are noted in this volume in the Canada study by Marchildon and Allin and the Netherlands study by Kruse and Jeurissen.

Also, there may be subversion of public policy goals by commercial enterprises seeking to maximize profits, such as successfully lobbying against the ability of the US federal government to bargain with drug companies under the 1997 law providing drug benefits under Medicare. Such companies both "game the system" and, as the past example indicates, "capture" the regulatory process (Angell 2004; Minow 2003; Smith 2021; Chapter 2 this volume).

Another abuse of the private part of the public/private mix is the example of the false information provided by pharmaceutical companies in the United States and internationally regarding the drug oxycodone, resulting in the opioid crises (Hoffman 2022), and/or the lobbyists for companies exercising significant influence (Pomey et al. 2007). With regard especially to the actions of commercial, for-profit enterprises in the healthcare system, it is important the healthcare market be subject to the oversight of reasonable regulations (Advisory Commission on Intergovernmental Relations 1984; Block and Polanyi 2003; Grogan 2015; Palley, Pomey, and Adams 2012; Rosenau 2003; Vladeck and Rice 2009; Vladeck 1981). And a recent study indicated that 21% of US nursing home residents receive antipsychotic drugs, which are dangerous for the health of many but reduces the need for helping personnel by supplying "chemical strait jackets" (Thomas, Gebeloff, and Silver-Greenberg 2021). Also, the need for greater public accountability for public spending with respect to pharmaceuticals is a current public policy issue in the United States (Gavulic and Dusetzina 2021).

With reasonable regulation, investments of the private commercial sector may expand the availability of modern hospitals with advanced technology (Palley, Pomey, and Adams 2012), but often too extensive reliance on private health insurance schemes results in institutionalized systemic class and regional inequities in national healthcare systems (Björkman and Venkat Raman 2020; Gusmano 2020; Pérez Durán 2020; Toth 2020), and they may also generate undue profits leaking out of the healthcare system and into the pockets of private—for-profit—actors as is indicated in Grogan's study in Chapter 2 of this volume. Also, in a study examining the choice of public or private insurance in Germany (1970–2016) and the Netherlands (1941–1986), Thomson and Mossialos concluded: "Due to market failures in health insurance and differences in regulatory frameworks governing public and private insurers, choices of public or private coverage creates strong incentives for private insurers to select [lower] risks and to risk segregation, thereby breaching equity in funding health care, heightening the financial risk borne by public insurers and lowering incentives to operate efficiently" (2016, 315).

Canada's Romanow report particularly questioned whether evidence could justify increasing private commercial delivery for healthcare in Canada as a mechanism replacing a degree of private not-for-profit or direct public provision of healthcare services. Romanow was particularly concerned with the need for the development of a public accountability process overseeing the pharmaceutical industry and other private healthcare providers in order to control costs and ensure access to needed services (Marchildon 2004). A similar skepticism regarding the significant role the private health insurance sector and other private entities in the US healthcare delivery system is expressed by Grogan in Chapter 2. And in France, where one has a complex mix of public and private actors in the healthcare system, the Pierre and Or study in Chapter 5 indicated that a high level of national public accountability results in a highly equitable health insurance system and a high level of quality of healthcare delivery. Nevertheless, they expressed concern that supplementary private insurance tends to be less adequate for the elderly and the poor, and that physician "extra-billing" may not be sufficiently "reigned in" by regulation and financial incentives.

Romanow, in discussing the "mixed" nature of the Canadian healthcare system, noted the complexity of the public/private mix. He observed:

People tend to think of the private sector involvement in health care as the direct delivery of services—such as eye and hernia clinics. But, there are also "private-for-profit" businesses whose revenues derive largely from the public system by providing important and expensive "second-line" items like medical supplies, lab and food supplies, laundry, IT, data processing, maintenance, security and so on. . . . The reality is that our health care system in a mixed bag of non-profit and "for-profit"; self practitioners and salaried professionals; unionized and non-unionized workers, and government and private financing mechanisms. (2002, xv–xvi)

Of course, such complexity is a characteristic of many national healthcare systems.

Variations in Organization and Delivery of Healthcare Services

The national healthcare studies in this volume demonstrate that the varieties of national healthcare funding and delivery of services produce a variety of outcomes regarding health equity and quality of care. Even in a national system, such as the Italian healthcare system, essentially funded by general taxation, extensive purchase of care arrangements may be made with private suppliers. For instance, in Italy about one-third of the services of the National Health Service is provided by private suppliers under special arrangements, and as Toth observed, there has been an increase of Italians purchasing private insurance, allowing quicker access to healthcare services and providing a choice of provider, which is not available in the national health service (also see Toth 2015 and 2021). Toth also noted that in spite of national efforts to achieve health equity throughout Italy, patients who can afford to, seek hospital care in more affluent middle and northern provinces, which they perceive has a higher quality of healthcare services.

Also in this volume, Lobato, Senna, and Burlandy (Chapter 11) and Duckett (Chapter 4) note the following in their respective studies of complementary: Comparing the provided private insurance alternatives to publicly provided health insurance and health services, the private alternatives may undermine the public system by creaming easier cases, referring more difficult and expensive cases to the public system and thereby undermining the funding of the public sector. In examining the mix of private insurance as an option as opposed to a publicly provided system, Bernales-Baksai and Velasquez (Chapter 9) determine that the Chilean system, which provides a greater degree of public subsidization for poorer individuals, provides better health equity than the Mexican system, where no such integration takes place. In Uruguay, the Ballert and Fuentes study (Chapter 10) indicates that where the level of public insurance is considerably publicly subsidized, the health insurance system provides a substantial level of health equity. And as Lobato et al. note in their examination of Brazil's health insurance system (Chapter 11), where the public system has been "defunded," issues of health inequity have been manifest.

And in Taiwan, while there is a single-payer insurance program with the regulatory system established by a national government, a majority of physicians practice in private clinics, and hospitals are mostly private, non-profit, Gusmano (Chapter 13) notes that the physician and hospital sector increasingly complain that the national government is underfunding the system and also that an effort to address the vulnerabilities of Taiwan's indigenous minorities was also underfunded (for earlier accounts, see Cheng 2010 and 2018). In the Russian Federation (see Chapter 12), the dominant public sector entitlements are underfunded, leading to high levels of deductibles that must be paid by patients—in spite of a few efforts to cover these costs through supplementary health insurance. While a few private health insurance policies have sought to deal with this problem, this area has seen only minor development.

As we have noted, national healthcare systems reflect a complex variety of financial structures; administrative and organizational systems; and political systems. This collection is concerned with how different varieties of public/private sector financing affect the delivery of healthcare services in different developed and "newly developed" nations. Very poor nations have been excluded from this study as their organizational, political, and resource issues are too distinctively different from the national healthcare systems under examination herein.

Variations with regard to the national healthcare systems' mix of public and private sectors are numerous. For example, the US complex mix of about 50% public and 50% private financing has contributed to a highly fragmented character of the healthcare services that serve different population groups and experience significant variations in healthcare delivery in terms of regions and income levels (Grogan 2015 and Chapter 2 this volume; Okma and Marmor 2020). Marchildon and Allin (Chapter 3) discuss the

Canadian system of about 70% public and 30% private financing, some-times labeled "narrow but deep," with universal access without financial barriers for hospital care and ambulatory medical services, which are pre-dominantly fee for service, but greater variation in coverage for prescrip-tion drugs and long-term care across provinces. They particularly note that there are instances regarding lack of public accountability with regard to nursing home care policies in provinces (also see Palley, Pomey, and Owen 2012; Marchildon and Allin 2016). In France, as has been noted, universal coverage goes hand in hand with significant private options in a complex system; financing is primarily through employer/employee payroll taxes and a nationally earmarked income tax, and delivery of services by physicians and hospitals is a complex mixture of public and private delivery of care with nationally determined standards and private supplementary insurance (Dutton 2007; Durand-Zaleski 2020; Pierre and Or, Chapter 5 this volume). The higher level of national accountability in France contrasts with the lower levels of such national accountability of private sector participants that are found in the United States and Australia and are discussed in this volume by Grogan (Chapter 2), Duckett (Chapter 4), and Lobato, Senna, and Burlandy (Chapter 11) in their contributions dealing with the United States, Australia, and Brazil, respectively.

Dutch healthcare policy presents a case of encouraging limited "market competition" while maintaining national norms of universal access to healthcare and national funding without undue individual burden. National funding is through a nationally defined, income-related premium contri-bution, a government grant for the insured below age 18, and community-rated insurance set by participating social insurers. As Krause and Jeurissen note (Chapter 7), basic benefits are nationally mandated, and insurers have some discretion regarding premiums and coinsurance features. Long-term care policy in the Netherlands is funded separately by a tax on earnings (Okma 2018b; Okma and Maarse 2010; and Krause and Jeurissen Chapter 7 this volume). This contrasts with the Swedish healthcare system, in which the broad concerns regarding care for inpatient, outpatient, hospital, and other health areas are financed, overseen, and implemented at the regional (county) council and municipal levels; these costs vary from jurisdiction to jurisdiction, and physicians may be private or public (40% of primary care practices are private). Out-of-pocket healthcare visit costs are very minor due to annual caps, and the out-of-pocket annual cost for prescription drugs for adults are also very limited due to such caps (Glenngård 2020; Glenngård Chapter 6 this volume). And social welfare services are funded separately at the regional and municipal levels. Within national constraints, the funding and implementation of Swedish healthcare are at the regional and municipality levels, particularly with regard to the primary care level examined in her study, revealing unevenness in the delivery of such healthcare services.

In the Russian Federation, Chubarova and Grigorieva (Chapter 12) note that public hospitals are the dominant healthcare institution, but a significant private fee system has developed for the payment of physicians. In the case of Brazil's healthcare system, as we have noted, parallel private and public healthcare systems have developed, leading to substantial inefficiencies and inequities. In Uruguay, the National Health Insurance Reform of 2007, while protecting the autonomy of physicians and the continuance of "multiple schemes" of private insurance, the government has assumed a more direct role as a regulator and increased the financial capacity of the national government to invest in the public health sector, which has reduced, although it has not eliminated, the discrepancies in healthcare existing on a class-based basis (Ballart and Fuentes 2019; Chapter 10 this volume).

As we observed in this chapter, Chile was better able to overcome healthcare equity issues in a healthcare system that was initially based on market competition (Leyer and Bernales-Baksai 2019; Paraje 2018; Bernales-Baksai and Velazquez, Chapter 9 this volume). While it is now a dual public/private system, it was able to reduce trends toward commodification in its public sector through an integrated employment-based coverage with a noncontributory subsidized coverage for lower income groups, while in Mexico families from all income groups must seek services from "scarcely regulated" providers that are characterized by low quality, limited access, and fragmentation of the health services, as indicated in the article by Bernales-Baksai and Velazquez (also see Leyer and Bernales-Baksai 2019). Furthermore, Bernales-Baksai and Velazquez also note that quality hospitals are concentrated in just the two metropolitan areas of Mexico City and Monterrey, and even basic primary care services are often unavailable in Mexico's south, where its indigenous population is concentrated.

Some Conclusions

The contributors in this volume examine from a variety of perspectives how public/private sector mix in healthcare delivery operates in different national systems. The various chapters demonstrate how the organizational structure and the level and system of financial support can affect healthcare delivery and the resultant policy outputs. As the contributions to this volume note, this results in a variety of complex outcomes with respect to health equity and the quality of healthcare. Also, the chapters in this volume examine a number of these issues in much greater depth than can be noted in this introduction. But two essential factors to achieving health equity are adequate funding necessary to achieve horizontal and vertical equity goals and to counteract the effects of marketization, sometimes referred to as "commodification" of healthcare delivery. Also, a workable system of public accountability for the spending of national revenues for both direct public services and privately provided services utilizing government revenues is needed to secure the goals of health equity and quality healthcare.

References

Adolino, Jessica, and Charles Blake. 2010. *Comparing Public Policies: Issues and Choices in Industrialized Countries*. Washington, DC: CQ Press.

Advisory Commission on Intergovernmental Relations. 1984. *Regulatory Federalism: Policy, Process, Impact and Reform*. Washington, DC: Advisory Commission on Intergovernmental Relations.

Angell, Marcia. 2004. *The Truth about the Drug Companies*. New York: Random House.

Ballart, Xavier, and Guillermo Fuentes. 2019. "Gaining Public Control on Health Policy: The Politics of Scaling Up to Universal Health Coverage in Uruguay." *Social Theory and Health* 17: 348–366. https://doi.org/10.1057/s41285-018-0080-7

Bevan, Gwyn, Sheelah Connolly, and Nicholas Mays. 2020. "The United Kingdom." In *Comparative Health Care Federalism*, edited by Katherine Fierlbeck and Howard A. Palley, 79–94. London: Routledge.

Björkman, James Warner. 2017. "Comparative Public Administration." In *Foundations of Public Administration*, edited by Joseph Raadschelder and Ronald Stillman, 57–74. Irvine, CA: Melvin and Leigh.

Björkman, James Warner. 2011. "Health Policy." In *International Encyclopedia of Political Science*, edited by Bertrand Badie, Dirk Berg-Schlosser, and Leonaro Morlino, 1061–1066. Los Angeles, CA: Sage.

Björkman, James Warner, and Juraj Nemec, eds. 2013. *Health Reforms in Central and Eastern Europe*. Hague, Netherlands: Eleven International.

Björkman, James Warner, and A. Venkat Raman. 2020. "India." In *Comparative Health Care Federalism*, edited by Katherine Fierlbeck and Howard A. Palley, 149–166. London: Routledge.

Blank, Robert H., Viola Burau, and Ellen Kuhlmann. 2018. *Comparative Health Policy*. London: Palgrave.

Block, Fred, and Karl Polanyi. 2003. "Karl Polanyi and the Writing of 'The Great Transformation.'" *Theory and Society* 32: 275–306.

Braverman, Paula. 2014. "What Are Health Disparities and Health Equity? We Need to Be Clear." *Public Health Report* Supplement 2(129): S5–S8.

Campbell, S. M., M. O. Rolland, and S. A. Buetow. 2000. "Defining Quality of Care." *Social Science and Medicine* 51 (11): 1611–1626.

Cheng, Tsung-Mei. 2010. "Taiwan's National Health Insurance System: High Value for the Dollar." In *Six Countries, Six Reform Models: The Healthcare Reform Experience of Israel, the Netherlands, Singapore, Switzerland and Taiwan,* edited by Kieke G. H. Okma and Luca Crivelli, 171–204. Singapore: World Scientific.

Cheng, Tsung-Mei. 2018. "Taiwan: Health System Reforms and Future Challenges." *American Affairs Journal* 2 (6). https://americanaffairsjournal.org/2018/02/health-care-reforms-across-world

Chubarova, Tatania, and Natalia Grigorieva 2020. "The Russian Federation." In *Comparative Health Care Federalism,* edited by Katherine Fierlbeck and Howard A. Palley, 195–212. London: Routledge.

Cohen, Alan B., Colleen M. Grogan, and Jedidiah M. Horwitt. 2017. "The Many Roads of Achieving Health Equity." *Journal of Politics, Policy and Law* 42(5): 739–748.

Costa-Font, Joan, and Scott L. Greer. 2013. *Federalism and Decentralization in European Health and Social Care.* New York: Palgrave Macmillan.

Dodds, Anneliese. 2018. *Comparative Public Policy.* New York: Macmillan.

Duckett, Stephen. 2020. "Australia." In *Comparative Health Care Federalism,* edited by Katherine Fierlbeck and Howard A. Palley, 79–94. London: Routledge.

Durand-Zaleski, Isabelle. 2020. "The French Health Care System." In *International Profiles of Health Care Systems,* edited by Roosa Tikkanen, Robin Osborn, Elias Mossiallos, Anna Djordjevic, and Geoge Wharton, 59–67. New York: Commonwealth Fund. https://www.researchgate.net

Dutton, Paul V. 2007. *Differential Diagnosis: A Comparative History of Health Care Problems and Solutions in the United States and France.* Ithaca, NY: Cornell University Press.

Fierlbeck, Katherine, and Howard A. Palley, eds. 2020. *Comparative Health Care Federalism.* London: Routledge.

Fischer, Frank, Gerald J. Miller, and Marc S. Sidney, eds. 2007. *Handbook of Public Policy Analysis.* Boca Raton, FL: CRC Press.

Flood, Colleen M., and Aeyal Gross, eds. 2014. *The Right to Health at the Public/Private Divide: A Global Comparative Study.* Cambridge, England: Cambridge University Press.

Fox, Justin, and Stuart V. Jordan. 2011. "Delegation and Accountability." *Journal of Politics* 73(3): 831–844.

Gavulic, Kyle A., and Stacie B. Dusetzina. 2021. "Prescription Drug Priorities under the Biden Administration." *Journal of Health Politics, Policy and Law* 46(4): 599–625.

Glenngård, Anna H. 2020. "The Swedish Health Care System." In *International Profiles of Health Care Systems,* edited by Roosa Tikkanen, Robin Osborn, Elias Moussialos, Ana Djorjevic, and George Wharton. New York: Commonwealth Foundation. https://www.researchgate.net

Glover, Lucinda. 2020. "The Australia Health Care System." In *International Profiles of Health Care Systems,* edited by Roosa Tikkanen, Robin Osborn, Elias Moussialos, Ana Djorjevic, and George Wharton. New York: Commonwealth Foundation. https://www.resarchgate.net

Grogan, Colleen M. 2015. "The Role of the Private Sphere in U.S. Healthcare Entitlements: Increased Spending, Weakened Public Mobilization and Reduced Equity." *The Forum* 13(1): 119–142.

Gusmano, Michael K. 2020. "China." In *Comparative Health Care Federalism,* edited by Katherine Fierlbeck and Howard A. Palley, 165–178. London: Routledge.

Hayek, Friedrich. 1944. *The Road to Serfdom*. Chicago: University of Chicago Press.

Hoffman, Jan. 2022. "Sacklers and Purdue Reach New Deal with States Over Opiods." *The New York Times*, March 4, A1.

Ingram, Helen, Anne Schneider, and Peter deLeon. 2007 "Social Construction and Policy Design." In *Theories of the Policy Process*, edited by Paul Sabatier, 93–128. New York: Westview Press.

Institute of Medicine (IOM). 2001. *Crossing the Quality Chasm: A New Health System for the 21st Century*. Washington, DC: National Academy Press.

Klein, Rudolf. 2010. "Foreword." In *Six Countries, Six Health Reform Models: Experience of Israel, the Netherlands, New Zealand, Singapore, Switzerland and Taiwan*, edited by Kieke G. H. Okma and Luca Crevelli, vii–x. Singapore: World Scientific.

Kohli, Atul. 2004. *State-Directed Development*. Cambridge, UK: Cambridge University Press.

Leyer, Ricardo Veláquez, and Pamela Brenales-Baksai. 2019. "In Search of the Authentic Universalism in Latin American Healthcare Systems: The Cases of Chile and Mexico." Unpublished manuscript.

Lobatto, Lenaura de V. C., and Mônica de C. M. Senna. 2020. "Brazil." In *Comparative Health Care Federalism*, edited by Katherine Fierlbeck and Howard A. Palley, 179–194. London: Routledge.

Maioni, Antonia, and Theodore R. Marmor. 2015. "Health Policy Reform in North America." In *The Palgrave International Handbook of Healthcare and Governance*, edited by Ellen Kuhlmann, Robert H. Blank, Ivy L. Bourgeault, and Claus Wendt, 222–237. New York: Palgrave Macmillan.

Marchildon, Gregory P. 2004. "The Public-Private Debate in the Funding, Administration and Delivery of Healthcare in Canada." *Healthcare Papers* 4(4): 61–68.

Marchildon, Gregory P., and Sara Allin. 2016. "The Public-Private Mix in the Delivery of Health Care Services: Its Relevance to Low Income Canadians." *Global Social Welfare* 3: 161–170.

Marmor, Theodore R., Richard Freeman, and Kieke G. H. Okma. 2005. "Comparative Perspective and Policy Learning in the World of Health Care." *Journal of Comparative Policy Analysis* 7(4): 331–348.

Minow, Martha. 2003. "Public and Private Partnerships: Accounting for the New Religion." *Harvard Law Review* 116: 1229–1270.

Nathanson, Constance A. 2007. *Disease Prevention as Social Change*. New York: Russell Sage Foundation.

Okma, Kieke G. H. 2018a. "Health Care Reforms across the World." *American Affairs Journal*, February. https://americanaffairsjournal.org/2018/02/health-care-reform-acr oss-the world/

Okma, Kieke G. H. 2018b. "The Netherlands: From Wholesale Change to Marginal Adjustments: Or, a Farewell to Health Reforms." *American Affairs Journal* 2(1). https:// americanaffairsjournal.org/2018/02/health-care-reforms-across-world/

Okama, Kieke G. H., and Luca Crevelli, eds. 2010. *Six Countries, Six Reform Models. The Healthcare Reform Experience of Israel, the Netherlands, Switzerland and Taiwan*. Singapore: World Publishing.

Okma, Kieke G. H., and Hans Maarse. 2010. "Change and Continuity in Dutch Health Care: Origins and Consequences of the 2006 Health Insurance Reforms." In *Six Countries, Six Reform Models: The Healthcare Reform Experience of Israel, the Netherlands, Switzerland and Taiwan, Singapore*, edited by Kieke G. H. Okma and Luca Crevelli, 43–82. Singapore: World Science.

Okma, Kieke G. H., and Theodore R. Marmor. 2020. In *Comparative Health Care Federalism*, edited by Katherine Fierlbeck and Howard A. Palley, 139–148. London: Routledge.

Olson, Laura Katz. 2016. *Elder Care Journey: A View from the Front Lines*. Albany, NY: State University of New York Press.

Palley, Howard A. and Julianne S. Oktay. 1983. *The Chronically-Limited Elderly: The Case for a National Policy for In-Home and Supportive Community-Based Services*. New York: Routledge.

Palley, Howard A., Marie-Pascale Pomey, and Owen B. Adams. 2012. *The Political and Economic Sustainability of Health Care in Canada: Private Sector Involvement in the Federal Provincial Healthcare System*. Amherst, NY: Cambria Press.

Paraje, Guillermo. 2018. "Chile: Early Adopter of Social Insurance." *American Affairs Journal* February 2 (4) https://americanaffairsjournal.org/2018/02/health-care-refo rms-across-world/

Pérez Durán, Ixchel. 2020. "Spain." In *Comparative Health Care Federalism*, edited by Katherine Fierlbeck and Howard A. Palley, 47–54. London: Routledge.

Pomey, Marie-Pascale, Pierre-Gerlier Forest, Howard A. Palley, and Elisabeth Martin. 2007. "Public/Private Partnerships for Prescription Drug Coverage: Policy Formulation and Outcomes in Quebec's Universal Drug Insurance Program, with Comparisons to the Medicare Prescription Drug Program in the United States." *Milbank Quarterly* 85(3): 469–498.

Riggs, Fred W. 1964. *Administration in Developing Countries: The Theory of Prismatic Society*. Boston, MA: 1964.

Roberts, Marc J. 2015 "Equity in Health Reform." In *The Palgrave International Handbook of Healthcare Policy and Governance*, edited by Ellen Kuhlmann, Robert H. Blank, Ivy L. Bourgeault, and Claus Wendt, 545–560. New York: Palgrave Macmillan.

Romanow, Roy. 2002. "Message to Canadians." In *Building on Values: The Future of Health Care in Canada*, xv–xvi. Ontario, ON, Canada: Commission on the Future of Health Care in Canada.

Rosenau, Pauline V. 2003. *The Competition Paradigm*. Lanham, MD: Rowman and Littlefield.

Sances, Michael W., and Jashua D. Clinton. 2019. "Who Participated in the ACA? Gains in Insurance Coverage by Political Partisanship." *Journal of Health Politics, Policy and Law* 44(3): 349–380.

Segatto, Catarina Ianni, Daniel Béland, and Gregory P. Marchildon. 2020. "Federalism, Physicians, and Public Policy: A Comparison of Health Care Reform in Canada and Brazil." *Journal of Comparative Policy Analysis* 22(3): 250–265. http://doi.org/10.1080/13876988.2019.1603357

Smith, Rachel E. 2021. "The Rhetorical Transformations and Policy Failures of Prescription Drug Pricing Reform under the Trump Administration." *Journal of Health Politics, Policy and Law* 46(6): 1053–1068.

Stone, Deborah. 2012. *Policy Paradox: The Art of Political Decision Making*. New York: Norton.

Thomas, Katie, Robert Gebeloff, and Jessica Silver-Greenberg. 2021. "False Diagnoses Conceal Drugging of Frail Seniors." *New York Times*, September 12, A1, A26.

Thomson, Sarah, and Elias Mossialos. 2016. "Choice of Public or Private Health Insurance: Learning from the Experience of Germany and the Netherlands." *Journal of European Social Policy* 16(4): 315–327.

Tikkanen, Rosa, Robin Osborn, Elias Mossialos, Ana Djordjevic, and George Wharton, eds. 2020. *International Profiles of Health Care Systems.*: New York: Commonwealth Fund.

Toth, Federico. 2020. "Italy." In *Comparative Health Care Federalism,* edited by Katherine Fierlbeck and Howard A. Palley, 63–77. London: Routledge.

Toth, Federico. 2021. "How Policy Tools Evolve in the Healthcare Sector. *Policy Studies* 42(3): 232–237. https://doi.org/10.1080/01442872.2019.1656182

Tuohy, Carolyn Hughes. 2009. "Canada Health Care Reform in Comparative Perspective." In *Comparative Studies and the Politics of Medical Care,* edited by Theodore R. Marmor, Robert Freeman, and Kieke G. H. Okma, 61–87. New Haven, CT: Yale University Press.

Tuohy, Carolyn Hughes. 2018. "Welfare State Eras, Policy Narratives, and the Role of Expertise: The Case of the Affordable Care Act in Historical and Comparative Perspective." *Journal of Health Politics, Policy and Law* 43(3): 427–454.

Venkat Raman, A., and James Warner Björkman. 2015. "Public-Private Partnerships in Health Care." In *The Palgrave International Handbook of Healthcare and Policy,* edited by Ellen Kuhlmann, Robert H. Blank, Ivy L. Bourgeault, and Claus Wendt, 376–392. New York: Palgrave Macmillan.

Vladeck, Bruce C., and Thomas Rice. 2009. "Market Failure and the Failure of Discourse Facing Up to the Power of Sellers." *Health Affair* 28(5): 1305–1315.

Vladeck, Bruce C. 1981. "The Market vs. Regulation: The Case for Regulation." *Health and Society* 92(2): 209–223.

Wilensky, Harold. 1997. "Social Science and the Public Agenda: Reflections on the Relation of Knowledge to Policy in the United States and Abroad." *Journal of Health Politics, Policy and Law* 22(5): 1241–1267.

2

The Dominance of Public Funding for Private Provision in the US Healthcare System

Colleen M. Grogan

The US healthcare system is a complex public/private sector system with significant implications for health equity, quality of care, and excessive health service and non–health service costs. The US system encompasses four major entitlement programs: Medicare, Medicaid, employer-based health insurance, and the subsidized marketplace enacted under the Patient Protection and Affordable Care Act (ACA) in 2010. Two policy designs are dominant under US healthcare entitlements: contracting with private actors to provide and administer publicly funded social benefits (Morgan and Campbell 2011) and providing "private benefits" through tax policy (Hacker 2002; Howard 1999). Because entitlements are structured to disburse benefits to private actors, who then provide services to beneficiaries, private actors also have the right—politically and legally—to make claims on the state. An important aspect of American healthcare exceptionalism is the extent to which private spending drives up the cost of US healthcare entitlements combined with the seemingly political impossibility to have any real discussions about establishing limits on private actors. Since the ACA further embeds the role of private actors, how private actors make claims on the state, and how the state reacts to these claims, becomes even more important because such claims significantly shape US healthcare entitlements. Unfortunately, although the ACA expanded access to health coverage to 20 million previously uninsured Americans, the most inequitable aspects of private healthcare benefits remain untouched by the ACA.

Colleen M. Grogan, *The Dominance of Public Funding for Private Provision in the US Healthcare System* In: *The Public/Private Sector Mix in Healthcare Delivery*. Edited by: Howard A. Palley, Oxford University Press. © Oxford University Press 2023. DOI: 10.1093/oso/9780197571101.003.0002

Brief History

Health Entitlements to Ensure Access
to Healthcare Coverage

Highlighting the importance of private benefits in welfare programs is not new. Social policy theorist Richard Titmuss pointed out in 1965 that the conceptual frameworks of welfare were too narrow, primarily focusing on benefits for the poor and only on *visible* government spending, which did not adequately account for how the state provided social benefits across the income distribution. Titmuss developed a theory of a three-tiered welfare system: the visible government spending under "social welfare"; beneath-the-surface "fiscal welfare," which includes income support to individuals and families through the tax code; and "occupational welfare," which offers tax-exempt fringe benefits to workers. Others have built on the work of Titmuss and highlighted the importance of this three-tiered welfare system for understanding US healthcare entitlements. In particular, the social welfare system is administered by the Department of Health and Human Services and includes Medicare and Medicaid; the fiscal welfare system by the Internal Revenue Service (IRS), which includes tax credits offered on the ACA marketplaces; and the occupational welfare system by individual firms, including the tax deduction for employer-based health insurance (EBHI) (Hacker 2002; Titmuss 1965; Abramovitz 2001). Hacker (2002) referred to benefits provided through the tax system (both fiscal and occupational welfare systems) as "private benefits," whereas benefits provided through Medicare and Medicaid were described as "public benefits" due to their clear and visible counting as government expenditures. These terms are highly imperfect because private benefits hides the role of public, which is often the strategic purpose of the policymakers of such tax designs and Hacker's point in naming them as such, but misleading when using the term to clarify the design structure (in the manner of Titmuss's **point**).

Moreover, the term *public benefits* is also misleading because it hides the role of private actors in these programs. Morgan and Campbell (2011) argued that the United States has become a "delegated welfare state" under which the state contracts with private actors to provide publicly funded social benefits. As discussed in more detail below, Medicare and Medicaid rely heavily on contracting with private health insurance plans to provide healthcare benefits. Indeed, the new ACA marketplaces rely on both private

2012). However, as Timothy Jost pointed out, "just because we lack constitutional guarantees to health care . . . does not mean that we lack legal healthcare entitlements" (Jost 2003, 30). Indeed, because healthcare entitlements are attached to various expectations regarding *earned* benefits, notions of deservingness and attachment to the labor force, there is a complex set of legal rules delineating the who, what, and how of benefits to which individuals are entitled. Thus, not only do Americans have legal healthcare entitlements, but due to years of litigation, which legally clarifies beneficiaries' statutory right to claim benefits, healthcare entitlements are framed in the United States not as social or political rights, but as legal claims (Jost 2003; Weir 2012).

Shep Melnick (1996) argued that the United States grants "programmatic" entitlements since benefits are made real by specific program requirements around eligibility and benefits (Melnick 1996). This is particularly true for means-tested targeted programs, especially Medicaid in the 1970s, when eligibility levels were strictly attached to the receipt of cash assistance. At this time and continuing today in the nonexpansion states, although recipients had statutory claim to eligible benefits, because the eligibility levels were so meager and could be increased or decreased each year at the whim of state legislatures, the substantive value of their claim was low. Given the power of government rules to shape the meaning of entitlements, Melnick (1996) argued further that "unlike the rights of free speech, religion, property, and privacy, which set limits on the power of government officials, programmatic rights require extensive public programs rather than private autonomy, a welfare state rather than limited government" (Melnick 1996, 327). While this description of the regime of programmatic rights makes clear the need for government funding to realize programmatic rights, Melnick's comment of an expanded "welfare state *rather* than limited government" fails to recognize how the US welfare state *expanded* under the rubric of limited government. Indeed, it is both the political framing of limited government and policy designs increasing the private sphere (through private benefits and private contracting), which allowed an expanded healthcare state.

Public Investments to Build a Private Healthcare Delivery System

The US government at all levels—federal, state, and local—has long played a central role in funding healthcare infrastructure. This applies to the development of the healthcare workforce as well as the development of healthcare facilities. Due to space constraints, I focus here on the development of the US hospital system, which illustrates the central role of the nonprofit sector, and government subsidies to support that sector in the US system. With the advent of many scientific advancements in the 1910s and 1920s, the modern scientific hospital was developed and recognized as a place for curative medicine rather than a place to die. This shift created demand across the country for public investment in hospital construction. Each decade witnessed phenomenal growth: In 1875 there were 661 hospitals in the United States, and by 1900 there were just over 2,000; in 1910 there were well over 4,000, and by 1928 there were almost 7,000 hospitals. From the very beginning there were different types of hospitals with distinct roles, purposes, and ownership status. Government-owned hospitals (or "state medicine" as it was called at the time) were considered acceptable for hard-to-treat conditions, notably persons with mental disease, tuberculosis, and other communicable diseases; and the care of military and naval personnel, inmates of prisons and other wards of the state, and indigent persons ("Medical Care for the American People: The Final Report of the Committee on the Costs of Medical Care, Adopted October 31, 1932" 1932). Whereas voluntary private nonprofit ownership was considered most appropriate for acute care general hospitals primarily for paying patients. Although these were private hospitals, government investment was substantial even in this early period.

For example, even in 1928, $5 billion had already been invested in hospitals and millions more spent each year to cover operating costs. Nearly three of every four occupied hospital beds in 1932 were government owned. This was largely due to long stays of mentally and physically disabled patients—with all of these stays paid for by federal, state, or local governments. In 1930, government paid $303 million for hospital operating costs, which represented almost half (46%) of the total operating costs of all hospitals. Nonetheless, even a substantial amount of short-term stays received government funding. While 60% of operating expenses went toward hospital care for those with tuberculosis and mental disease, the remainder, $118 million, went toward general hospital service (Corwin and Commonwealth 1946).

Besides direct government outlays, many cities and counties also paid voluntary hospitals for hospital services rendered to the poor. However, the real hidden story was the government's role in hospital capital investment. Even in 1928, before the Depression hit, 91% of capital investment was provided in equal amounts by government and nonprofit associations, representing a total capital investment of more than $3 billion (Rorem 1930, 10). From the very beginning capital expenditures represented a trend toward heavy emphasis on hospital improvements (e.g., acquiring new technology and private room amenities) rather than *significantly* expanding access to new hospitals. From 1908 to 1928, there was an average per year increase of 20,000 beds; however, most of this increase came from existing hospitals expanding bed supply. Of the 85 hospital construction projects conducted in 1929, only 24 represented new hospital construction. Importantly, this investment in hospital intensity did not occur equally across all types of hospitals. Not surprisingly, the increase was concentrated in acute care general hospitals where, as noted previously, the capital investment costs per bed were significantly higher among voluntary hospitals ($6,202) compared to government-owned hospitals ($3,613) (Rorem 1930, 26).

Government's role in capital investment is crucially important to understand for two reasons. First, although the government played a substantial financial role in building up the hospital industry, no government body ever asked for a clear accounting from nonprofit hospitals on what value was gained from higher priced beds (Rorem 1930, 22). Second, despite rhetoric even in this early period that nonprofit hospitals were benevolent and provided charity care, the government never specified what level of "charity" should be required, especially in light of public subsidies. Nonprofit hospitals enjoyed tax-exempt status in most states then (and now), but states remained silent on what obligations this status might entail. Without any requirements, medical historian Rosemary Stevens's research on hospitals confirmed:

> Many, if not most, of the new hospitals were not predominantly "charitable" if the term is limited to the provision of free care. . . . The state acted as if it were a modern foundation. It acknowledged the public role of hospitals and a willingness to fund requests. However, it took no responsibility for the provision of hospital care throughout the state. . . . There was no incentive to plan, to control, or to regulate. (Stevens 1982, 287)

Third, the government accepted proposals from leaders of voluntary hospitals to connect capital investment to hospital charges. Because capital investments supported expensive high-intensity care, this method led to inflationary charges in the hospital industry, which the government supported and subsidized for years to come.

For example, when nonprofit voluntary hospitals were the hardest hit during the Depression, the federal government responded to the crisis. The Public Works Administration (PWA) and the Works Progress Administration (WPA) provided hospital construction funds as part of its reemployment programs. In 1933 alone, the PWA provided 51,000 hospital beds. The program also provided grants to local government bodies for hospital construction. From 1933 to 1936, the PWA allocated $75 million for hospital construction. The WPA also focused on hospital construction, mostly by providing labor; 101 new hospitals were built and 1,422 renovated from 1935 to 1938. The Lantham Act was passed in 1941 as another public works program administered by the Federal Works Agency, which provided federal assistance to build hospitals and health centers in defense areas. Over 5 years, from 1941 to 1946, $121 million was spent on 874 hospital and health-related projects (Stevens 1989, 209).

Although this legislation was limited, it also set a precedent that the *federal* government[1] would continue to support the private voluntary hospital sector beyond the New Deal emergency relief programs to enable growth in this sector. And, yet, it also set an important precedent that the federal government would allow the private sector complete autonomy to define what obligations—if any—were tied to this notion of a "community nonprofit hospital." Therefore, when Congress passed the Hill-Burton Act in 1946, it allowed the federal Public Health Service (PHS) to grant funding to local communities for hospital construction *almost* carte blanche.[2] Over the next 25 years, the federal government disbursed nearly $4 billion, asking for no commitment in return to ensure access to health or hospital care for the American people.

In the 1960s, state governments began to offer nonprofit hospitals more favorable lending conditions under the tax-exempt bond, which catapulted nonprofit hospitals into the capital credit markets. Debt financing increased from 38% of total financing for hospital construction in 1968 to 69% in 1981 (Cohodes and Kinkead 1984, 25–26).[3] The dollar volume of healthcare debt issues in the tax-exempt market went from $22 billion (5.7% of total issues) in 1974 to $75 billion (12.3%) in 1982. In just 1 year, from 1980 to 1981, hospitals and other healthcare institutions borrowed more than $5 billion in the long-term tax-exempt bond market. This represented a 40% increase from the 1980 level.

The increased reliance on private capital markets played a central role in creating a fundamental transformation toward the corporatization of the

American healthcare system (Ermann and Gabel 1984; Institute of Medicine Committee on Implications of For-Profit Enterprise in Health 1986). The implications of this shift toward corporatization were threefold. First, reliance on private capital encouraged the formation of multihospital systems. The percentage of US community hospitals affiliated with systems increased from 31% in 1979 to 53% in 2001 (Bazzoli 2004, 889). Because large organizations could support the overhead necessary to develop sophisticated financial strategies, investment advisers and bond-rating agencies viewed multihospital systems as more financially stable (Brown and Saltman 1985, 123). Because the credit rating of multi-institutional systems tended to be higher than single-facility hospitals, there was strong motivation to join multihospital systems. For example, while 23% and 38% of multihospital systems had AA± and A+ ratings, respectively, only 2% and 16% of single-facility hospitals had such ratings (Institute of Medicine 1983). It is important to note that these mergers and acquisitions occurred regardless of ownership: Nonprofit voluntary hospitals also experienced a growing number of corporate mergers and large-scale joint ventures (Institute of Medicine 1983).[4]

Second, the shift toward reliance on private capital created explosive growth of proprietary hospital chains. The number of short-term acute care hospitals owned by for-profit hospital chains rose from 6% in 1977 to 10% in 1982. The five largest chains more than doubled their total beds during the same time period (Ermann and Gabel 1984; Institute of Medicine 1983; Relman 1980). In 1990, for-profit systems owned 33% of system hospitals (about one in four hospital beds) (Bazzoli 2004).

Third, the reliance on capital markets further bifurcated the US healthcare system. While public subsidies to access tax-exempt bonds were made easier for nonprofit hospitals in the post-1965 period, public hospitals were unable to take comparable advantage of subsidies attached to the tax-exempt bond markets. Because public hospitals had a higher proportion of Medicaid patients among their payer mix, even private investors in the tax-exempt bond market with more lax rules saw them as a greater risk (Cleverley and Nutt 1984). This lower risk rating was clearly biased against a larger minority patient base and where many public hospitals were situated—in poorer minority neighborhoods in urban centers. While nonprofit hospitals serving predominantly White patients were welcomed into the capital markets, public hospitals (and other community hospitals with large Medicaid populations) were deemed a "bad risk" (Kinney and Lefkowitz 1982, 653).

Once they were deemed a bad risk, public hospitals found it very difficult to change their risk rating. Because public hospitals had much lower capital investment, their level of payments based on debt principal was low. As a result, it was difficult to build up an internal revenue base to use as leverage. Instead, public hospitals used a large portion of their discretionary funds to cover operating deficits, especially to meet the requirements of their mission to care for nonpaying patients. This stopgap measure led to future problems; since there was little capital investment, the amount of reimbursement continued to decline, and, as a result, discretionary funds continued to dwindle, and a downward cycle ensued. By the mid-1980s, several studies confirmed that public and nonprofit voluntary hospitals that served a disproportionate number of Black, Latino, and poor residents were much less likely to have access to capital markets than those hospitals that served predominantly White residents with private insurance (Cleverley and Nutt 1984; Kinney and Lefkowitz 1982; Feder, Hadley, and Urban Institute 1984; Schatzkin 1984).

At the same time that states opened up the capital markets to nonprofit hospitals through the tax-exempt bond, in 1969 the IRS enacted a major change in interpreting charitable care for tax-exempt hospitals. As a result of the passage of Medicare and Medicaid, the IRS accepted the American Hospital Association's claim that "they couldn't find patients to whom to give free care" (Fox and Schaffer 1991, 262). As part of its 1969 ruling, the IRS applied a far broader definition of "charitable" to hospitals, wherein the promotion of health is considered to be a charitable purpose. The IRS concluded that a hospital could be tax exempt "even though the class of beneficiaries eligible to receive a direct benefit from its activities does not include . . . indigent members of the community" (Fox and Schaffer 1991, 258). This IRS ruling legally allowed nonprofit hospitals access to state-subsidized capital markets to invest in hospital renovations and new technology to distinguish themselves (as much as they could) as hospitals for the middle and upper class (by primarily accepting those with private insurance and Medicare), while leaving (and in many cases pushing) the poor and uninsured on to public hospitals.

While all nonprofit hospitals enjoy tax-exempt status and can technically take advantage of the 1969 IRS ruling, not all do. Many small community-based nonprofit hospitals—especially those located in communities with high poverty rates and a high proportion of residents of color or in rural areas—maintain a mission that predominantly serves the un- and under-insured and Medicaid beneficiaries. Like public hospitals, these nonprofit community-based hospitals have difficulty accessing the capital markets and taking advantage of tax-exempt bonds. Thus, over time, a strict demarcation emerged between the "have-not" safety net hospitals, which include public and some nonprofit hospitals, and the "have" hospitals, which include for-profit and some nonprofit hospitals with access to capital markets.

Current Organization of Healthcare Delivery

The passage of the ACA in 2010 represented the most significant healthcare reform in the United States since the passage of Medicare and Medicaid in 1965. It expanded health insurance coverage to 20 million Americans; it included $15 billion for a new Prevention and Public Health Fund that expanded community and clinical prevention services and primary care workforce development. In 2011, there were 350 new community health center sites established, making preventive and primary care services available to nearly twice as many people *regardless* of their insurance status. The medical and administrative personnel used to staff this expanding network of clinics across the country continues to be almost entirely by public funds.

Nonetheless, despite these substantial expansions, the ACA built on the existing healthcare system, and therefore kept the pattern of substantial public funding for private provision intact. First, the two main coverage expansions—the Medicaid Expansion and subsidies for the purchase of private marketplace insurance—center private insurance provision. The marketplace subsidies are a perfect example of programmatic entitlements where specific eligibility rules apply: A person (1) must not be eligible for employer-based health insurance; (2) must be a US citizen or lawful resident of the United States; (3) must not be incarcerated; and (4) must have income levels between 100% and 400% of poverty (Health Policy Brief: Premium Tax Credits 2013). Under the ACA marketplace, citizens are now obligated to act as consumers purchasing private health insurance—similar to private tax benefits offered through EBHI. Yet, while the generosity of marketplace subsidies are hotly contested, the subsidies people enjoy under EBHI are hidden, and the benefits are viewed as earned rights. Yet, the lost revenue in EBHI subsidies added up to $300 billion in 2018 (Congressional Budget Office [CBO] 2018). EBHI tax-exemption subsidies to middle- and upper income Americans persist and continue to increase, but remain hidden from public scrutiny.

Under the ACA, Medicare and Medicaid also continue to move in the direction of offering beneficiaries the choice of private plans. Perhaps predictably, since Medicare is a social insurance program with a strong political constituency, Medicare beneficiaries are allowed a *choice* between a private plan with a more generous benefit package and lower premium but more restricted set of providers and the traditional Medicare program. In stark contrast, the vast majority of the 50 state Medicaid programs *mandate* that low-income families enrolled in Medicaid must chose a private health plan and are automatically assigned to one if they fail to do so.

Although the majority of Medicare beneficiaries remain in the traditional program, 42% were enrolled in private health plans through the Medicare Advantage program in 2021. This percentage has increased dramatically since the early 2000s, when only 13% were enrolled in 2003. The CBO projects that the share will continue to increase, estimating that the majority of Medicare beneficiaries (51%) will be enrolled in private plans by 2030 (Freed et al. 2021). And, not surprisingly, since the majority of states mandate managed care enrollment, nearly 70% (69%) of all Medicaid enrollees were enrolled in private plans in 2018. As of July 2019, forty states, including Washington, DC, contracted with private managed care plans (Hinton et al. 2021). The ACA encouraged the continued conversion to Medicaid managed care, and most of the newly Medicaid-eligible population under the ACA were placed in private healthcare plans. What this means is that private spending through contracting with private health insurance plans remains a central characteristic of all four US healthcare entitlements.

The public/private patterns in the healthcare delivery system also remained largely untouched by the ACA. Despite enormous subsidies to the healthcare system—funding at least 60% of total national health expenditures (Grogan 2023; Pauly 2019)—the government's role in planning the healthcare system is largely restricted to antitrust rulings in the courts, and those decisions have largely turned in favor of mergers and acquisitions in the last three decades (Capps et al. 2019). While the number of multihospital systems increased from the 1970s to 2000, the growth in health system consolidations since 2000 has been enormous. Between 1998 and 2015, there were 1,410 hospital mergers and acquisitions in the United States (Pope 2019). By 2010, the top five hospitals or systems accounted for 88% of market power (Cutler and Scott Morton 2013). Since 2010 average annual hospital merger volume has surged by 50% compared to the prior decade (Crnovich, Clarin, and O'Riordan 2018), and by 2018 91 percent of hospital beds were in system-affiliated hospitals—an increase from 88 percent in 2016 (Furukawa et al. 2020).

Assessment of America's Exceptional Public/Private Mix

Health Equity

There are multiple ways to approach achieving health equity: from focusing on creating a more inclusive and fair decision-making process to improve health equity to focusing on direct investments in vulnerable communities to create a more equal distribution of health outcomes. What should be fully appreciated about the ACA is that it indeed included provisions for improving health equity through creation of a fairer process and a more equal distribution of health outcomes; it also invested across multiple levels within the healthcare system. This is crucially important because you cannot begin to achieve a goal unless you place that goal in legislation and create concrete implementation plans to begin the hard work. The ACA did that. And, yet, because it built on the existing unequal system, and most of the health equity reforms were process reforms (C. M. Grogan 2017), the ACA has not been able to move the dial much on creating more health equity.

Access to Coverage. The ACA provides subsidized coverage to private insurance on the marketplace and allowed states to expand Medicaid eligibility to nonelderly adults with incomes up to 138% of the federal poverty level (about $16,650 for individuals or $33,950 for a family of four in 2017). The main way Americans gained access to coverage was through state Medicaid expansion programs. For states that expanded Medicaid, the overwhelming evidence suggests that expansion is linked to gains in coverage and improvements in access, financial security, and selected health outcomes (Mazurenko et al. 2018; Antonisse et al. 2019).

Although there were (and remain) concerns about whether Medicaid would have sufficient capacity to serve the increased number of enrollees, and the findings on provider capacity are mixed, the majority of studies confirmed that access to care and utilization of services has increased substantially in expansion states (Mazurenko et al. 2018; Antonisse et al. 2019). Even very vulnerable "hard-to-reach" populations have gained access to coverage in Medicaid expansion states, including people with substance use disorders, people with HIV, and low-income adults diagnosed with depression or cancer (Antonisse et al. 2019; Zewde and Wimer 2019). The Medicaid expansion has also been able to fulfill a fundamental goal of insurance coverage: to protect individuals from financial liability when care is needed. Several studies demonstrated that financial security has improved among Medicaid enrollees in expansion states, and as a result, positive spillover effects are also realized: reductions in the poverty rate, personal bankruptcy, and evictions (Antonisse et al. 2019; Zewde and Wimer 2019). Fewer studies have been able to assess health outcomes, but self-reported health status has also improved (Allen and Sommers 2019; Antonisse et al. 2019; Zewde and Wimer 2019).

Given these findings of improved access to care and financial well-being for poor and low-income individuals, it is all the more appalling that millions of Americans remain uninsured in states that have refused to expand the Medicaid program. This gap in coverage left over 3 million Americans uninsured when the Medicaid expansion would have been fully enacted in 2014 (Garfield et al. 2015) and still nearly 2.2 million in 2020 (Garfield, Rudowitz, and Damico 2020). This lack of coverage means different things to different people, but if you are sick and uninsured, it almost certainly means that you do not have adequate access to the care you need. Especially in the midst of the opioid epidemic, for example, this means that people in nonexpansion states are less likely to get life-saving treatments (C. M. Grogan et al. 2020).

Another trend in Republican-led states—whether they adopted the Medicaid expansion or not—has been the implementation of policy reforms that focus on individual behaviors of particular Medicaid recipients, with the intent to increase personal responsibility, rooted in questions about whether certain low-income Americans deserve public coverage (C. M. Grogan, Singer, and Jones 2017; Vulimiri et al. 2019). As of November 2019, seven states had approved work requirements, which require work as a condition of eligibility for Medicaid; ten states required premium payments, including receipt of payment before coverage begins or a lockout period (e.g., 6 months in Indiana) if premiums are not paid; and seven states have received waivers to increase copays above previously allowed levels and/or healthy behavior incentives tied to premiums or cost sharing ("Approved Section 1115 Medicaid Waivers" 2019).

Early data suggest these policy designs result in many individuals losing their Medicaid coverage. After Arkansas implemented its work requirement, 18,000 people were disenrolled from the program (Rudowitz, Musumeci, and Hall 2019). Other studies found cost-related barriers due to Indiana's lockout period if required payments were not deposited in health savings accounts. Although coverage has expanded in the state, its coverage gains are significantly less than in traditional expansion states because of these restrictions (Freedman, Richardson, and Simon 2018; Sommers et al. 2018). There are also serious concerns about how states will consider work requirements for people who are not officially classified as "disabled" but have behavioral health issues, such as opioid use disorder, or other chronic health conditions that make work requirements particularly challenging to fulfill (Wen, Saloner, and Cummings 2019).

Delivery Model Reforms and Quality. Although researchers have long identified social factors such as income, education, and housing as crucially affecting health outcomes (Alderwick, Hood-Ronick, and Gottlieb 2019), only in the last decade, with the onset of the Medicaid expansion, have states begun to invest in social needs. Addressing social needs such as education, housing, and income support has a direct impact on advancing healthcare outcomes, especially for those with high levels of vulnerability. States realize that Medicaid is uniquely positioned to support social needs given its central role in providing coverage to low-income Americans (Alderwick et al. 2019). Under current Medicaid policy, states have the option to provide basic social supports, such as food or housing resources, to Medicaid enrollees. Many states—Republican and Democrat alike—are using their contracts with managed care organizations (MCOs) to encourage or require referrals to address patients' social needs. In particular, 16 states required MCOs to screen enrollees for social needs in 2018, and an additional 10 states encouraged the screening. Moreover, a survey of Medicaid MCOs revealed that over three-fourths of plans were undertaking activities to address housing needs, 73% were addressing nutrition, 51% education, and 31% employment needs (Hinton et al. 2021).

States can also apply for 1115 waivers to use Medicaid funds to invest in more intensive social interventions that often utilize health and social service partnerships. Several states have received such waivers to address patients' social needs ("Approved Section 1115 Medicaid Waivers" 2019). Early evidence of these initiatives in Oregon and Colorado suggested improvements in quality, controlling costs and reducing health disparities (McConnell et al. 2017; Muoto et al. 2016).

Title IV of the ACA also created community transformation grants administered by the CDC (Centers for Disease Control and Prevention), with the expressed purpose of creating healthy communities that would prioritize strategies to "to reduce health gaps and expand services to prevent and manage chronic diseases." In the first year alone (2011), the CDC provided 61 grants across 36 states (CDC Community Transformation Grants Website). Most grants funded private/public partnerships across multiple sectors, including schools, transportation, private businesses, and faith-based and nonprofit community-based organizations (https://www.cdc.gov/nccdphp/dch/programs/ctgcommunities/ctg-communities.htm).

Similar to state investments in social needs, Medicaid waivers allowed under the ACA have also ushered in major delivery model reforms attempting to coordinate care, improve quality, and lower costs. Every state in the nation is experimenting with some type of Medicaid delivery model reform, such as accountable care organizations, primary care medical homes, and health homes (Kaiser Family Foundation 2019a, 2019b, 2019c). While the attention to reforming the delivery system for Medicaid is unprecedented, there is little evidence to date on the outcomes of these reform efforts.

A long-standing concern about the Medicaid program is that many providers refuse to participate in the program. Although the proportion of primary care physicians' patient panels made up of adult Medicaid patients increased in expansion states, from 10% to nearly 14% (Neprash et al. 2018), most Medicaid patients still utilize the healthcare safety net for their care. In 2015, of primary care physicians, 20% saw 60% of Medicaid patients (Neprash et al. 2018). While Medicaid patients might prefer to see safety net providers, especially federally qualified health centers that offer wraparound services, such as language translation and transportation, audit studies also confirmed that relatively few private providers are available for new Medicaid patients (Polsky et al. 2018). In addition, so-called narrow networks—plans that employ 30% or fewer physicians in their market—are much more common among Medicaid MCOs than among employer-based MCOs or MCOs on the ACA marketplaces (Ndumele et al. 2018). Although the percentage of Medicaid MCOs with narrow networks has declined, from a high of 42% in 2011 to 27% in 2015, still one in four Medicaid MCOs offered to enrollees has a limited number of providers available and high turnover rates, raising concerns about continuity of care in addition to lack of choice (Ndumele et al. 2018). In sum, the hope of providing so-called mainstream medical care to Medicaid recipients has never been realized, and the ACA has not substantially changed that reality of an inequitable dual system of care.

Distribution of Financing Burden. One would hope, especially given the name of the ACA—the *Affordable* Care Act—that the legislation would enable a more equitable distribution of the cost of health insurance premiums, making them more equally affordable across the income distribution. The inclusion of private plans in Medicare has introduced substantial variation in the average premiums paid among the elderly by region, by type of plan chosen, and whether the person stays in traditional Medicare and purchases supplemental insurance (or Medigap coverage)—to name just a few of the varying factors. Even if we leave Medicare (and therefore people aged 65 and over) out of the analysis, the average cost at different income levels still varies substantially depending on which program an individual is eligible for and whether the individual lives in an expansion or nonexpansion state

The ACA did not reform prices in the EBHI system, which means employee contributions remain extremely regressive: As income rises, employees pay a smaller share of their income. On average, the amount workers are asked to contribute in low-wage firms (defined as firms with 35% or more employees earning $23,000 or less, which is the poverty level for a family of four) is extremely high relative to their incomes: 28%. Even in high-wage firms (defined as firms with 35% or more employees earning $57,000 or more), workers, on average, contribute 8% of their income toward premiums. Very few firms adjust the share they ask employees to pay according to salary levels. Only 10% of high-wage firms and 3% of low-wage firms offer progressively rated premium shares where high salary employees are asked to pay a higher share of their premiums than low salary individuals (Kaiser Family Foundation 2014). As a result, when a fixed premium share is distributed across different income levels, the distribution of burden is highly regressive.

There are two ways to finance the cost of a coverage expansion: the amount individuals are asked to contribute (the premium share) when they purchase (or select) a plan, as discussed above, and the amount taxpayers are asked to contribute to pay for the subsidies. On the revenue side, the ACA made the tax system more progressive; in particular: "It requires higher federal taxes for individuals with incomes above $200,000 per year and for families above $250,000 per year—about 2% of taxpayers. [And], for these [same] groups, it raises Medicare payroll taxes by 0.9% and taxes on unearned income (largely investments) by 3.8%" (Rice 2011, 492). These new taxes are estimated to cover about 17% of the total funding needed to pay for the ACA in 2019 (Dorn, Garrett, and Holahan 2014). While this amount is sizable and important from a revenue perspective, when calculated as a percentage of this high-income group's average income, it only represents 0.3%. When adding this figure to the average 2% high-income groups pay for premiums, their total contribution (2.3%) is still much lower than those earning less (Dorn et al. 2014; C. M. Grogan 2017).

Finally, the other way health costs are paid for is through the implementation of user fees. User fees impose out-of-pocket costs on individuals when they utilize healthcare services and, of course, are the flip side of progressivity; they place a more significant burden on lower income families for two reasons: first, cost-sharing amounts represent a higher share of their income; and, second, because low-income people tend to be sicker than higher income people (with higher rates of chronic disease), they have higher out-of-pocket costs. In short, the gains in equity due to progressively rated premiums are reversed when high user fees are imposed.

The ACA allows user fees in all its metal tiers (bronze, silver, gold, platinum) offered on the marketplace. There is a logical trade-off between the premium amount and the cost-sharing rate: Premiums are lowest under the bronze plan, where cost-sharing levels are very high (individuals pay 40% of healthcare costs), and conversely premiums are highest in the platinum plans, where cost-sharing rates are lowest (individuals pay 10% of healthcare costs). There are progressively rated cost-sharing subsidies for people who earn up to 250% of poverty on the marketplace (from 6% to 27% cost-sharing levels) (James 2013). And, the ACA does set limits on the total out-of-pocket costs for marketplace plans ($6,600 for an individual plan and $13,200 for a family plan for 2015). However, especially for those between 250% and 400% of the poverty rate and those who continue in the EBHI system under high cost-sharing plans, affordability is a concern. Especially among those with a chronic condition, out-of-pocket costs can be very high. In 2011, for example, 23% of people with diabetes faced high out-of-pocket burdens, defined as costs that exceed 10% of income (Li et al. 2014), and, in 2014, among those with at least one chronic condition 17% faced high out-of-pocket burdens (Collins et al. 2014). Looking at the entire population, 13% of the public faced high out-of-pocket costs in 2014 (Collins et al. 2014). Note that the ACA limit on out-of-pocket costs of $13,200 for a family of four at 400% poverty is 14% of their income. Combine this with the premium limit of 9.5% of income, and families at 400% of income are expected to cover 23.5% of income before subsidies and limits kick in.

In sum, analyzing the distribution of cost burdens across income levels reveals that ACA coverage programs clearly increased equity. However, several concerns remain: First, after 400% of poverty, US healthcare entitlements are extremely regressive; second, because the premium levels vary by location as well as the out-of-pocket cost burdens—because healthcare prices vary drastically—individuals will have higher or lower burdens simply because they live in a particular place; third, the out-of-pocket costs are regressive, and studies suggested that many low-income Americans continue to face high out-of-pocket cost burdens consuming more than 10% of their incomes.

Healthcare Costs and Lack of Transparency

One area of extreme weakness in the ACA is its inability to control costs. The cost-control provisions were weak and experimental. And, as hospital consolidations increased significantly after 2010, there is growing evidence that hospital and provider organizations have garnered monopoly-like power and are able to command significantly higher prices from commercial insurers (Cooper et al. 2019; MedPac 2020). The main way hospitals are profitable is to charge high prices to private insurance, which is why they prefer privately insured patients over publicly insured patients (Ly and Cutler 2018).

As such, health system consolidations since 2010 have also exacerbated inequities. There are now not only "have" but also "must-have" hospitals that are able to obtain among the highest rates of payments from commercial payers, often exceeding 250% of Medicare's allowed payment (Berenson 2015). In a study of 13 healthcare markets, there was evidence of a wide gap between the highest and lowest priced hospitals; in three markets, the highest priced hospital was paid well above twice as much as the lowest priced hospital for inpatient services (White, Bond, and Reschovsky 2013). And, with these high prices, as Robert Berenson explained: "These prestigious organizations are able to set aside huge reserves and compensate their executives quite generously" (Berenson 2015, 713). As such, the wealthy health systems with monopoly-like power have contributed significantly to not only the enormous healthcare expenditure problem in the United States but also further bifurcation in the system (Berenson 2015; Rosenthal 2019). Of course, as the data above attest, many of these large, consolidated healthcare systems were quite wealthy before the pandemic hit. The median US hospital has more than 53 days of cash on hand, but some of the largest and wealthiest not-for-profit hospital systems had two to three times the amount of cash on hand (Liss 2020). Moody's Investors Service rated the bonds of 284 hospitals in 2018, and 50% had enough cash on hand to cover at least 6 months of operating costs with no revenues (Rau 2020). In contrast, the poorest 25% of all hospitals in the United States (including public, nonprofit, and for-profit hospitals) had only enough cash on hand to pay for a week (7.6 days) of their operating expenses (Khullar, Bond, and Schpero 2020).

Nonprofit hospitals also have many partnership arrangements with for-profit entities that may change their incentive structure (MedPac 2020). For example, they have purchase-of-care arrangements with for profits for many of the following services: emergency room practices, laundries, restaurants, and debt collectors. Because these arrangements increase debt liability, there is concern that nonprofits shift their focus to paying off their loans and emphasizing profitable services such as tertiary care over unprofitable services such as early preventive interventions.[5]

There is also concern that, with little state oversight, for-profit commercial MCOs operating in the Medicaid program are earning significant profit margins (Herman 2016). The for-profit sector in Medicaid is substantial. By 2009, already 41% of Medicaid MCO members were enrolled in publicly traded plans (McCue 2012). While the profit levels are concerning, there is almost no evidence to date about how Medicaid recipients fair in for-profit MCOs (especially post-ACA) relative to nonprofit plans.

The increase in public ACA funding has meant significant profits for not only many private organizations in the healthcare industry but also private equity (PE) investors as well. Total healthcare assets under PE management have increased by $600 billion since 2006 (PitchBook 2019). In 2018, the value of PE healthcare assets under management reached nearly $1.5 trillion (Baker 2019; PitchBook 2019). By 2020, PE firms had moved into almost every facet of healthcare. Apollo Global Management, a $330 billion investment firm owns RCCH Healthcare Partners, an operator of 88 rural hospital campuses in West Virginia, Tennessee, Kentucky, and 26 other states. Cerberus Capital Management, a $42 billion investment firm, owns Steward Health Care; it runs 35 hospitals and a swath of urgent care facilities in 11 states. Warburg Pincus owns Modernizing Medicine, an information technology company that helps healthcare providers ramp up profits through medical billing and, to a lesser degree, debt collections. The Carlyle Group owns MedRisk, a leading provider of physical therapy cost-containment systems for US workers' compensation payers, such as insurers and large employers (Morgensen and Saliba 2020).

When PE firms acquire businesses, they can overhaul how the company is managed. Because PEs role behind the acquired company is hidden, it can often force cost-cutting management reforms that are otherwise not popular or acceptable for public companies, such as massive layoffs. While the evidence is somewhat mixed on whether PE contributes to layoffs more than other publicly owned companies (there is no comparison to nonprofit or a specific look in the healthcare field), a recent article suggested PE-acquired companies contribute to job polarization, which means it eliminates midlevel jobs and contributes to shrinking of the middle class (Olsson and Tåg 2017). Recent research also suggested that companies acquired through leverage buyouts are more likely to depress worker wages and cut investments and have a higher risk of bankruptcy. PE firms charge a 20% fee on profits above a certain level, which is known as "carried interest" and it is particularly important because it receives favorable tax treatment, while the [acquired] company is left to grapple with often debilitating debt (Kelly 2019; Kaplan and Rauh 2013).[6]

But, why is the healthcare industry so attractive to PE investment firms? The same reason that healthcare was an attractive industry in the early 2000s, continued to be even truer after 2010 due to the passage of the ACA. Murphy and Jain of *Bain Insights*, asked in *Forbes* (2017): "If healthcare is in so much turmoil, why do private equity investors like it so much?" Their answer was: "Healthcare is a safe-haven investment—that is, one with a proven resilience to economic volatility. . . . [This] holds true even when the uncertainty affects the industry itself, as it has with the acrimonious debate over the future of the ACA." Indeed, healthcare has ranked among the top three industries in terms of return on investment for PE firms every year since 2011 (Kaplan and Rauh 2013; Associates).

Just as the reliability of Medicare dollars created a profitable market for specialty hospitals and Medicaid dollars in the nursing home industry made early PE investments profitable in the 2000s, publicly funded expansions under the ACA have been a particularly lucrative target for PE in the last decade. For example, due to new benefit requirements under the ACA, insurance coverage of behavioral health services—especially Medicaid coverage—has expanded enormously since 2010. Industries where Medicaid is the major funder of care (e.g., long-term care and home healthcare services, and behavioral health) have been a particularly lucrative target. For example, Medicaid is the largest payer for addiction treatment (Andrews et al. 2018), and PE investments in behavioral health increased 24% in deal volume in just 1 year, amounting to $2.9 billion investments in treatment facilities in 2016 (Whalen and Cooper 2017). This coverage expansion came at the same time the United States was still experiencing the opioid epidemic; thus, as coverage expanded, there was also a dramatic increase in demand for behavioral health services, and PE firms pounced on the opportunity.

Private equity investment in the nursing home industry resulted in many facilities in large for-profit chains closing and laying off employees, while PE executives and investors received substantial earnings (Appelbaum and Batt 2014; Bos and Harrington 2017; Gupta, Howell, and Yannelis 2021; Baker 2019). Despite some murmurings of the need to regulate the PE markets, especially as they have impacted needed medical facilities and services, the industry remains almost completely unregulated (Appelbaum and Batt 2014; Bos and Harrington 2017; Baker 2019).

As reporter Heather Perlberg from *Bloomberg Businessweek* recently explained: "Wall Street investors invade its every corner, engineering medical practices and hospitals to maximize profits as if they were little different from grocery stores. At the center of this story are private equity firms, which saw the explosive growth of health-care spending and have been buying up physicians staffing companies, surgery centers, and everything else in sight" (Perlberg 2020). The key phrase in her quotation is they "saw the explosive growth in health-care spending." This growth in spending is fueled by government taxpayers because PE is earning large returns in an industry that is primarily funded with taxpayer dollars. The PE industry capitalizes on fragmentation and the growth of public healthcare funding (even of private health insurance) and yet is able to hide its role. As *Bloomberg Businessweek* reported, PE itself is a hidden industry: "One of PE's superpowers is that it's hard for outsiders to see and understand the industry" (Kelly 2019).

Indeed, we know very little about the outcomes of PE investments in healthcare, because these financial mechanisms are unregulated and remain intentionally obscured by the industry. However, what we do know is alarming. PE firms have been involved in closing many rural hospitals; major layoffs among staff working in the long-term care industry, where one recent study showed higher mortality rates among PE-backed nursing homes; and the surprise billing phenomenon (where insured patients receive large out-of-network bills) from emergency and ambulatory care services (Appelbaum and Batt 2020; Gupta et al. 2021; Baker 2019). In the meantime, PE investments have also produced a major shift in several sectors, such as behavioral health, from predominantly nonprofit to for profit (Baker 2019).

In 2019, *Bloomberg Businessweek* wrote in an aptly titled article, "Everything Is Private Equity Now": "Private equity managers won the financial crisis. A decade since the world economy almost came apart, big banks are more heavily regulated and scrutinized. . . . But the firms once known as leveraged buyout shops are thriving. Almost everything that's happened since 2008 has tilted in their favor" (Kelly 2019). In October 2019, just 6 months before the pandemic hit, the PE industry had trillions of dollars in assets under management (Barron 2019), and healthcare was still its most active area of investment deals, valuing at $79 billion, and where the returns on investment were highest. And, even during the COVID-19 pandemic, when the rest of the economy was experiencing one of the worst downturns since the Great Depression, PE profits continued apace because the US healthcare system fuels the industry (Morgensen and Saliba 2020).

Conclusion: Privileging Private While Hiding Public

The ACA's public/private design is sufficiently complex that an extensive information campaign was necessary to help the public understand how to access the available benefits. The intent of those informational ads, from state and federal exchanges and the plans themselves, was both to inform and to encourage eligible individuals to sign up. But these ads also sent messages about the public and private elements of enrollment, such as an ad from the federal government's Department of Health and Human Services emphasizing that through healthcare.gov consumers purchase "plans from brand-name companies." The framing of such ads may have important consequences for how citizens perceive the role of government.

In the past, state-level ads attempting to increase enrollment in the Children's Health Insurance Program avoided using the "Medicaid" name and highlighted instead a user-friendly state name (e.g., AllKids in Illinois or Husky Care in Connecticut) and the use of private insurance plans. Underlying these campaign strategies was a belief that Medicaid is associated with public insurance and therefore stigmatizing, and that access to private plans would be viewed more favorably. There is some evidence, albeit weak, that such advertising strategies might have reduced not only stigma but also knowledge about and support for Medicaid—when the term *Medicaid* is used.[7]

The Need for Public Accountability

The question of how information about US healthcare entitlements is conveyed and how this influences public knowledge and claims on the state is crucially important in a democratic society where citizens are expected to hold elected officials accountable. If elected officials are creating social programs with public funds, it is important for citizens to know that it is government that should be held accountable. Thus, it follows that the multiple ways in which government benefits are hidden through private actors is particularly concerning if it results in misinformation and induces citizens to act against their own intentions and self-interest. For example, citizens could be led to believe that their social benefits paid for with substantial public taxpayer dollars are private benefits largely financed through their own premium contribution. In turn, that might mean they would be happy with the program but support reductions in government funding due to a lack of knowledge about the extent to which they rely on public subsidies. Thus, the problem is that citizens charged with the power of democratic accountability may be misled. If the public is unaware of the extent of the government's role behind US healthcare entitlements with a private insurer face, we may find an increase in private claims on private insurers through grievance processes, but not an increase in social and political claims on the state as one might expect from such a huge increase in government healthcare investment.

Particularly concerning is when "private" frames and the role of the state are intentionally hidden, and public funds received from the federal government are strategically obscured in the US healthcare system. While Medicaid is defined as "public" and conservatives use old welfare tropes to describe enrollees on Medicaid, the healthcare system that middle- and upper income Americans are said to rely on is repeatedly described as "predominantly private"—despite $300 billion in tax-exempt subsidies for EBHI in 2018 (CBO 2018). In reality, the US healthcare system reflects a complete interdependence between private and public sectors. Even Pauly (2019), writing for the conservative American Enterprise Institute, calculated that nearly 80% of healthcare dollars are government directed in some way, which fuels the growth in private-sector delivery and administration. Thus, labeling a program as public or private is a political construction and should be understood as part of a political struggle in the US context. As such, it is important to reveal some basic truths: first, the extent to which all Americans—across the income distribution—rely on public subsidies to obtain healthcare coverage; and second, the extent to which the for-profit sector and the financial industry is profiting off of the American healthcare system, while many Americans continue to struggle to access quality healthcare and pay their medical bills.

Notes

1. A precedent had already been set for state and local governments' investment in hospital construction for quite some time (see Stevens 1989.
2. In return for subsidized hospital construction, the federal government required communities to survey existing healthcare facilities (including hospitals and health centers) and, based on this survey, to present an organized plan for facility construction. But, there was no follow-up to ensure that communities actually followed through with any community health planning, and indeed few communities did follow through.
3. Data source from "AHA Survey of Sources of Funding for Hospital Construction, 1968, 1981"; reported in Cohodes and Kinkead as published in *Journal of Hospital Capital Finance*, First Quarter, 1986, 8.
4. See also Richard B. Siegrist, "Wall Street and the For-Profit Hospital Management Companies," in same volume.
5. Confidential interview with person who gave expert testimony at meetings of the State of Delaware Health Facilities Authority (Horwitz and Nichols 2022; July 27, 2021).
6. For evidence on the enormous wealth gains of PE owners, see Phalippou, Ludovic, *An Inconvenient Fact: Private Equity Returns & The Billionaire Factory* (June 10, 2020). University of Oxford, Said Business School, Working Paper. Available at SSRN: https://ssrn.com/abstract=3623820 or http://dx.doi.org/10.2139/ssrn.3623820
7. Grogan and Park 2017.

References

Abramovitz, M. 2001. "Everyone Is Still on Welfare: The Role of Redistribution in Social Policy." *Social Work* 46(4): 297–308. https://doi.org/10.1093/sw/46.4.297

Alderwick, H., C. M. Hood-Ronick, and L. M. Gottlieb. 2019. "Medicaid Investments to Address Social Needs in Oregon and California." *Health Affairs (Millwood)* 38(5): 774–781. https://doi.org/10.1377/hlthaff.2018.05171

Allen, H., and B. D. Sommers. 2019. "Medicaid Expansion and Health: Assessing the Evidence after 5 Years." *JAMA* 322(13): 1253–1254. https://doi.org/10.1001/jama.2019.12345

Andrews, Christina M., Colleen M. Grogan, Bikki Tran Smith, Amanda J. Abraham, Harold A. Pollack, Keith Humphreys, Melissa A. Westlake, and Peter D. Friedmann. 2018. "Medicaid Benefits for Addiction Treatment Expanded After Implementation of the Affordable Care Act." *Health Affairs* 37(8): 1216–1222. https://www.healthaffairs.org/doi/10.1377/hlthaff.2018.0272

Antonisse, Larisa, Rachel Garfield, Robin Rudowitz, and Madeline Guth. 2019. "The Effects of Medicaid Expansion under the ACA: Updated Findings from a Literature Review." https://files.kff.org/attachment/Issue-brief-The-Effects-of-Medicaid-Expansion-under-the-ACA-Findings-from-a-Literature-Review (accessed August 15).

Appelbaum, Eileen, and Rosemary Batt. 2014. *Private Equity at Work: When Wall Street Manages Main Street*. Russell Sage Foundation.

Appelbaum, Eileen, and Rosemary Batt. 2020. "Private Equity Buyouts in Healthcare: Who Wins, Who Loses?" Working Papers Series. Center for Economic and Policy Research Institute for New Economic Thinking. https://ideas.repec.org/p/thk/wpaper/118.html

"Approved Section 1115 Medicaid Waivers." 2019. Cambridge Associates. Kaiser Family Foundation. State Health Facts. "Approved Section 1115 Medicaid Waivers." Website: https://www.kff.org/other/state-indicator/approved-section-1115-medic aid-waivers/?currentTimeframe=0&sortModel=%7B%22colId%22:%22Locat ion%22,%22sort%22:%22asc%22%7D (accessed on July 14, 2022).

Baker, Jim. 2019. "Adverse Reaction: How Will the Flood of Private Equity Money into Health Care Providers Impact Access to, Cost, and Quality of Care?" Private Equity Stakeholder Project. https://pestakeholder.org/wp-content/uploads/2019/11/Adverse-Reaction-PE-Investment-in-Health-Care-PESP-110619.pdf

Barron, Jesse. 2019. "How America's Oldest Gun Maker Went Bankrupt: A Financial Engineering Mystery." *New York Times Magazine.* May 1. Website: https://www.nyti mes.com/interactive/2019/05/01/magazine/remington-guns-jobs-huntsville.html (accessed on July 14, 2022).

Bazzoli, Gloria J. 2004. "The Corporatization of American Hospitals." *Journal of Health Politics, Policy and Law* 29(4–5): 885–906. https://doi.org/10.1215/03616878-29-4-5-885

Berenson, R. 2015. "Addressing Pricing Power in Integrated Delivery: The Limits of Antitrust." *Journal of Health Politics, Policy and Law* 40(4): 711–744. https://doi.org/ 10.1215/03616878-3150026

Bos, Aline, and Charlene Harrington. 2017. "What Happens to a Nursing Home Chain When Private Equity Takes Over? A Longitudinal Case Study." *Inquiry: A Journal of Medical Care Organization, Provision and Financing* 54. https://doi.org/10.1177/00469 58017742761

Brown, J. B., and R. B. Saltman. 1985. "Health Capital Policy in the United States: A Strategic Perspective." *Inquiry* 22(2): 122–131.

Capps, Cory, Laura Kmitch, Zenon Zabinski, and Slava Zayats. 2019. "The Continuing Saga of Hospital Merger Enforcement." *Antitrust Law Journal* 82(2): 441–496.

Cleverley, W. O., and P. C. Nutt. 1984. "The Decision Process Used for Hospital Bond Rating—and Its Implications." *Health Services Research* 19(5): 615–637.

Cohodes, Donald R., and Brian M. Kinkead. 1984. *Hospital Capital Formation in the 1980s.* Baltimore: Johns Hopkins University Press.

Collins, Sara R., Petra W. Rasmussen, Michelle M. Doty, and Sophie Beutel. 2014. "Too High a Price: Out-of-Pocket Health Care Costs in the United States. Findings from the Commonwealth Fund Health Care Affordability Tracking Survey, September–October 2014." Commonwealth Fund. https://www.commonwealthfund.org/sites/default/files/ documents/___media_files_publications_issue_brief_2014_nov_1784_collins_too_ high_a_price_out_of_pocket_tb_v2.pdf

Congressional Budget Office (CBO). 2018. "Reduce Tax Subsidies for Employment-Based Health Insurance." Website: https://www.cbo.gov/budget-options/54798 (Accessed August 2, 2021).

Cooper, Z., S. V. Craig, M. Gaynor, and J. Van Reenen. 2019. "The Price Ain't Right? Hospital Prices and Health Spending on the Privately Insured." *Quarterly Journal of Economics* 134(1): 51–107. https://doi.org/10.1093/qje/qjy020

Corwin, E. H. L., and Commonwealth Fund. 1946. *The American Hospital.* New York: Commonwealth Fund.

Crnovich, Paul, Dan Clarin, and Jason O'Riordan. 2018. "2018 State of Consumerism in Healthcare: Activity in Search of Strategy." Kaufman Hall. https://www.kaufmanhall. com/sites/default/files/legacy_files/kh_soc-report-2018-press_k2_Rebrand.pdf

Cutler, D. M., and F. Scott Morton. 2013. "Hospitals, Market Share, and Consolidation." *JAMA* 310(18): 1964–1970. https://doi.org/10.1001/jama.2013.281675

Derthick, Martha. 1979. *Policymaking for Social Security*. Brookings Institution Press.

Dorn, Stan, Bowen Garrett, and John Holahan. 2014. "Redistribution Under the ACA Is Modest in Scope." Urban Institute. https://www.urban.org/sites/default/files/publicat ion/22271/413023-redistribution-under-the-aca-is-modest-in-scope.pdf

Ermann, Dan, and Jon Gabel. 1984. "Multihospital Systems: Issues and Empirical Findings." *Health Affairs* 3(1): 50–64. https://doi.org/10.1377/hlthaff.3.1.50

Feder, Judith M., Jack Hadley, and Urban Institute. 1984. *Cutbacks, Recession and Care to the Poor: Will the Urban Poor Get Hospital Care?* Washington, DC: Urban Institute.

Fox, D. M., and D. C. Schaffer. 1991. "Tax Administration as Health Policy: Hospitals, the Internal Revenue Service, and the Courts." *Journal of Health, Politics and Policy Law* 16(2): 251–279. https://doi.org/10.1215/03616878-16-2-251

Freed, Meredith, Jeannie Fuglesten Biniek, Anthony Damico, and Tricia Neuman. 2021. "Medicare Advantage in 2021: Enrollment Update and Key Trends." Kaiser Family Foundation. June 21. Website: https://www.kff.org/medicare/issue-brief/medicare-advantage-in-2021-enrollment-update-and-key-trends/ (accessed August 2, 2021).

Freedman, S., L. Richardson, and K. I. Simon. 2018. "Learning from Waiver States: Coverage Effects under Indiana's HIP Medicaid Expansion." *Health Affairs (Millwood)* 37(6): 936–943. https://doi.org/10.1377/hlthaff.2017.1596

Furukawa, M. F., L. Kimmey, D. J. Jones, R. M. Machta, J. Guo, and E. C. Rich. 2020. "Consolidation of Providers into Health Systems Increased Substantially, 2016–18." *Health Affairs (Millwood)* 39(8): 1321–1325. https://doi.org/10.1377/hlthaff.2020.00017

Garfield, Rachel, Anthony Damico, and Robin Rudowitz. 2021. "Taking a Closer Look at Characteristics of People in the Coverage Gap." Kaiser Family Foundation. https://www.kff.org/policy-watch/taking-a-closer-look-at-characteristics-of-people-in-the-coverage-gap/

Garfield, Rachel, Anthony Damico, Jessica Stephens, and Saman Rouhani. 2015. "The Coverage Gap: Uninsured Poor Adults in States that Do Not Expand Medicaid—An Update." Kaiser Family Foundation. Accessed February 22, 2015.

Garfield, Rachel, Robin Rudowitz, and Anthony Damico. 2020. "How Many Uninsured Adults Could Be Reached If All States Expanded Medicaid?" Kaiser Family Foundation. https://www.kff.org/uninsured/issue-brief/how-many-uninsured-adults-could-be-reached-if-all-states-expanded-medicaid/

Graetz, Michael J., and Jerry L. Mashaw. 1999. *True Security: Rethinking American Social Insurance*. New Haven, CT: Yale University Press.

Grogan, C. M. 2017. "How the ACA Addressed Health Equity and What Repeal Would Mean." *Journal of Health, Politics and Policy Law* 42(5): 985–993. https://doi.org/10.1215/03616878-3940508

Grogan, C. M., C. S. Bersamira, P. M. Singer, B. T. Smith, H. A. Pollack, C. M. Andrews, and A. J. Abraham. 2020. "Are Policy Strategies for Addressing the Opioid Epidemic Partisan? A View from the States." *Journal of Health, Politics and Policy Law* 45(2): 277–309. https://doi.org/10.1215/03616878-8004886

Grogan, C. M., P. M. Singer, and D. K. Jones. 2017. "Rhetoric and Reform in Waiver States." *Journal of Health, Politics and Policy Law* 42(2): 247–284. https://doi.org/10.1215/03616878-3766719

Grogan, C., and E. Patashnik. 2003. "Between Welfare Medicine and Mainstream Entitlement: Medicaid at the Political Crossroads." *Journal of Health, Politics and Policy Law* 28(5): 821–858. https://doi.org/10.1215/03616878-28-5-821

Grogan, Colleen M. Forthcoming, 2023. *Grow and Hide: The History of the American Health Care State*. Oxford, UK: Oxford University Press.

Grogan, Colleen M. 2013. "Medicaid: Designed to Grow." In *Health Politics and Policy*, 5th ed., edited by Daniel Ehlke and James Morone, 142–163. Stamford, CT: Cengage Learning.

Grogan, Colleen M., and Sunggeun (Ethan) Park*. 2017. "The Politics of Medicaid: Most Americans are Connected to the Program, Support Its Expansion, and Do Not View It as Stigmatizing." *The Milbank Quarterly* 95(4): 749–782.

Gupta, Atul, Sabrina T. Howell, and Constantine Yannelis, and Abhinav Gupta. 2021. "Does Private Equity Investment in Healthcare Benefit Patients? Evidence from Nursing Homes." National Bureau of Economic Research Working Paper Series No. 28474. https://doi.org/10.3386/w28474. http://www.nber.org/papers/w28474

Hacker, Jacob S. 2002. *The Divided Welfare State: The Battle over Public and Private Social Benefits in the United States*. Cambridge: Cambridge University Press.

Health Policy Brief. 2013. "Premium Tax Credits." *Health Affairs* August 1, 2013.

Herman, B. 2016. "Medicaid's Unmanaged Managed Care." *Modern Healthcare* 46(18): 16–18.

Hinton, Elizabeth, Robin Rudowitz, Lina Stolyar, and Natalie Singer. 2021. "10 Things to Know about Medicaid Managed Care." Kaiser Family Foundation. February 23. Website: https://www.kff.org/medicaid/issue-brief/10-things-to-know-about-medic aid-managed-care/ (accessed on July 14, 2022).

Hoffman, Beatrix Rebecca. 2012. *Health Care for Some: Rights and Rationing in the United States since 1930*. Chicago, IL: University of Chicago Press.

Horwitz, J. R., and Nichols, A. 2022. "Hospital Service Offerings Still Differ Substantially By Ownership Type: Study Examines Service Offerings by Hospital Ownership Type." *Health Affairs* 41(3): 331–340.

Howard, Christopher. 1999. *The Hidden Welfare State: Tax Expenditures and Social Policy in the United States*. Princeton, NJ: Princeton University Press.

Institute of Medicine. 1983. In *The New Health Care for Profit: Doctors and Hospitals in a Competitive Environment*, edited by B. H. Gray. Washington, DC: National Academies Press.

Institute of Medicine Committee on Implications of For-Profit Enterprise in Health Care. 1986. In *For-Profit Enterprise in Health Care*, edited by B. H. Gray. Washington, DC: National Academies Press.

James, Julia. 2013. "Patient Engagement." *Health Affairs Health Policy Brief*. https://www.healthaffairs.org/do/10.1377/hpb20130214.898775/full/

Jost, Timothy S. 2003. *Disentitlement?: The threats facing our public health-care programs and a rights-based response*. New York, NY: Oxford University Press.

Kaiser Family Foundation. 2014. "2014 Employer Health Benefits Survey." https://www.kff.org/report-section/ehbs-2014-section-one-cost-of-health-insurance/

Kaiser Family Foundation. 2019a. "Mapping Medicaid Delivery System and Payment Reform." https://www.kff.org/interactive/delivery-system-and-payment-reform/

Kaiser Family Foundation. 2019b. "States' Positions in the Affordable Care Act Case at the Supreme Court." [Interactive]. https://www.kff.org/health-reform/state-indica tor/state-positions-on-aca-case/?currentTimeframe=0&selectedDistributions= state-positions-on-aca-case&sortModel=%7B%22colId%22:%22Location%22,%22s ort%22:%22asc%22%7D

Kaiser Family Foundation. 2019c. "Status of State Medicaid Expansion Decisions: Interactive Map." https://www.kff.org/medicaid/issue-brief/status-of-state-medicaid-expansion-decisions-interactive-map/

Kaplan, Steven N., and Joshua Rauh. 2013. "It's the Market: The Broad-Based Rise in the Return to Top Talent." *Journal of Economic Perspectives* 27(3): 35–56. https://www.aea web.org/articles?id=10.1257/jep.27.3.35

Kara Murphy, and Nirad Jain, Bain and Company. June 20. "How Private Equity Picks Healthcare Winners" https://www.forbes.com/sites/baininsights/2017/06/20/how-private-equity-picks-healthcare-winners/#57db2fc12490 (accessed 12/10/17).

Katz, Michael B. 1986. *In the Shadow of the Poorhouse: A Social History of Welfare in America.* New York: Basic Books.

Kelly, Jason. 2019. "Everything Is Private Equity Now. *Bloomberg Businessweek*, October 8. Website: https://www.bloomberg.com/news/features/2019-10-03/how-private-equ ity-works-and-took-over-everything (accessed on September 8, 2020).

Khullar, D., A. M. Bond, and W. L. Schpero. 2020. "COVID-19 and the Financial Health of US Hospitals." *JAMA* 323(21): 2127–2128. https://doi.org/10.1001/jama.2020.6269

Kinney, E. D., and B. Lefkowitz. 1982. "Capital Cost Reimbursement to Community Hospitals under Federal Health Insurance Programs." *Journal of Health, Politics and Policy Law* 7(3): 648–666. https://doi.org/10.1215/03616878-7-3-648.

Li, R., L. E. Barker, S. Shrestha, P. Zhang, O. K. Duru, T. Pearson-Clarke, and E. W. Gregg. 2014. "Changes over Time in High Out-of-Pocket Health Care Burden in U.S. Adults with Diabetes, 2001–2011." *Diabetes Care* 37(6): 1629–1635. https://doi.org/10.2337/dc13-1997

Liss, Samantha. 2020. "Nonprofit Health Systems—Despite Huge Cash Reserves—Get Billions in CARES Funding." *HealthcareDive*, June 23. Website: https://www.healthc aredive.com/news/nonprofit-health-systems-despite-huge-cash-reserves-get-billi ons-in-car/580078/ (accessed on July 14, 2022).

Ly, D. P., and D. M. Cutler. 2018. "Factors of U.S. Hospitals Associated with Improved Profit Margins: An Observational Study." *Journal of General Internal Medicine* 33(7): 1020–1027. https://doi.org/10.1007/s11606-018-4347-4

Marmor, Theodore R., Jerry L. Mashaw, and Philip Harvey. 1992. *America's Misunderstood Welfare State: Persistent Myths, Enduring Realities.* Basic Books.

Mazurenko, O., C. P. Balio, R. Agarwal, A. E. Carroll, and N. Menachemi. 2018. "The Effects of Medicaid Expansion under the ACA: A Systematic Review." *Health Affairs (Millwood)* 37(6): 944–950. https://doi.org/10.1377/hlthaff.2017.1491

McConnell, K. J., S. Renfro, B. K. Chan, T. H. Meath, A. Mendelson, D. Cohen, J. Waxmonsky, D. McCarty, N. Wallace, and R. C. Lindrooth. 2017. "Early Performance in Medicaid Accountable Care Organizations: A Comparison of Oregon and Colorado." *JAMA Internal Medicine* 177(4): 538–545. https://doi.org/10.1001/jamain ternmed.2016.9098

McCue, M. 2012. "Financial Performance of Health Plans in Medicaid Managed Care." *Medicare Medicaid Res Rev* 2(2): E1–E10. https://doi.org/10.5600/mmrr.002.02.a07

"Medical Care for the American People: The Final Report of the Committee on the Costs of Medical Care, Adopted October 31, 1932." 1932. In *Publication (Committee on the Cost of Medical Care)*, edited by Care Committee on the Cost of Medical (213). Chicago: University of Chicago Press.

MedPac (Medicare Payment Advisory Commission). 2020. "Report to the Congress: Medicare Payment Policy." https://www.medpac.gov/document/http-www-medpac-gov-docs-default-source-reports-mar20_entirereport_sec-pdf/

Melnick, R. Shep. 1996. "Federalism and the New Rights." *Yale Law and Policy Review* 14(2): 325–354.

Morgan, Kimberly J., and Andrea Louise Campbell. 2011. *The Delegated Welfare State: Medicare, Markets, and the Governance of Social Policy.* Oxford University Press.

Morgensen, Gretchen, and Emmanuelle Saliba. 2020. "Private Equity Firms Now Control Many Hospitals, ERs and Nursing Homes. Is It Good for Health Care?" *NBC News.* Website: https://www.nbcnews.com/health/health-care/private-equity-firms-now-control-many-hospitals-ers-nursing-homes-n1203161 (accessed September 8, 2020).

Muoto, I., J. Luck, J. Yoon, S. Bernell, and J. M. Snowden. 2016. "Oregon's Coordinated Care Organizations Increased Timely Prenatal Care Initiation and Decreased Disparities." *Health Affairs (Millwood)* 35(9): 1625–1632. https://doi.org/10.1377/hlth aff.2016.0396

Ndumele, Chima D., Becky Staiger, Joseph S. Ross, and Mark J. Schlesinger. 2018. "Network Optimization and the Continuity of Physicians in Medicaid Managed Care." *Health Affairs* 37(6): 929–935. https://www.healthaffairs.org/doi/abs/10.1377/hlth aff.2017.1410

Neprash, H. T., A. Zink, J. Gray, and K. Hempstead. 2018. "Physicians' Participation in Medicaid Increased Only Slightly Following Expansion." *Health Affairs (Millwood)* 37(7): 1087–1091. https://doi.org/10.1377/hlthaff.2017.1085

Olsson, Martin, and Joacim Tåg. 2016, May 1. "Private Equity, Layoffs, and Job Polarization." IFN Working Paper no. 1068. *SSRN.* https://ssrn.com/abstract=2596651

Pauly, Mark V. 2019. "Will Health Care's Immediate Future Look a Lot Like the Recent Past? More Public-Sector Funding, But More Private-Sector Delivery and Administration." American Enterprise Institute. June 7. Website: https://www.aei.org/research-produ cts/report/health-care-public-sector-funding/ (accessed on July 14, 2022).

Perlberg, Heather. 2020. "How Private Equity Is Ruining American Health Care." *Bloomberg Businessweek.*May 20. Website: https://www.bloomberg.com/news/featu res/2020-05-20/private-equity-is-ruining-health-care-covid-is-making-it-worse (accessed on September 8, 2020)

Polsky, Daniel, Molly K. Candon, Paula Chatterjee, and Xinwei Chen. 2018. "Scope of Primary Care Physicians' Participation in the Health Insurance Marketplaces." *Health Affairs* 37(8): 1252–1256. https://www.healthaffairs.org/doi/abs/10.1377/hlth aff.2018.0179

Pope, Chris. 2019. "The Cost of Hospital Protectionism." *National Affairs Winter,* (52: Summer). Website: https://www.nationalaffairs.com/publications/detail/the-cost-of-hospital-protectionism (accessed on July 14, 2022).

Rau, Jordan. 2020. "Amid Coronavirus Distress, Wealthy Hospitals Hoard Millions." *Kaiser Health News,* April 28. Website: https://khn.org/news/amid-coronavirus-distr ess-wealthy-hospitals-hoard-millions/ (accessed on July 14, 2022).

Relman, A. S. 1980. "The New Medical-Industrial Complex." *New England Journal of Medicine* 303(17): 963–970.

Rice, T. 2011. "A Progressive Turn of Events." *Journal of Health, Politics and Policy Law* 36(3): 491–494. https://doi.org/10.1215/03616878-1271144

Rorem, Clarence Rufus. 1930. *The Public's Investment in Hospitals.* Chicago: University of Chicago Press, xxii, 251.

Rosenbaum, Sara, and Timothy M. Westmoreland. 2012. "The Supreme Court's Surprising Decision on the Medicaid Expansion: How Will the Federal Government and States Proceed?" *Health Affairs* 31(8): 1663–1672. https://doi.org/10.1377/hlthaff.2012.0766

Rosenthal, Elizabeth. 2019. "Analysis: How Your Beloved Hospital Helps to Drive Up Health Care Costs." *Kaiser Health News*, September 5. Website: https://khn.org/news/analysis-how-your-beloved-hospital-helps-to-drive-up-health-care-costs/ (accessed on July 14, 2022).

Rudowitz, Robin, MaryBeth Musumeci, and Cornelia Hall. 2019. "February State Data for Medicaid Work Requirements in Arkansas." Kaiser Family Foundation. March 25. Website: https://www.kff.org/medicaid/issue-brief/state-data-for-medicaid-work-requirements-in-arkansas/ (accessed on July 14, 2022).

Schatzkin, A. 1984. "The Relationship of Inpatient Racial Composition and Hospital Closure in New York City." *Medical Care* 22(5): 379–387. https://doi.org/10.1097/00005650-198405000-00002

Sommers, B. D., C. E. Fry, R. J. Blendon, and A. M. Epstein. 2018. "New Approaches in Medicaid: Work Requirements, Health Savings Accounts, and Health Care Access." *Health Affairs (Millwood)* 37 (7):1099–1108. https://doi.org/10.1377/hlthaff.2018.0331

Stevens, Rosemary. 1982. "'A Poor Sort of Memory': Voluntary Hospitals and Government before the Depression." *Milbank Memorial Fund Quarterly. Health and Society* 60(4): 551–584. https://doi.org/10.2307/3349691

Stevens, Rosemary, and American Council of Learned Societies. 1989. *In Sickness and in Wealth: American Hospitals in the Twentieth Century*. Baltimore, MD: Johns Hopkins University Press.

Titmuss, Richard M. 1965. "The Role of Redistribution in Social Policy." *Social Security Bulletin* 28(6): 14–20.

Vulimiri, M., W. K. Bleser, R. S. Saunders, F. Madanay, C. Moseley, H. F. McGuire, P. A. Ubel, A. McKethan, M. McClellan, and C. A. Wong. 2019. "Engaging Beneficiaries in Medicaid Programs that Incentivize Health-Promoting Behaviors." *Health Affairs (Millwood)* 38(3): 431–439. https://doi.org/10.1377/hlthaff.2018.05427

Weir, Margaret. 2012. "Entitlements." In *Oxford Companion to American Politics*, edited by David Coates, 346–347. New York: Oxford University Press.

Wen, Hefei, Brendan Saloner, and Janet R. Cummings. 2019. "Behavioral and Other Chronic Conditions among Adult Medicaid Enrollees: Implications for Work Requirements." *Health Affairs* 38(4): 660–667. https://doi.org/10.1377/hlthaff.2018.05059

Whalen, Jeanne, and Laura Cooper. 2017. "Private-Equity Pours Cash into Opioid Treatment Sector." *Wall Street Journal*. September 2. Website: https://www.wsj.com/articles/opioid-crisis-opens-opportunities-for-private-equity-firms-1504353601 (accessed on July 14, 2022).

White, C., A. M. Bond, and J. D. Reschovsky. 2013. "High and Varying Prices for Privately Insured Patients Underscore Hospital Market Power." Center for Studying Health System Change. *Research Brief September* (27): 1–10. Website: https://www.heartland.org/_template-assets/documents/publications/high_and_varying_prices_for_privately_insured_patients_underscore_hospital_market_power.pdf (accessed on July 14, 2022).

Zewde, N., and C. Wimer. 2019. "Antipoverty Impact of Medicaid Growing with State Expansions over Time." *Health Affairs (Millwood)* 38(1): 132–138. https://doi.org/10.1377/hlthaff.2018.05155

3

Public and Private Interfaces in Canadian Healthcare

Health Equity and Quality of Healthcare Services Implications

Gregory P. Marchildon and Sara Allin

Introduction

The public/private mix in the financing and delivery of healthcare is, almost everywhere, a subject of hot dispute for obvious reasons. Since health spending in high-income countries such as Canada forms such a significant portion of the economy, there is always considerable tension on whether the money comes from public or private sources and whether private rather than public providers deliver these services as well as the source, manner, and extent of their payment for these. Canadian health economist Robert Evans once pointed out that the revenues assembled for healthcare from whatever source "must exactly equal the expenditures to fund providers of care, and these in turn must equal the total incomes earned by individuals from the provision of care" (Evans 2004, 142). Of course, Evans was referring to not only the direct providers of care but also financial intermediaries such as insurance firms as well as health system and organization leaders and managers. Evans's purpose was to illustrate the fact that in every high-income country in which healthcare is one of the largest sectors of the economy, there is going to be constant contestation over who should control, and benefit from, health spending, in terms of provider remuneration and corporate profits.

Universal health coverage (UHC)—or Medicare as it is popularly known in Canada—involves both of the constitutionally recognized, federal and provincial, orders of government. The federal government sets high-level requirements on the provincial governments in terms of how they determine

Gregory P. Marchildon and Sara Allin, *Public and Private Interfaces in Canadian Healthcare* In: *The Public/Private Sector Mix in Healthcare Delivery.* Edited by: Howard A. Palley, Oxford University Press. © Oxford University Press 2023.
DOI: 10.1093/oso/9780197571101.003.0003

and manage the access of their respective residents to medically necessary hospital, diagnostic, and physician services as well as inpatient prescription drugs. These requirements, known as the five criteria of public administration, comprehensiveness, universality, portability, and accessibility in the *Canada Health Act*, are basically access rules that ensure that all Canadians receive coverage by virtue of their residence in a province; that this coverage is free at the point of service; that it is portable when Canadians are visiting, or moving to, other parts of the country; and that the coverage is uniform across the country. In addition, the criteria of public administration means that provincial health ministers must hold ultimate accountability for the expenditure of public funds on Medicare services: It does not mean that these services must be delivered through the public sector. While these rules focus on equity, it is important to note that they do not impose any standards concerning the quality of healthcare services or the timeliness of their delivery—these issues are entirely in the hands of individual subnational governments in Canada.

These five criteria of the Canada Health Act can be enforced through the threat of potential withdrawals of federal transfer money that flow annually to the provincial governments through the Canada Health Transfer. Enforcement is rare, however, due to the lack of surveillance and the unwillingness of some federal government administrations to challenge provincial governments on their practices (Choudhry 1996; Flood, Lahey, and Thomas 2017).

Beyond the criteria of the Canada Health Act, provincial governments are free to decide on the management and delivery of Medicare services, including whether they are financed or delivered by public or private actors. Indeed, the federal government does not have the constitutional jurisdiction to dictate the manner in which provincial healthcare services are delivered (Marchildon 2018).

Since the basket of Medicare services is fairly narrow in Canada relative to what is included in UHC in other high-income countries in Europe and Australasia, it needs to be emphasized that there are no federal access rules on other health services, including outpatient prescription drug therapies, long-term care (LTC), home care, rehabilitation services, dental care, and vision care. Provincial governments can decide whether to provide coverage, and, if so, the degree and type of coverage. In fact, all provincial governments have prescription drug plans that attempt to fill the gaps left by private employer-based health insurance plans, and all provide some funding and services for LTC and home care. However, there has been minimal provincial involvement in dental and vision care (Marchildon, Allin, and Merkur 2020).

The objective of this chapter is to describe the evolution of the public/private mix, highlighting major shifts over time. To keep this within the confines of a single chapter, we focus on three health service sectors: (1) hospitals and acute care; (2) physicians and medical care, including ambulatory care; and (3) long-term, facility-based care. The first two sectors are included in the basket of Medicare services, while the third sector is excluded and therefore not subject to the Canada Health Act. However, it should be noted that this chapter does not address important public-private debates and cleavage in other sectors, such as pharmaceuticals—the second largest category of spending after hospital care and for which about half of financing is from private sources, as well as home care, and dental care, which are covered elsewhere by the authors and others (Allin, Farmer, et al. 2020; Allin, Rudoler, et al. 2020; Boothe 2018).

The first two areas involve services, institutions, and professional bodies that are core to UHC in Canada. Historically, these Medicare services, although entirely financed through the general tax revenues of federal and provincial governments, were privately delivered by private not-for-profit hospitals and professional for-profit doctors working independently and paid by governments on a fee-for-service basis. As will be seen, while there has been a major shift in the ownership and control of hospitals from the not-for-profit sector to the public sector in most provinces, the position of doctors as private professionals remains largely the same today.

The third area of LTC has involved a mixture of public and private finances since provincial governments began to implement programs in the 1970s. Today, most of the financing of residential, or facility-based, LTC comes from provincial governments, but the delivery—the mix of which varies considerably across jurisdictions—is divided among public, private for-profit, and private not-for-profit, although tilted more heavily toward private delivery if for-profit and not-for-profit sectors are combined (Marchildon and Allin 2016; CIHI [Canadian Institute for Health Information] 2021b). On average across Canada, over half of LTC homes are privately owned, of which about 54% are for profit (CIHI 2021b). As noted further in this chapter, the ratio of public-private LTC homes varies across the country: In Saskatchewan, Quebec, Newfoundland, and Labrador and the three northern territories, the large majority (or all) are publicly owned, while in others (e.g., British Columbia, Ontario, and Nova Scotia) the majority are privately owned. We have selected this sector in part because of the weaknesses of the for-profit sector that were exposed by the COVID-19 pandemic (Tuohy 2021; Stall et al. 2020).

The chapter's second objective is to consider the implications of the public-private division on the equity objectives of Canadian healthcare and on the issue of the quality of services, including the question of wait times, a major challenge in the Canadian system (Martin et al. 2018). We insert our observations on the equity and quality dimensions in our analysis of the public-private divide for hospitals and acute care followed by the medical care sector that involves physician care embracing both primary and specialist care, and finally for facility-based LTC.

What does quality healthcare entail? Unfortunately, there is no commonly accepted definition of quality among health system scholars (Busse, Panteli, and Quentin 2019). However, one of the more commonly accepted definitions was developed by the Institute of Medicine (IOM) in the United States. The IOM considers six domains, or aims, of quality of care—safe, effective, patient centered, timely, efficient, and equitable, or broadly "the degree to which health services for individuals and populations increase the likelihood of desired health outcomes and are consistent with professional knowledge" (IOM cited in Busse, Panateli, and Quentin 2019, 6) These desired health outcomes go beyond health status and quality-of-life measures to include patient satisfaction.

Equity is both an aim of quality, whereby quality should not vary based on patient characteristics such as gender, geography, socioeconomic status, race, and ethnicity, as well as a stand-alone goal. Put simply, equity requires individuals with the same levels of need to be treated the same (horizontal equity) and individuals with different levels of need to be treated differently, in according to their needs (vertical equity). Thus, we observe inequity in healthcare if access to or quality of care varies systematically by characteristics other than need. It is important to note that, although outside the scope of this chapter, a significant source of inequity in health and access to care in Canada has its origins in the colonization and cultural genocide inflicted on indigenous peoples. There is a growing body of literature that documents the causes and magnitude of these inequities and proposes solutions (Allan and Smylie 2015; Inuit Tapiriit Kanatami 2014; Turpel-Lafond 2020)

In order to provide an analytical structure to the review, it is first necessary to rethink the simple public-private dichotomy. Aside from government and the for-profit private sector, there is an active civil society involvement in the delivery, and at times the financing, of healthcare in Canada. This sector does not operate according to the rules, processes, and assumptions underpinning government and the private sector. For this reason, a new conceptual framework is introduced in order to address the confusion that is common to discussions about public and private financing and delivery of healthcare as well as better identify the various "public-private" interfaces in the Canadian health system.

A Conceptual Framework of Public-Private Interfaces

There is perpetual confusion between the concepts of private financing versus private delivery of health services. Public finance is at the core of UHC, known as Medicare in Canada; however, private delivery, especially physician care, has always been a major component of the Canadian system, to the point that one noted history of the emergence of Medicare was titled *Private Practice, Public Payment* (Naylor 1986). Indeed, the origin of the phrase "single payer" is directly linked to the difference between Canada's approach compared to National Health Service (NHS) style systems, such as that in the United Kingdom, where the majority of both finance and delivery is public (Tuohy 2009). This private delivery component forms the main difference between National Health Insurance health systems (e.g., the Canadian system) and NHS systems such as those in the United Kingdom and the Nordic countries (Böhm et al. 2013; Cuadrado et al. 2019).

The second area of confusion involves the appropriate definition of public and private, in part because of the gray areas between governmental finance and delivery at one end of the extreme and delivery by pure private-for-profit actors at the other end (Deber 2004). Table 3.1 attempts to address both areas of confusion by separating finance and delivery and by introducing a category that captures nonprofit financing and delivery by cooperatives or religious and other civil society organizations motivated by a sense of mission rather than profit to serve their members or the poor and marginalized. Table 3.1 depicts nine discrete cells, each with a unique interface between public, civil society or private financing and public, civil society or private delivery.

Cell I, the private financing and private delivery interface, describes the situation before Medicare was introduced in Canada in the 1950s and 1960s, when the majority of the financing of physician services came from individuals or families paying out of pocket or through private health insurance

Table 3.1. Nine possible public-private interfaces in Canada

		Delivery of healthcare		
		Private for profit (corporate and professional)	Private not for profit (civil society, religious, or mutual)	Public (government, direct, or arm's length)
Financing of healthcare	Private (out of pocket and private insurance)	I—Physician care before universal medical care coverage introduced in 1960s	II—Most hospital care before Medicare	III
	Nongovernmental (mission based or charitable donations)	IV	V—Contribution to hospital capital budgets in Ontario, including expensive imaging technologies	VI—Contributor to hospital capital budgets, including expensive imaging technologies
	Public through provincial governments as the single payers of Medicare services and through targeted funding of LTC	VII—Almost all doctors and hospitals financed publicly	VIII—Hospitals from 1960s to 1990s (and continuing in Ontario to the present)	IX—Since 1990s, most hospital operating budgets, acute care, and LTC (except Ontario)

paid for through premiums; this is not discussed further in this chapter. Cell I would also apply to the majority of dental care in Canada; the reliance on private finance and private delivery in this sector contributes to inequity of access to dental care (Grignon et al. 2010). Since the vast majority of hospitals in Canada have always been private not for profit, cell II describes the situation for hospital care before public hospital financing was introduced over a decade before physician coverage.

Cell V largely describes the private contribution, largely through charities, of hospital infrastructure, including expensive medical technologies, information technology, and the research enterprises in teaching hospitals, a contribution that may exceed 20% of total hospital capital spending (Teja et al. 2020). Admittedly, however, the lion's share of capital funding for hospital care comes from public sources, putting this into cell IX and, in Ontario, into cell VII. Cell VI covers considerable activity within Canadian Medicare, including the significant relationship between the provincial governments as the single payers of Medicare and doctors as independent private contractors.

Hospitals and Acute Care

The introduction of Medicare through universal hospital coverage in the late 1940s and the 1950s followed by universal medical care coverage in the 1960s and early 1970s fundamentally altered the public/private mix in healthcare financing in Canada. Prior to Medicare, individuals paid for all healthcare services out of pocket or through private insurance. Once Medicare was implemented, all finances for UHC services originated from the general taxes of the federal and provincial governments, and all hospital and physician bills were paid directly by provincial governments through their single-payer administrations. What did not change, at least immediately, was the predominant nature of private delivery through Canada. Hospitals were owned and operated by religious denominations, foundations, and, in some cases, municipal governments and local residents, while physicians remained independent contractors. Although their bills were paid by government, hospitals were nonetheless independent of the provincial government with their own boards and managed their own operations on a nonprofit basis.

The one area that has changed most in recent decades in Canada is hospital ownership and control. In the early to mid-1990s, nine provincial governments introduced regional health authorities (RHAs) to manage the majority of both Medicare and non-Medicare services. Created under provincial statute as arm's-length public bodies answerable to the provincial ministers of health, the new RHAs received the mandate to organize and manage the delivery of acute care, LTC, home care, and public health services within their respective geographic boundaries. Provincial governments also took ownership of the majority of private not-for-profit hospitals; the ownership and control was then placed in the hands of the RHAs. This effectively shifted the public-private interface from space 8 to space 9 in Table 3.1, thereby making both delivery and financing public.

In the last 15 years, there has been a trend to greater public centralization through a reduction in the number of RHAs in some provinces, and in others, notably the provinces of Alberta, Saskatchewan, and Nova Scotia, the absorption of all RHAs a single provincial health authority (Marchildon 2016b; Fierlbeck 2019). However, this centralization has not altered the public-private interface in that regionalization pushed hospitals into interface 9 (Table 3.1), and the centralization of RHAs into single provincial health authorities does not alter the public financing and public delivery aspect of most hospital care in Canada, with the exception of Ontario, which kept its private hospitals.

Ontario's 151 private non-for-profit and six private-for-profit hospitals and their respective boards of directors have remained independent of the provincial government (Wilson, Mattison, and Lavis 2016). There are also a few exceptions to the public hospital ownership in other provinces such as the private not-for-profit Roman Catholic hospitals in the four Western Canadian provinces. However, these hospitals, as well as all Ontario hospitals and obviously all the hospitals owned by health authorities, receive all (or almost all) their operating funding through the provincial single-payer Medicare systems. As a consequence, all hospitals, irrespective of ownership, must operate under the Medicare laws and rules established by the provincial governments, including the rule that access must be based on medical necessity rather than ability to pay.[1] None of these hospitals, including the private hospitals in Ontario, are permitted to charge user or facility fees for such services.

In contrast to operating expenses, the source of hospital capital infrastructure, including new buildings, research facilities, and endowments, and expensive imaging technologies is more varied. While some hospital capital financing comes from provincial governments via provincial and regional health agencies, there remains an important share that comes from nongovernmental sources, mainly charities associated with hospitals or nonprofit foundations. These private contributions are in part a consequence of insufficient and erratic capital funding of hospitals by provincial governments, which tend to defer major capital investments to a future electoral cycle "in order to avoid an increase in deficits in the current electoral cycle or in hope of greater future tax revenues" (Teja et al. 2020, E680).

The practical consequence of this is that those hospitals less supported through charitable contributions, such as nonteaching hospitals in poorer urban neighborhoods or outside of major cities, can have less satisfactory facilities and technologies. This has clear equity implications, whereby access to advanced technology and the amenities that may improve patient experience vary by factors other than need (notably geography and socio-economic status). Moreover, this can also pose a challenge to the aspiration of a single-tier system where all citizens are expected to have access, on uniform conditions, to the same Medicare services (Marchildon 2018). Despite the equity implications, this problem has not been researched or flagged as a policy problem by Medicare activists (CBC 2017).

One interesting dimension of Canadian hospitals is the fact that most physicians that work within these hospitals are not employed by the hospitals or the provincial health authorities that own and manage hospitals. Instead, they remain independent contractors paid directly on a (mainly) fee-for-service basis by provincial governments. This peculiar governance and payment arrangement can, at times, create some difficulties in terms of the relationship between hospital-based physicians, hospital and health authority management, and employees, including other clinicians such as nurses who are working directly for the organizations managing the hospitals (Marchildon and Sherar 2018). At the same time, however, hospital-based physicians are expected to work within federal and provincial Medicare rules and are expected to treat patients based on a medical necessity order of priority and are not permitted to extra-bill the patients they treat in such facilities. As a special case, physicians and the care they provide outside hospitals are discussed further below.

Physicians and Medical Care, Including Ambulatory Care

Physicians ran their practices as small professional businesses, a mode of practice that organized medicine insisted on when universal medical care coverage was first introduced, and that remains in place today (Naylor 1986; Marchildon 2016a). Indeed, there has been almost no change in terms of the public-private interface. If anything, the private nature of physician practices has been further entrenched by the rapid growth in physicians, both specialists and general practitioners, incorporating their practices to facilitate preferred tax treatment (Nielsen and Sweetman 2018).

In recent years, primary care reforms have encouraged doctors to set up group practices, including some multiprofessional practices. While in some cases payment systems have changed, ownership remains firmly in the hands of private practice physicians rather than public authorities, emphasizing the historic private practice and public finance divide in Canadian

Medicare (Church, Skrypnek, and Smith 2018; Sullivan 2018; Marchildon and Hutchison 2018).

All physicians who have not opted out of their provincial Medicare plans are subject to federal and provincial Medicare rules. While they have wide latitude in selecting patients for their practices, they cannot extra-bill these patients, all of whom are expected to receive medically necessary or required services free at the point of delivery. The one province that has seen a recent growth in the number of opted-out physicians is Quebec, due in part to the provincial government's clamping down, in 2017, on physicians providing elective interventions who engaged in what became known as double billing. This practice involved billing the provincial government for Medicare services but charging their clients directly for extra items, including anesthetics, record management, and even eye drops used in ophthalmological interventions (Contandriopoulos and Law 2021). The obvious equity implication is that the more opted-out physicians in a province, the fewer available physician services for Medicare patients, thereby increasing wait times for elective procedures or specialist consultations.

In more urbanized provinces, some opted-out surgical specialists have established ambulatory surgical centers to perform day surgeries. A private market exists in some of Canada's largest cities for such surgeries due to the number of visitors from other countries and resident foreigners, especially Americans and other foreigners who play on professional sports teams based in those centers. In addition, there are a few Canadians who are willing to pay to avoid the public queue for elective procedures. However, the most prevalent reason for this private market is the funding that emanates from provincial worker compensation boards (WCBs). These WCBs are willing to pay a premium to have their beneficiaries placed ahead of the public Medicare queue for elective surgery. Although recommendations were made to re-examine this separate public tier of funding competing with Medicare by the federal Royal Commission on the Future of Health Care in Canada two decades ago, there has been no effort by the federal or provincial governments to reconsider the interaction between WCBs and provincial Medicare systems (Romanow 2002; Healey 2007).

This clash between WCBs and Medicare is of relatively recent origin and was not an issue until the early and mid-1990s when provincial government budget cuts led to a lengthening of wait times for elective surgery. Budget cuts also led to some shortages in the health workforce, expensive imaging equipment, and limits on operating room time (Tuohy 2002). The end result was increased rationing through wait times, including long wait times for nonurgent surgery; difficulties for patients in finding a family doctor; congested emergency departments in large urban centers; and long wait times on patient referrals to specialists. Although provincial governments had reinvested heavily in their health systems in the years that followed, they found reducing wait times—particularly for elective surgeries—a major challenge that continues to this day (Martin et al. 2018; Marchildon, Allin and Merkur 2020).

Some non-Medicare surgeons have also treated Medicare patients in an effort to get provincial governments to relax or eliminate their rules on dual practice that prevents such opted-out physicians from billing provincial Medicare plans. The restriction was originally put in place by provincial governments to prevent the public cross-subsidy of non-Medicare practices and to prevent a situation in which dual-practice physicians would always have an incentive to give priority to private-paying patients (Garcia-Pardo and Gonzalez 2011; Thomas 2020). Dr. Brian Day, an orthopedic surgeon who is an owner and operator of a private clinic in Vancouver, has been the most active in trying to change the provincial Medicare rules on dual practice.

In 1995, Day established the private-for-profit Cambie Surgery Center that catered to WCB patients, resident foreigners, nonresident visitors, and those provincial residents willing to pay out of pocket for orthopedic surgeries to avoid public wait times. In 2009, Day filed a legal claim on behalf of his clinic, and some of his patients challenged the British Columbia government's ban on private health insurance for Medicare services. The case went on for years, eventually resulting in a trial that saw dozens of health experts being examined and cross-examined on the merits and demerits of single-payer and single-tier Medicare and the rules on dual practice. In 2020, the trial judge delivered an 880-page decision rejecting the argument that wait-lists for elective surgical procedures deprived Day's patients of life, liberty, or security of person (Section 7 of the Charter of Rights and Freedoms) and therefore could not justify the court declaring that British Columbia's Medicare laws and regulations contravened the Constitution Act 1982 (CBC 2020; Supreme Court of British Columbia 2020).

Although Day was not yet successful in arguing that lengthy wait times for elective surgery could be addressed with dual practice for physicians, the challenge of wait times persists throughout the health system and may contribute to inequities. Studies of inequity in access to care have shown that, despite Medicare virtually eliminating financial barriers to accessing physician services in Canada, individuals with higher income are more likely to access a physician, particularly a specialist, and are less likely to report unmet need for care than those with lower income (Marchildon, Allin, and Merkur 2020). Access to primary and specialist care also varies by other characteristics, such as immigration status, which may relate to language barriers and to lower likelihood of holding private insurance that covers the cost of prescription drugs among new immigrants (Sanmartin and Ross 2006; Antonipillai et al. 2021). Inequities in access to primary care may relate to the continued challenge of ensuring all residents have a regular healthcare provider; most recent data from 2017 to 2018 suggested about 15% of Canadians do not have a regular healthcare provider (CIHI 2021c) and, therefore, may face difficulties seeking routine care and getting referrals to more specialized care. These inequities in access and use of primary and specialist services may also relate to different referral patterns by primary care physicians, different levels of health literacy and ability to advocate for a prompt appointment or a referral, and differences in wait times.

The presence of inequity in wait times is not widely researched because data are not routinely collected and reported at the individual level in the provincial or national data systems. Yet, a recent analysis of Commonwealth Fund survey data found higher income Canadians reported significantly shorter wait times to see their primary care provider (by about 1 to 1.8 days) (Martin, Siciliani, and Smith 2020). However, wait times data are not disaggregated by those with a regular healthcare provider compared to those without. These wait times serve to not only reduce the quality of care for many Canadian patients but also undermine their confidence in Medicare as a system. As a result, some pro-Medicare scholars and doctors have urged governments to make wait times a priority (Martin et al. 2018). Analysis of administrative data in one region of British Columbia found that individuals in higher income neighborhoods waited a similar time for general elective surgery, but were in better health (on average) prior to surgery, than those in lower income neighborhoods (Sutherland et al. 2019), which suggests possible inequity in prioritization of patients on wait-lists with lower thresholds of clinical need used for higher income individuals.

The challenges of inequity in access and the impact of wait times on the quality of care received by patients can be better understood in the context of the public-private interface in physician care. Physicians in Canada are free to choose where to practice, but with limits based on residency openings.

They tend to congregate in urban areas, in part because this is where large teaching hospitals are located and in part because they desire the amenities of urban life. Physicians also manage their own wait-lists, though there have been numerous calls for centralized wait-lists or "single-entry" models as more efficient and equitable use of wait-lists to manage scarce resources (Urbach and Martin 2020). As sole funders of private practicing physicians, governments have used, to varying degrees, financial incentives to address geographical and other inequities in access to care; however, these have had limited impact. As a consequence, access barriers, and wait times, persist.

Facility-Based Long-Term Care

Medicare in Canada is generally defined as deep (no user fees) but narrow due to the narrowness of the basket of services covered under UHC. Among the services excluded are outpatient prescription drugs and social care services, including LTC. We have chosen to focus on LTC, defined for purposes of this chapter as facility-based care in which there is access to 24-hour nursing care. This sector exhibited major weaknesses during the COVID-19 pandemic, such that LTC residents represented 80% of all deaths during the first year of the pandemic (Tuohy 2021).

The fact that LTC is not included in Medicare means that such services are not covered under the national standards set in the Canada Health Act. Provincial governments alone determine such standards as well as any policies on funding, regulation, and ownership. While regionalization did result in the taking over of some private LTC facilities by health authorities, far less changed in this sector than the hospital sector. This means that there is considerable variation across the 10 provinces when it comes LTC policies, regulation, financing, administration, and ownership. As a result, there is no general rule on the ownership of LTC facilities except that there is a mixture of public, private not-for-profit, and private for-profit in all 10 provinces.

The current ownership breakdown of LTC homes in Canada averages as follows: 46% are publicly owned; 28% are private-for-profit homes; and 23% are private not-for-profit homes (CIHI 2021b). This average obscures major variations across the country. In Ontario, which has the largest private for-profit LTC sector in Canada, 57% of its 626 LTC homes are owned by private for-profit organizations, while 27% are owned by private not-for-profit organizations, and only 16% are under public ownership. At the other end of the spectrum, 86% of Quebec's 437 LTC homes are publicly owned and operated, while only 14% are privately owned, either for profit or not for profit (CIHI 2021b).

Despite these large differences among provinces, there are some common elements. One is that all provincial governments finance the majority of LTC in Canada that has around-the-clock nursing supervision. These LTC homes, historically separated from assisted living and retirement homes with minimal to no nursing supervision, respectively, tend to be more highly regulated by the provinces because they receive patients who have been assessed by provincial authorities as having a relatively high level of physical or cognitive disability and therefore in need of such care. Irrespective of ownership, LTC facilities with 24-hour nursing care that are deemed by law or regulation eligible to receive publicly subsidized patients are mainly funded by provincial governments.

A second common feature is that the subsidization of LTC is means based. While the nursing and medical care of LTC residents is paid for by provincial governments, individuals with the means—calculated on the basis of income and/or wealth—are expected to contribute to their accommodation and living expenses. These means tests are variably assessed across provinces, some on income, some on assets, and still others on a combination of wealth and income.

A third common element is that the demand for beds in provincially approved LTC facilities outstrips provincial supply, and as a consequence, private facilities with nursing assistance have been filling some of gap in demand (Roblin et al. 2019; Um and Iveniuk 2020). Indeed, due to the reluctance of provincial governments to invest in this sector because of funding pressures for hospital and physician care, the gap between supply and demand has been growing. Similar to some provincial wait-lists for elective surgery, the reality of the LTC wait-list is that a number of elder individuals with physical or cognitive disabilities are unable to gain access to publicly financed LTC facilities, and, unless they or their respective families have sufficient money, cannot consider private LTC as an option. In addition to being inequitable for the individual needing LTC care, this can place undue hardship on the families and friends of such individuals in their roles as unpaid caregivers.

Limited investment in LTC, as evidenced by the lengthy and growing wait-lists, is well known to researchers, LTC workers, and advocates. However, the disproportionate impact of the COVID-19 pandemic on long-term care residents and workers highlighted the many weaknesses in the sector: In the first wave of the pandemic, COVID-19 deaths in Canada made up 66% of all deaths, and nearly a third of all LTC homes experienced an outbreak (CIHI 2021a).

In Ontario, resident deaths from COVID-19 were significantly higher among for-profit LTC homes relative to public and private not-for-profit homes, a pattern that can be explained by older design standards and chain ownership of the for-profit homes (Stall et al. 2020) and greater likelihood of for-profit homes to have resident overcrowding (shared bedrooms and bathrooms) (Brown et al. 2021). Similar findings have been shown in the United States, with for-profit ownership associated with higher COVID-19 mortality, in part due to lower staffing levels (McGregor and Harrington 2020). The issues with inadequate staffing and outdated designs with multiperson rooms require urgent attention, as do lengthy wait times and supply shortages. Also, there is inadequate oversight and enforcement of the provincial regulations that are meant to ensure minimum standards. The government-commissioned report on the experience of COVID-19 in LTC homes in Ontario found that inspection processes were inadequate, the number of inspections performed dropped significantly in 2019, and the significant drop in the number of inspections performed in 2019 with a move from a universal to "a complaint- and critical incident approach to inspections" all contributed to the dire outcomes observed during the pandemic (Commissioners of Ontario's Long-Term Care COVID Commission 2021).

The continued reliance on the for-profit delivery model in LTC in Ontario in particular is now being contested vigorously as a consequence of the COVID-19 pandemic, and unless the provincial government can significantly improve its regulation and enforcement of quality standards, there is likely to be sustained pressure for more public and private not-for-profit delivery of LTC care. However, the major concerns with poor quality of care will persist in any delivery model if levels of funding and oversight of legislative standards remain inadequate (Béland and Marier 2020). For example, in Quebec, most LTC facilities are publicly owned and managed—perhaps the most "public" LTC system in Canada—yet the monitoring of quality standards is inadequate (Palley, Pomey, and Fleury 2012). This history of inadequate inspection of public facilities was one of the contributing factors in the LTC crisis during the COVID-19 pandemic and the high rate of deaths in LTC facilities in that province (Beaulieu, Genesse, and St-Martin 2021).

Conclusions

There are a number of public-private interfaces in the Canadian health systems, some of which have been contested for years, such as the public funding and private physician delivery interface. This is exemplified in the restrictions on dual practice and the growth (e.g., Quebec) in the opting out of Medicare by physicians. In fact, waiting times for elective procedures in the public system have created a market for physicians who opt out to serve those who choose to pay out-of-pocket in order to bypass public queues.

At the same time, with the exception of Ontario, the majority of hospitals shifted from private nonprofit to public ownership in the 1990s with limited controversy. This would have created a NHS-style system in those provinces except for the fact that hospital-based physicians remained apart from the reform and are not paid—even as independent contractors—by the provincial or regional health authorities that own and manage these hospitals. These doctors, however, are expected to conform to federal and provincial Medicare rules that prohibit extra-billing and requires that services be provided on the sole criterion of medical necessity.

Due to the COVID-19 pandemic revealing serious deficiencies in LTC, especially in the homes owned by private for-profit enterprises, this publicly funded but privately delivered space has become hotly contested. As the province most dependent on for-profit LTC homes, Ontario is on the front line of this debate and will likely be forced to make major changes in the wake of the pandemic, regulating the private sector much more effectively, making a major investment in new public LTC facilities, or both simultaneously given the fact that the shortage of publicly supported LTC lies at the root of the problem. Due to the scale of the failure of LTC in not only Ontario but also other provinces, this is the one area where the federal government has been called on by numerous interest groups to set national quality standards through its use of the spending power with the provinces (Marchildon and Tuohy 2021).

Note

1. These rules do vary. For example, in most provinces, abortion is considered a medically necessary service but was very restricted in provinces such as New Brunswick and Prince Edward Island due to a more socially conservative political culture and history

(Johnstone 2018). In Western Canada, abortions are provided in facilities other than Roman Catholic hospitals.

References

Allan, Billie, and Janet Smylie. 2015. "First Peoples, Second Class Treatment: The Role of Racism in the Health and Well-Being of Indigenous Peoples in Canada." Toronto: Wellesley Institute. https://www.wellesleyinstitute.com/publications/first-peoples-second-class-treatment/

Allin, Sara, Julie Farmer, Carlos Quiñonez, Allie Peckham, Gregory Marchildon, Dimitra Panteli, Cornelia Henschke, Giovanni Fattore, Demetrio Lamloum, Alexander Holden, and Thomas Rice. 2020. "Do Health Systems Cover the Mouth? Comparing Dental Care Coverage for Older Adults in Eight Jurisdictions." *Health Policy* 124(9): 998–1007. https://doi.org/10.1016/j.healthpol.2020.06.015

Allin, Sara, David Rudoler, Danielle Dawson, and Jonathan Mullen. 2020. "Experiences with Two-Tier Home Care in Canada: A Focus on Inequalities in Home Care Use." In *Is Two-Tier Health Care the Future?*, edited by Colleen M. Flood and Bryan Thomas, 123–144. Ottawa: University of Ottawa Press.

Antonipillai, Valentina, Emmanuel Guindon, Arthur Sweetman, Andrea Baumann, Olive Wahoush, and Lisa Schwartz. 2021. "Associations of Health Services Utilization by Prescription Drug Coverage and Immigration Category in Ontario, Canada." *Health Policy* 125(9): 1311–1321. https://doi.org/10.1016/j.healthpol.2021.06.007

Beaulieu, Marie, Julien Cadieux Genesse, and Kevin St-Martin. 2021. "High Death Rate of Older Persons from COVID-19 in Quebec (Canada) Long-Term Care Facilities: Chronology and Analysis." *Journal of Adult Protection* 23(2): 110–115. https://doi.org/10.1108/JAP-08-2020-0033

Béland, Daniel, and Patrik Marier. 2020. "COVID-19 and Long-Term Care Policy for Older People in Canada." *Journal of Aging and Social Policy* 32(4–5): 358–364. https://doi.org/10.1080/08959420.2020.1764319

Böhm, Katharina, Achim Schmid, Ralf Götze, Claudia Landwehr, and Heinz Rothgang. 2013. "Five Types of OECD Healthcare Systems: Empirical Results of a Deductive Classification." *Health Policy* 113(3): 258–269. https://doi.org/10.1016/j.healthpol.2013.09.003

Boothe, Katherine. 2018. "Pharmaceutical Policy Reform in Canada: Lessons from History." *Health Economics, Policy and Law* 13(3-4): 299–322. https://doi.org/10.1017/s1744133117000408

Brown, Kevin A., Aaron Jones, Nick Daneman, Adrienne K. Chan, Kevin L. Schwartz, Gary E. Garber, Andrew P. Costa, and Nathan M. Stall. 2021. "Association between Nursing Home Crowding and COVID-19 Infection and Mortality in Ontario, Canada." *JAMA Internal Medicine* 181(2): 229–236. https://doi.org/10.1001/jamainternmed.2020.6466

Busse, Reinhard, Dimitra Panteli, and Wilm Quentin. 2019. "An Introductions to Healthcare Quality: Defining and Explaining Its Role in Health Systems." In *Improving Healthcare Quality in Europe: Characteristics, Effectiveness and Implementation of Different Strategies*, edited by Reinhard Busse, Niek Klazinga, Dimitra Panteli, and Wilm Quentin, 3–17. Copenhagen: World Health Organization on behalf of the European Observatory on Health Systems and Policies.

CBC. 2017. "Canada's Public Health Care System Relies an Awful Lot on Private Money." Last updated December 13, 2017. https://www.cbc.ca/news/opinion/private-health-care-donations-1.4444679

CBC. 2020. "Private Vancouver Clinics Loses Constitutional Challenge of Public Health-Care Rules." Last updated September 10, 2020. https://www.cbc.ca/news/canada/british-columbia/cambie-surgeries-case-trial-decision-bc-supreme-court-2020-1.5718589

Choudhry, Sajit. 1996. "The Enforcement of the Canada Health Act." *McGill Law Journal* 41(2): 462–509.

Church, John, Rob Skrypnek, and Neale Smith. 2018. "Improving Physician Accountability through Primary Care Reform in Alberta." *Healthcare Papers* 17(4): 48–55. https://doi.org/10.12927/hcpap.2018.25576

CIHI (Canadian Institute for Health Information). 2021a. "Long-Term Care and COVID-19 in the First 6 Months." Ottawa: Canadian Institute for Health Information. https://www.cihi.ca/en/long-term-care-and-covid-19-the-first-6-months

CIHI (Canadian Institute for Health Information). 2021b. "Long-Term Care Homes in Canada: How Many and Who Owns Them?" Ottawa: Canadian Institute for Health Information. https://www.cihi.ca/en/long-term-care-homes-in-canada-how-many-and-who-owns-them

CIHI (Canadian Institute for Health Information). 2021c. "Your Health System Has a Regular Provider." Ottawa: Canadian Institute for Health Information. https://yourh ealthsystem.cihi.ca/hsp/inbrief?lang=en#!/indicators/074/has-a-regular-health-care-provider/;mapC1;mapLevel2;/

Commissioners of Ontario's Long-Term Care COVID Commission. 2021. *Long-Term Care COVID-19 Commission: Final Report.* Toronto: Queen's Printer for Ontario. http://www.ltccommission-commissionsld.ca/report/pdf/20210623_LTCC_AODA_EN.pdf

Contandriopoulos, Damien, and Michael R. Law. 2021. "Policy Changes and Physicians Opting Out from Medicare in Quebec: An Interrupted Time-Series Analysis." *CMAJ* 193(7): E237–E241. https://doi.org/10.1503/cmaj.201216

Cuadrado, Cristóbal, Francisca Crispi, Matias Libuy, Gregory Marchildon, and Camilo Cid. 2019. "National Health Insurance: A Conceptual Framework from Conflicting Typologies." *Health Policy* 123(7): 621–629. https://doi.org/10.1016/j.health pol.2019.05.013

Deber, Raisa B. 2004. "Delivering Health Care: Public, Not-for-Profit, or Private?" In *The Fiscal Sustainability of Health Care in Canada*, edited by Gregory P. Marchildon, Thomas McIntosh, and Pierre-Gerlier Forest, 233–296. Toronto: University of Toronto Press.

Evans, Robert G. 2004. "Financing Health Care: Options, Consequences and Objectives." In *The Fiscal Sustainability of Health Care in Canada*, edited by Gregory P. Marchildon, Thomas McIntosh, and Pierre-Gerlier Forest, 139–196. Toronto: University of Toronto Press.

Fierlbeck, Katherine. 2019. "Amalgamating Provincial Health Authorities: Assessing the Experience of Nova Scotia." *Health Reform Observer—Observatoire des Réformes de Santé* 7(3): article 3. https://doi.org/10.13162/hro-ors.v7i3.4046

Flood, Colleen M., William Lahey, and Bryan Thomas. 2017. "Federalism and Health Care in Canada: A Troubled Romance." In *The Oxford Handbook of the Canadian Constitution*, edited by Peter Oliver, Patrick Macklem, and Nathalie des Rosiers, 449–474. New York: Oxford University Press.

Garcia-Pardo, Ariadna, and Paula Gonzales. 2011. "Whom Do Physicians Work For? An Analysis of Dual Practice in the Health Sector." *Journal of Health Politics, Policy and Law* 36(2): 265–294. https://doi.org/10.1215/03616878-1222721

Grignon, Michel, Jeremiah Hurley, Li Wang, and Sara Allin. 2010. "Inequity in a Market-Based Health System: Evidence from Canada's Dental Sector." *Health Policy* 98(1): 81–90. https://doi.org/10.1016/j.healthpol.2010.05.018

Healy, Teresa. 2007. "Health Care Privatization and the Workers' Compensation System in Canada." Unpublished conference paper, Canadian Political Science Association Annual Meeting, June 1, 2007. https://www.cpsa-acsp.ca/papers-2007/Healy.pdf

Inuit Tapiriit Kanatami. 2014. "Social Determinants of Inuit Health in Canada." Ottawa: Inuit Tapiriit Kanatami. https://www.itk.ca/wp-content/uploads/2016/07/ITK _Social_Determinants_Report.pdf

Johnstone, Rachael. 2018. "Explaining Abortion Policy Developments in New Brunswick and Prince Edward Island." *Journal of Canadian Studies* 52(3): 765–784.

Marchildon, Gregory P. 2016a. "Legacy of the Doctors' Strike and the Saskatoon Agreement." *CMAJ* 188(9): 676–677. https://doi.org/10.1503/cmaj.151360

Marchildon, Gregory P. 2016b. "Regionalization: What Have We Learned?" *Healthcare Papers* 16(1): 8–14. https://doi.org/10.12927/hcpap.2016.24766

Marchildon, Gregory P. 2018. "Health Care in Canada: Interdependence and Independence." In *Federalism and Decentralization in Health Care: A Decision Space Approach*, edited by Gregory P. Marchildon and Thomas J. Bossert, 43–70. Toronto: University of Toronto Press.

Marchildon, Gregory P. 2020. "Private Finance and Canadian Medicare: Learning from History." In *Is Two-Tier Health Care the Future?*, edited by Colleen M. Flood and Bryan Thomas, 15–35. Ottawa: University of Ottawa Press.

Marchildon, Gregory P., and Sara Allin. 2016. "The Public-Private Mix in the Delivery of Health-care Services: Its Relevance for Lower-Income Canadians." *Global Social Welfare* 3(3): 161–170. https://doi.org/10.1007/s40609-016-0070-4

Marchildon, Gregory P., Sara Allin, and Sherry Merkur. 2020. "Canada: Health System Review." *Health Systems in Transition* 22(3): 1–194.

Marchildon, Gregory P., and Brian Hutchison. 2018. "Primary Care in Ontario, Canada: New Proposals after 15 Years of Reform." *Health Policy* 120(7): 732–738. https://doi.org/10.1016/j.healthpol.2016.04.010

Marchildon, Gregory P., and Michael Sherar. 2018. "Doctors and Canadian Medicare: Improving Accountability and Performance." *Healthcare Papers* 17(4): 14–26. https://doi.org/10.12927/hcpap.2018.25580

Marchildon, Gregory P., and Carolyn H. Tuohy. 2021. "Expanding Health Care Coverage in Canada: A Dramatic Shift in the Debate." *Health Economics, Policy and Law* 16(3): 371–377. https://doi.org/10.1017/S1744133121000062

Martin, Danielle, Ashley P. Miller, Amélie Quesnel-Vallée, Nadine R. Caron, Bilkis Visandjée, and Gregory P. Marchildon. 2018. "Canada's Universal Health-care System: Achieving its Potential." *The Lancet* 391(10131): 81–88.

Martin, Steve, Luigi Siciliani, and Peter Smith. 2020. "Socioeconomic Inequalities in Waiting Times for Primary Care across Ten OECD Countries." *Social Science & Medicine* 263: 113230. https://doi.org/10.1016/j.socscimed.2020.113230

McGregor, Margaret J., and Charlene Harrington. 2020. "COVID-19 and Long-Term Care Facilities: Does Ownership Matter?" *CMAJ* 192 (33) E961–E962. https://doi.org/ 10.1503/cmaj.201714

Naylor, C. David. 1986. *Private Practice, Public Payment: Canadian Medicine and the Politics of Health Insurance, 1911–1966*. Montreal: McGill-Queen's University Press.

Nielsen, Lars, and Arthur Sweetman. 2018. "Measuring Physicians' Incomes with a Focus on Canadian-Controlled Private Corporations." *Healthcare Policy* 17(4): 77–86. https://doi.org/10.12927/hcpap.2018.25572

Palley, Howard A., Marie-Pascale Pomey, and Marie-Josée Fleury. 2012. "Long-Term Care for the Elderly in Quebec: Considerations of Appropriateness and Quality of Care." *Association of Canadian Studies in the United States: Occasional Papers on Public Policy Series* 4(1): 1–8.

Roblin, Blair, Raisa Deber, Kerry Kuluski, and Michelle Pannor Silver. 2019. "Ontario's Retirement Homes and Long-Term Care Homes: A Comparison of Care Services and Funding Regimes." *Canadian Journal of Aging* 38(2): 155–167. https://doi.org/10.1017/S0714980818000569

Romanow, Roy J. 2002. *Building on Values: The Future of Health Care in Canada*. Saskatoon: Commission on the Future of Health Care in Canada.

Sanmartin, Claudia, and Nancy Ross. 2006. "Experiencing Difficulties Accessing First-Contact Health Services in Canada: Canadians without Regular Doctors and Recent Immigrants Have Difficulties Accessing First-Contact Healthcare Services. Reports of Difficulties in Accessing Care Vary by Age, Sex and Region." *Healthcare Policy* 1(2): 103–119.

Stall, Nathan A., Aaron Jones, Kevin A. Brown, Paula A. Rochon, and Andrew P. Costa. 2020. "For-Profit Long-Term Care Homes and the Risk of COVID-19 Outbreaks and Resident Deaths." *CMAJ* 192(33): E946–E955. https://doi.org/10.1503/cmaj.201197

Sullivan, Terry. 2018. "Physician Compensation, Accountability and Performance in Canada: Changing the *Pas de Deux*." *Healthcare Papers* 17(4): 4–12.

Supreme Court of British Columbia. 2020. "Hon. Justice Steeves Reasons for Judgment, Supreme Court of British Columbia in the Cambie Surgeries Corporation v. British Columbia (Attorney General), Sept. 10, 2020." https://www.bccourts.ca/jdb-txt/sc/20/13/2020BCSC1310.htm

Sutherland, Jason, M., Zuzanna Kurzawa, Ahmer Karimuddin, Katrina Duncan, Guiping Liu, and Trafford Crump. 2019. "Wait Lists and Adult General Surgery: Is There a Socioeconomic Dimension in Canada?" *BMC Health Services Research* 19(161): article 161. https://doi.org/10.1186/s12913-019-3981-9

Teja, Bijan, Imtiaz Daniel, George H. Pink, Adalsteinn Brown, and David J. Klein. 2020. "Ensuring Adequate Capital Investment in Canadian Health Care." *CMAJ* 192(25): E677–E683. https://doi.org/10.1503/cmaj.191126

Thomas, Bryan. 2020. "Contracting Our Way around Two-Tier Care? The Use of Physician Contracts to Limit Dual Practice." In *Is Two-Tier Health Care the Future?*, edited by Colleen M. Flood and Bryan Thomas, 315–333. Ottawa: University of Ottawa Press.

Tuohy, Carolyn H. 2002. "The Costs of Constraints and Prospects for Health Care Reform in Canada." *Health Affairs* 21(3): 32–46. https://doi.org/10.1377/hlthaff.21.3.32

Tuohy, Carolyn H. 2009. "Single-Payer, Multiple Systems: The Scopes and Limits of Subnational Variation under a Federal Health Policy Framework." *Journal of Health Politics, Policy and Law* 34(4): 453–496. https://doi.org/10.1215/03616878-2009-011

Tuohy, Carolyn H. 2021. "Federalism as a Strength: A Path Toward Ending the Crisis in Long-Term Care." IRPP Insight no. 36. Montreal: Institute for Research on Public Policy. https://centre.irpp.org/research-studies/federalism-as-a-strength-a-path-toward-ending-the-crisis-in-long-term-care/#study-tab-text

Turpel-Lafond, Mary-Ellen. 2020. "In Plain Sight: Addressing Indigenous-Specific Racism and Discrimination in B.C. Health Care." Vancouver: Addressing Racism Review. https://engage.gov.bc.ca/app/uploads/sites/613/2020/11/In-Plain-Sight-Full-Report.pdf

Um, Seong-gee, and James Iveniuk. 2020. "Waiting for Long-Term Care in the GTA: Trends and Persistent Disparities." Toronto: Wellesley Institute. https://www.wellesleyinstitute.com/wp-content/uploads/2020/09/Waiting-for-Long-Term-Care-in-the-GTA.pdf

Urbach, David R., and Danielle Martin. 2020. "Confronting the COVID-19 Surgery Crisis: Time for Transformational Change." *CMAJ* 192(21): E585–E586. https://www.cmaj.ca/content/cmaj/192/21/E585.full.pdf

Wilson, Michael G., Cristina A. Mattison, and John N. Lavis. 2016. "Delivery Arrangements 1: Infrastructure." In *Ontario's Health System: Key Insights for Engaged Citizens, Professionals and Policymakers*, edited by John N. Lavis, 122–174. Hamilton, ON: McMaster Health Forum. https://www.mcmasterforum.org/docs/default-source/ohs-book/one-page-per-sheet/ch4_delivery-arrangements-1-infrastructure-ohs.pdf?sfvrsn=f3aa55d5_2

4

Australia's Health Insurance System and Its Two-Level Hospital System—A Result of Muddled and Contested Objectives

Stephen Duckett

Australia has given the world some unique animals with unusual characteristics; Egg-laying mammals, such as the platypus, are is a notable example (Richardson 2005). Equally unique is Australia's health system, where public and private systems exist in a symbiotic relationship. Public funding for the public hospital system is constrained, resulting in long waiting times for care. Perversely, there is a parallel system of private care that is also publicly subsidized—through subsidies for private health insurance (PHI) —so public funding is also provided to bypass these public hospital constraints.

These government subsidies to PHI create a two-level hospital system where those with private health insurance enjoy quicker access to care—a selling point for PHI (Ellis and Savage 2008), but more private care does not speed up care for those without PHI, despite the arguments of subsidy advocates; rather, the reverse is the case (Duckett 2005, 2018). The role of PHI in Australia is muddled and contested. This chapter first briefly describes the key elements of the Australian healthcare system, then analyzes the espoused role of PHI, particularly focusing on arguments advanced to subsidize PHI, and critique the case for subsidized insurance in Australia.

The Australian Healthcare System

Australia's healthcare system is a complex mix of public and private financing and public and private service provision, operating within a federal system where the Commonwealth (national) government and the eight states and territories (hereafter, states) have roles in healthcare policy. It

Stephen Duckett, *Australia's Health Insurance System and Its Two-Level Hospital System—A Result of Muddled and Contested Objectives* In: *The Public/Private Sector Mix in Healthcare Delivery*. Edited by: Howard A. Palley, Oxford University Press. © Oxford University Press 2023. DOI: 10.1093/oso/9780197571101.003.0004 comprises the universal public health insurance scheme known as Medicare and a voluntary PHI system. Under Medicare, all Australians are entitled to taxpayer-funded access to public hospitals, without a direct patient payment; subsidized medical services provided by private medical practitioners (about 85% of all family physician [general practice] visits are provided without any direct payment by the patient); and subsidized prescribed medicines. There is a separate private hospital system, mostly owned by private companies or, in the case of smaller facilities such as day procedure centers, by medical practitioners.

Medicare's universality means that there are no financial barriers to access hospital care in public hospitals, but underfunding of public hospitals results in waits for elective procedures; a marketing emphasis of PHI is to bypass these waits through care in a private hospital.

Responsibility for the health system (both funding and provision) is shared between the Commonwealth and state governments. The states are responsible for public health services, including funding of public and community health services and patient transport services. Public hospitals are jointly funded by the Commonwealth and the states but managed by the states. Private hospitals are owned and operated by the private sector but licensed and regulated by state governments.

Australia's universal health insurance scheme system has meant that a key element of equity, financial barriers to access, has been addressed, albeit imperfectly as discussed below. Unfortunately, other aspects of equity are not addressed well, in particular Indigenous Australians have a life expectancy about a decade shorter than nonindigenous Australians (Thompson, Talley, and Kong 2017), and outcomes for Indigenous Australians are poorer on almost every other process or outcome measure (Dwyer et al. 2016). Although governments espouse policies to address these inequities, including through development of Aboriginal controlled community health organizations (Bartlett and Boffa 2001, 2005), progress on improving equity in this area has been glacial.

Quality, especially hospital safety, has been a focus of policy since identification of relatively high rates of adverse events in hospitals in the 1990s (Wilson et al. 1995). Quality is a multidimensional construct (Donabedian 2002), and Australian policies address many aspects of quality. Safety of hospital care remains a critical issue, with scandals erupting in each state every decade or so (McLean and Walsh 2003; Eagar 2004; van der Weyden

2005; Selvaratnam et al. 2021); policy attention has also focused on other dimensions of quality, including appropriateness of care.

Timeliness—an important dimension of quality—for both elective procedures and emergency care in public hospitals is an area of concern. All states have adopted strategies, including prioritization of elective procedure waiting times, targets, and penalties (Willcox et al. 2007), but sustained improvement has proven elusive. In 2019–2020 the median waiting time for cataract extraction in public hospitals was more than 3 months, with 10% waiting almost 1 year; the median waiting time for hip replacements was 4 months, with the 90th percentile also almost a year. The situation was much better for coronary artery bypass grafts, typically assigned to the top priority for admission, with high penalties for failure to admit within 30 days, with a median wait of 18 days and 90th percentile wait of 76 days (Australian Institute of Health and Welfare 2020b, Table 4.6).

Emergency performance is also under challenge (Judkins 2021). Although patients in the highest triage category are all seen within an appropriate time (Australian Institute of Health and Welfare 2020c), achievement of triage time targets stand at 67% for category 3 (seen within 30 minutes, target 75%) and 76% for category 4 (60 minutes, 70%), and 93% for category 5 (120 minutes, 70%).

Who Pays for Care?

Together, the Commonwealth and the states fund 70% of health expenditure, including subsidies to PHI, which account for 3% of the total spending (Australian Institute of Health and Welfare 2020d). Individuals fund a significant proportion of healthcare from their own pocket: Out-of-pocket payments are 17% of total health spending. High rates of out-of-pocket payments create inequity—including that many people defer or do not obtain care because of costs. In 2019–2020, about 3.7% of the population deferred or did not obtain family physician (general practice) care because of cost, and 8% deferred or did not obtain care from a medical specialist because of cost (Australian Bureau of Statistics 2020).

A further 9% of expenditure is funded through PHI premiums, with the remaining 4% coming from other sources, including accident compensation schemes.

The Commonwealth government is responsible for about 43% of all health spending, with states responsible for about 26%. However, government spending is highly concentrated: Government spends over 90% of public hospital spending (state governments about 52%, Commonwealth about 40%), but only 23% of dental spending (state 8%, Commonwealth 15%).

PHI provides two main types of coverage. The first, hospital insurance, provides cover against the costs of fees charged for accommodation and medical fees in private hospitals or, if admitted as a private patient, in public hospitals. The second, general insurance, provides cover for a range of nonmedical services offered by health professionals other than medical practitioners, including dental, optical, and allied health. About 44% of the population has hospital insurance, and slightly more than half the population has general insurance. PHI is statutorily barred from covering out-of-hospital medical expenses.

Physicians in larger public hospitals are mostly paid on a full or part-time salary basis, in contrast to specialists in private hospitals and smaller public hospitals, who are paid a fee for service. Fee-for-service remuneration is generally more lucrative per hour than salaried payments. Medicare covers 75% of the official fee ("scheduled" fee, as listed in the government-determined Medicare Benefits Schedule) for in-hospital services, with PHI mandated to pay the 25% balance. However, doctors in Australia are allowed to charge what they wish, and only 25% of in-hospital services are billed at the official fee. PHI is allowed to cover fees above the official rate, but there are limits to what PHI is prepared to pay, and some consumers are left with significant out-of-pocket payments for doctors' bills (Duckett and Nemet 2019b).

There is a strong income gradient in PHI coverage (see Figure 4.1). Only about one-third of people living in the most disadvantaged neighborhoods have taken out PHI, less than half the rate of the wealthiest neighborhoods.

About two-thirds of private hospital income comes through PHI, including the PHI rebate.

Private Health Insurance Coverage has been Trending Down

Before its universal healthcare system was introduced, Australia had relatively high levels of PHI coverage: About 80% of the population had some type of coverage for hospital treatment. This quickly dropped to about 50%

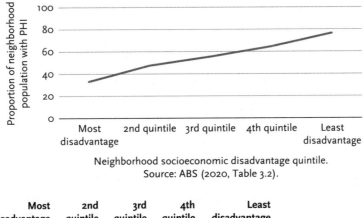

Neighborhood socioeconomic disadvantage quintile.
Source: ABS (2020, Table 3.2).

Most disadvantage	2nd quintile	3rd quintile	4th quintile	Least disadvantage
33.2	47.5	55.4	64.5	76.5

Figure 4.1 Take-up of PHI is inequitable.

after Medicare was introduced in 1984—because people no longer had to insure for public hospital care—and continued to fall to about 30% by the mid-1990s.

In a voluntary insurance system, any decline creates the risk of an "adverse selection" spiral, where higher-risk people purchase insurance and lower-risk people do not (Zweifel and Frech 2016). This in turn increases the average risk profile of the remaining insured population, premiums rise, more healthy people drop out, and the cycle continues.

The Commonwealth government has introduced a range of incentives and penalties designed to encourage people to take out insurance (Hall, De Abreu Lourenco, and Viney 1999; Robson and Paolucci 2012). These include an age-adjusted, means-tested subsidy for PHI premiums ("the rebate"), tax penalties for higher-income earners who do not take out insurance, and premium surcharges for people who take out PHI after age 30 (see Table 4.1). The tax penalties result in the bizarre situation where for higher-income earners some PHI products are essentially free because the tax that would have been paid is more than the product cost.

Formally the rebate is paid at the end of the financial year as part of a person's tax return. However, contributors to PHI declare their eligibility and anticipated level of rebate when paying their PHI premiums, and this reduces their upfront payments. If they have estimated their eligibility incorrectly, it is adjusted in calculating their year-end tax liability. The PHI rebate costs the

Table 4.1. Private health insurance rebate and Medicare levy surcharge by income and age, March 2021–April 2022

	Income ranges for rebate and surcharge			
Singles	≤$90,000	$90,001–105,000	$105,001–140,000	≥$140,001
Families	≤$180,000	$180,001–210,000	$210,001–280,000	≥$280,001
Rebate (subsidy for PHI premiums)				
<65 years	24.608%	16.405%	8.202%	0%
65–69 years	28.710%	20.507%	12.303%	0%
70 years or more	32.812%	24.608%	16.405%	0%
Medicare levy surcharge (additional tax payable by those without health insurance)				
All ages	0.0%	1.0%	1.25%	1.5%

Source: https://www.ato.gov.au/Individuals/Medicare-and-private-health-insurance/Private-health-insurance-rebate/Income-thresholds-and-rates-for.-the-private-health-insurance-rebate/, 2022.

Commonwealth government about $6 billion a year (all expenditure in this chapter is in Australian dollars). In addition, the Commonwealth spends an extra $3 billion on private inpatient medical services through an additional rebate for in-hospital fees.

The current levels of PHI have been maintained largely due to these incentives and penalties. Over the past two decades, PHI coverage has been basically stable. But in recent years there has been a slight overall downturn, particularly driven by relative declines among younger people. In the 5 years March 2015 to March 2021, the number of 20- to 29-year-olds with hospital cover fell by 6%. By contrast, the number of individuals 65+ years old with hospital cover increased by 22% (Duckett and Moran 2021). Overall, the 20- to 29-year-old share of the insured population dropped from 24% to 22%, while the 65+ share increased from 16% to 20%. This changed age profile leads to adverse selection as more young people drop out or do not take up insurance and then a "death spiral"—of increasing premiums and more younger people dropping out—ensues (Duckett and Nemet 2019a).

Despite the rebates and subsidies, the cost of insurance private health insurance has continued to increase significantly faster than wages (Duckett and Cowgill 2019; Duckett and Nemet 2019a; Duckett and Moran 2021). In Australia, and overseas, healthcare spending is rising much faster than inflation. PHI premium increases must be approved by the Commonwealth minister for health as part of an annual process where each fund submits its proposed increases for approval. Nevertheless, premiums have gone up even faster than healthcare spending and faster than wages every year over the past decade. From 2000 to 2020, premiums increased 179%, faster than inflation at 62%, health inflation at 143%, and wages at 114% (Duckett and Moran 2021).

Insurers have responded by offering consumers a broader range of products, including products with "excesses" or "deductibles"—where a consumer must pay the first $500 or more of the cost of a hospital treatment—and products that have exclusions—where a procedure is not covered by the policy.

The proportion of policies with excesses or deductibles and/or exclusions (limited coverage) has increased. Twenty years ago, only one-third of policies had an excess or exclusion. Today, more than 85% of policies have some form of excess or exclusion. This shift is starting to unwind the principle of community rating. Healthy people are more likely to take out cheaper policies with more deductibles or exclusions, creating horizontal inequity within the insured population.

The Role of Private Health Insurance is Contested

Private health insurance has served a dual role in Australia's muddled healthcare system. On the one hand, it provides a source of private funding for healthcare that *complements* (tops up) public funding for services, facilities, and amenity beyond that available under the publicly funded system. For example, hospital insurance can cover the extra benefits available in some private hospitals—such as single rooms and different food choices—and treatment by a specific, chosen specialist. "Choice of doctor" has been a key differentiator of public and private care, despite the fact that choice is often illusory given there are no comparative websites in Australia comparing outcomes or costs of specialists.

A second type of complement is where there is no public universal program that provides unrestricted access to the services covered by private insurance, such as dental, chiropractic, physical therapy, and optical services. Health insurance may also cover admission to a private hospital for services that would not be provided in some circumstances by the universal system, such as when the patient's condition is less severe. The result of this last type of complement is higher rates of low-value care in private hospitals (Badgery-Parker et al. 2019; Chalmers et al. 2019).

On the other hand, PHI provides a source of funding that *substitutes* (replaces) public funding of services by duplicating the coverage in the public system. For example, it can cover treatment in a private hospital that might otherwise have occurred in a public hospital.

Of course, the distinction between services being a complement or a substitute is not clear cut. Some hospital admissions are a substitute with complementary elements (e.g., a necessary hip replacement in a private hospital with better amenities).

The emphasis on each of these roles has varied over time, reflecting attitudes to the role and size of government at the time. The argument for a public subsidy is strongest if PHI is a substitute and the cost of the subsidy is below the cost of the public provision displaced, and it is very weak if it is a complement or the cost of the subsidy is relatively high.

Conservative governments—known in Australia as the Liberal-National Coalition—have directly supported PHI as both a substitute for and a complement to the public system. Former Commonwealth Health Minister Tony Abbott declared: "Private health insurance is in our DNA" (Dunlevy 2012). Some conservative governments have also expressed a view that public funding and provision should be available only to people who could not afford PHI, contrary to the universality principle of Australia's Medicare scheme. According to this view, access to publicly funded and provided services should be means tested because they are meant to provide only a "safety net" for the disadvantaged.

Labor governments have tended to focus on supporting the public system, while allowing PHI to operate alongside as a complement. Labor has tended to promote a universal, public insurance model and public provision of hospital services.

The basic design of the health system has become less contested over time. At least since 1996, Australia's two major political parties have both been overtly committed to public hospital care accessible to all without means testing, but for people to have access to an option for PHI with at least some level of government subsidy.

But, as the parties have converged toward today's healthcare system, it has become riddled with inconsistencies and perverse incentives. It is increasingly unfair, costly, and confusing. For people with PHI, premiums and out-of-pocket costs if they use their insurance have gone up faster than inflation.

Meanwhile, government began footing a large share of the PHI bill to try to make insurance more attractive to consumers and introduced an increasing array of penalties for those without insurance. Despite all this, the long-term viability of the PHI industry is bleak.

Successive governments have failed to define the role of PHI in the funding and delivery of healthcare in the context of Medicare, Australia's widely supported scheme for universal access to public hospital care and physician services out of hospital.

The Critical Question: What is Private Health Insurance in Australia for?

Private health insurance has served dual roles, at times with competing and overlapping objectives. Immediately after the introduction of Medicare in 1984, PHI was seen as peripheral to the public system, providing access to services (predominantly nonmedical) not offered publicly. It also offered coverage for wider dimensions of service and amenities, including choice of doctor, choice of hospital, better accommodation, and shorter waiting times. These additional dimensions—generally perceived to be indicators of quality—were sometimes available in both public and private hospitals (e.g., to private patients in public hospitals).

The downward trend in PHI associated with the introduction of universal insurance was generally not seen as an issue warranting intervention by Labor governments in office from 1984 to 1996. Conservative governments took the opposite view and initiated a series of policy changes, starting with a means-tested subsidy shortly after its election in 1996. The subsidies were revised and increased but had little impact on PHI take-up. The major increase in coverage—a 50% increase from about 30% to 45% population coverage—was from introduction of the policy of lifetime health cover, implemented in 2000, which penalizes people who join PHI after they turn 31 (Butler 2002). The lifetime cover policy increases premium cost by 2% for each year after 30 that contributors first takes out PHI.

Private health insurance coverage has drifted down despite the extensive government aid provided to the sector. That support has significant budgetary and social costs, and this has prompted questions about the justification for providing support and whether the resources currently supporting private care could be used more efficiently.

Government intervention in the health system and health insurance has generally been justified on the basis of broader social objectives, such as promoting equal access to healthcare, better health outcomes for the population, and ensuring the budgetary sustainability of the public health system. Neither of the first two arguments can be used to justify support for PHI, so public arguments in Australia rely on the third, together with an appeal to the value of "choice."

The cost to government of providing this support has been significant and now represents almost 8% of Commonwealth government health expenditure. From its introduction in 1997, the cost of the rebate, in constant dollar terms, increased from $0.6 billion to a peak of $5.9 billion in 2012. The cost of the rebate per head of population over this period increased by more than 500%. And by 2012, premiums were growing faster than overall health expenditure. The Labor government at the time responded by capping, from 2014, rebate growth to the lesser of the Consumer Price Index and the annual average increase in premiums. Since then, government expenditure on the rebate has been constant in real terms, with the rebate percentage subsidizing premiums declining to affect the overall expenditure capping policy.

There are also social costs—in terms of both inefficiency and inequity—to supporting PHI. A competing private sector, underpinned by PHI, may drive up costs for public hospitals. Private insurers are often constrained in how they fund providers, and so cannot fully drive efficiency in the costs of providers, resulting in significant funding inefficiencies in private care. PHI facilitates queue-jumping for people who can afford it, providing access to healthcare based on PHI status rather than patient need.

If PHI is Solely a Complement to Public Funding, the Case for Subsidies is Weak

One of the key roles of PHI in the current system in Australia is to complement public funding. PHI complements public funding and provision by providing access to services not covered by Medicare and by providing access to a different type of service from that provided in the public system. These complementary roles include

- subsidizing access to services that give people a choice of treating doctors;

- providing improved access to private services that are not reimbursed under Medicare, which are predominantly nonmedical services, such as dental, physical therapy, and other allied health services;
- providing access to facilities and amenities beyond what is otherwise available under the public system, such as single rooms and better accommodation; and
- subsidizing faster access to care by bypassing public hospital waiting lists.

Total spending on public hospitals is determined by a complex formula under which the Commonwealth provides base funding and shares (paying 45%) of the cost of growth in activity or costs. But majority funding is the responsibility of state governments, and state governments drive public hospital behavior in their state. The mechanics differ from state to state, but in essence the state government sets a maximum spending cap for each public hospital. In most states, demand for admission exceeds funded activity levels, so waiting lists for elective procedures are created, which can be many months, especially for elective procedures ranked lower priority (Australian Institute of Health and Welfare 2020b). Bypassing those waits—through admission to a private hospital—is a key selling point for PHI.

The Irrationality of the Choice Argument

Central to the PHI value proposition is the idea of choice. A former conservative health minister, Michael Wooldridge, identified that "the essence of the [PHI] rebate is choice." Implicit in this is the assumption that you cannot have access to private health care without PHI.

The current system of PHI "carrots and sticks" is to some extent the opposite of choice: Some people are effectively coerced into PHI because of tax penalties; others are encouraged through the rebate that subsidizes PHI; and yet others, who may want to choose private hospital care, cannot because of the uneven geographical distribution of private hospitals. Private hospitals are mostly located in metropolitan areas—and in the wealthiest suburbs within those cities—with few private hospitals in smaller regional centers or remote Australia. The rate of private hospital admissions is therefore skewed toward major cities (see Table 4.2).

Although consumers may regard some choice as better than none, the choice provided by PHI may be worth relatively little because in the absence of full information about options of treating doctors and their fees and

Table 4.2. Residents of regional centers and remote Australia are much less likely to use private hospitals, 2019–2020

	Major cities	Inner regional	Outer regional	Remote	Very remote	Total
Private hospital admission rate per thousand population	169.4	135.6	104.6	87.9	131.4	156.3

Source: Australian Institute of Health and Welfare (2021, Table 3.5).

complication rates, patients (and referring doctors) are rarely able to make an informed choice based on the relative merits of hospitals or practitioners.

And not everyone with PHI gets the choice they want. As pointed out above, choice is limited for people in regional areas. Benefit restrictions—because some people do not have coverage for all types of care—and benefit caps limit the choices people with PHI can make. Industry attempts to manage cost pressures through preferred provider or contracted arrangements also diminish people's choices.

Choice does not necessarily result in better-informed decisions by patients or lead to better health outcomes (Schram and Sonnemans 2011). The complex nature of products often leads patients to irrational choices, such as selecting a product with a higher deductible when an equivalent product with a lower deductible is available for the same price (Bhargava, Loewenstein, and Sydnor 2017).

Under the universal Medicare scheme, all Australians are entitled to receive care in the public system. Subsidizing people who choose to take out PHI and seek treatment as a private patient because they prefer the additional dimensions of service provided in private care seems illogical. If private care is solely a complement to public care, it seems more logical that people who prefer more than the care provided under the public system should bear the full cost of that choice. A person's right to choose private care remains, with or without a subsidy. Therefore, it would be more equitable for the costs to be borne by those who make that choice and get the benefits of that choice.

Restrict Public Provision, Yet Subsidize Getting Around Those Restrictions?

Private health insurance as a complement occurs because the public sector does not provide or fund a service, does not provide a service at a consumer's desired amenities level, or service constraints mean the care is not provided within the time frame a consumer wants. All of these are inherent and expected consequences of priority setting.

Assuming government has made a rational choice about the scope of the public benefits package and the characteristics of public provision in terms of amenities and waiting times, it seems illogical in the extreme for government to subsidize some consumers to bypass the consequences of the constraints that its policies have created. If physical therapy or dental care is not to be include in the public benefit package, for example, it makes no sense to subsidize physical therapy or dental care indirectly through insurance—especially when it is a product with an inequitable income incidence.

PHI is Inequitable

People with higher incomes are more likely to take out PHI (Doiron, Jones, and Savage 2008). Therefore, even though the subsidy is means tested, it tends to disproportionately benefit people with middle to higher incomes. Yet, people with middle to higher incomes are the people whose decision to take up PHI is least likely to be influenced by the government subsidy.

People with PHI also gain greater access to hospitals and health services, which undermines the principle of access to service based on clinical need. To the extent that PHI facilitates faster access to care by encouraging queue-jumping and allowing people to bypass public hospital waiting lists based on PHI status and ability to pay, this is inequitable and also may result in unequal quality of healthcare services. It raises the question of whether a better use of public funding is to expand public access directly, and to the extent that it reduces the availability of doctors in public hospitals, subsidization undermines the principles of a universal public system. The admission rate for people with PHI is higher than those without, further contributing to a perceived inequity—although because the incidence of low-value care is greater in private hospitals compared to public hospitals, whether a higher admission rate is a real benefit is a moot point.

General insurance (for ancillary services and extras, e.g., dental care) is only a complement—there are no government programs that provide unfettered access to the services covered by private insurance.

If the purpose of PHI is merely to complement the public system by providing people with improved access and choice of services, facilities, and amenities beyond those considered necessary under the publicly funded system, the argument for subsidizing PHI is weak. Complementary insurance is by definition for services over and above the government-prescribed standard. If government is not prepared to provide those additional services universally, it is illogical to subsidize for a subset of the population through PHI, especially when that subset is not the most disadvantaged in the community.

If PHI is a Substitute for Public Funding, the Case for Subsidies is Stronger

In 2019–1920, there were more than 11 million admissions to hospitals in Australia, 40% to private hospitals (see Table 4.3). Private hospitals tend to focus on less-complex elective procedures, such as knee and hip replacements for people without additional diagnoses ("comorbidities"). Two-thirds of all elective surgery is undertaken in private hospitals, but emergency care shows the opposite picture: Only 1 in 12 emergency patients is admitted to a private hospital.

Public hospitals in Australia are perceived to be high quality: The more complex care is provided there, and all major trauma is also treated in public hospitals. Academic medical centers in Australia are all public hospitals.

Private care is not a direct substitute for public care. Complex procedures requiring specialized equipment or skills are rarely available in private hospitals. Private hospitals engage in "cream skimming" and tend to refer out complex patients to public hospitals and receive referrals for less-complex patients from public hospitals (Brameld, Holman, and Moorin 2006; Cheng, Haisken-DeNew, and Yong 2015).

Particularly for less-complex elective procedures, people who have the means to pay for a private hospital admission—either because of their PHI coverage or by paying for the admission out of their own pocket—may have a choice of public hospital care or admission to a private hospital, depending on the procedure.

The substitution-based argument for a subsidy is stronger if it results in a cost saving for government or private provision is economically more efficient than services that are provided universally through the public system. But the evidence suggests this is not so: Patients in private hospitals tend to stay longer than patients in public hospitals. For 20 common reasons for admission (classified according to their diagnosis related group), the

Table 4.3. Types of treatments in public and private hospitals, 2019–20

	Public hospitals			Private hospitals			Total hospital activity
	Episodes	Percentage of public hospital activity	Percentage of total hospital activity	Episodes	Percentage of private hospital activity	Percentage of total hospital activity	Episodes
Elective							
Surgical	713,632	11	6	1,436,211	33	13	2,149,843
Medical	1,871,641	28	17	2,054,761	47	18	3,926,402
Subtotal	2,585,273	38	23	3,490,972	79	31	6,076,245
Emergency							0
Surgical	318,132	5	3	49,442	1	0	367,574
Medical	2,532,078	38	23	199,404	5	2	2,731,482
Subtotal	2,850,210	42	26	248,846	6	2	3,099,056
Other	1,294,589	19	12	668,122	15	6	1,962,711
Total	6,730,072	100	60	4,407,940	100	40	11,138,012

Note: Includes same-day facilities.

Source: Australian Institute of Health and Welfare 2020a; Australian Institute of Health and Welfare 2021, Tables 4.2, 6.16, and 6.18.

(unweighted) average length of stay for patients in private hospitals was 40% longer than for patients in public hospitals; in only two cases, both involving primarily same-day admissions (appendectomy and tonsillectomy) was the average length of stay shorter in private hospitals than public hospitals (Australian Institute of Health and Welfare 2021, Figure 2.3).

There may be a number of reasons for this pattern, perhaps because there is less pressure on private hospital beds or perhaps because financial incentives to reduce length of stay are not so strong in private hospitals. But longer length of stay may be because the value proposition to the customer of the private product may involve a more relaxed attitude to discharge (e.g., in maternity care), and here comparative inefficiency is built into the private hospital model.

Differences in institutional arrangements, case mix, and treatment complexity make it hard to compare the efficiency of the two sectors. Because private hospitals mostly specialize in elective, scheduled procedures, they avoid the overheads of emergencies and the need to staff for uncertainties. One study that did control for case mix found that, for a similar case mix, public hospitals were 10% less costly than private hospitals (Duckett and Jackson 2000). An Australian government economic advisory body has undertaken two studies on the relative efficiency of public and private hospitals. One found there was virtually no difference; the other found private hospitals were less costly (Productivity Commission 2009, 2010), but both were methodologically flawed as neither of these studies used good measures to control for differences in case mix.

Any advantages of PHI subsidies must be weighed against any adverse impact on the public system, including additional costs to the public system; reductions in quality in the public system; and adverse impacts on the principle of universal access.

Does Private Healthcare Save Costs Overall?

Subsidies probably induce some people to take out PHI and rely less on the public hospital system. Of course, a significant number of people, particularly high-income earners and high users of healthcare services—the elderly and people suffering from chronic health conditions—would probably retain insurance and continue to rely on private hospitals even if there were no subsidy. The natural—unreimbursed and uncoerced—level of PHI may be about

25% to 30% of the population, the level PHI dropped to by the end of Labor's period in office in 1996. Thus, the dead weight of subsidies might be about the two-thirds of those with PHI who would probably be insured if the subsidy and other carrots and sticks had not been introduced.

Even without PHI, it is unlikely that public hospitals would need to accommodate all private hospital activity and stays (Doiron and Kettlewell 2018; Yu et al. 2019) because of the higher incidence of low-value care in private hospitals and because average length of stay is longer in private hospitals.

Nevertheless, without PHI there would be more patients in the public sector. The cost of their admissions would have to be paid in full by the public sector rather than paid only in part through a subsidy. However, on balance the savings on the subsidy would probably pay for the expansion in the public sector necessary to accommodate the additional transferring patients. More public-sector patients might also require new capital stock, but additional demand might also be met by increasing the use of private hospitals under contract to the public sector, thus avoiding new builds and capital expenditure by state governments to accommodate any shift in admission patterns.

For those who care a lot about minimizing the size of government, PHI would be justified if it saved the government money. But for those unconcerned about the size of government, this is not enough. For them, PHI would be justified only if it reduced total spending on health, even if government spending were higher because there were more public and fewer private services.

If private hospitals are more efficient overall than public hospitals, then encouraging people to use private hospitals would contribute to the overall efficiency of the health system, but the evidence suggests the contrary: that private hospitals are less efficient than public hospitals.

It is therefore unlikely that PHI reduces total spending on health. Stays are longer, and it pays for some services that would not meet thresholds of "clinical need" in the public system (Badgery-Parker et al. 2019; Chalmers et al. 2019).

The Medicare principles specify that access to public hospital services is to be based on clinical need. If PHI did not increase total health spending, then patients would be admitted to private hospitals based on the same standards of clinical need as applied in public hospitals.

But in practice, thresholds for admission in private hospitals are often lower than for public hospitals because there is more demand for public hospital care relative to capacity. Patients can be admitted to a private hospital for a procedure that the patient and the treating doctor think is clinically desirable even if it would not meet the thresholds for admission to a public hospital. A study by Brameld et al. (2006), which looked at the effect of having PHI on hospital use in Western Australia, found that for all major diagnostic categories, other than treatment on an emergency basis, privately insured patients had a higher rate of surgical procedures. The study suggests that the higher level of intervention for privately insured patients may be a result of lower thresholds for treatment in the private sector. These treatments may well have been in the patient's interests, but it is possible that some were not and were the result of supplier-induced demand, as evidenced by the higher proportion of low-value care in private hospitals.

Private hospital use increased after the PHI incentives were introduced. Private hospital patients were more likely to receive more in-hospital medical services than patients in public hospitals. It is unclear how much of the additional activity in private healthcare is due to the unmet needs of patients in public hospitals and how much is the result of medical specialist-induced demand, based on patients' ability to pay rather than their clinical needs (Richardson and Peacock 2006; Peacock and Richardson 2007).

Some of the additional activity funded by PHI may not improve patient outcomes. And, because of the higher incidence of low-value care in private hospitals, private healthcare is adding cost but not improving outcomes. Private maternity patients are more likely to have cesarean sections (Einarsdóttir et al. 2013; Eldridge, Onur, and Velamuri 2017), and private patients are likely to have more rehabilitation days than public hospital patients, and yet the outcomes are no different (Schilling et al. 2018).

Apart from the volume of services, private healthcare may also increase the price paid for services (in economic terms, it transfers surplus from consumers to producers). The limited incentives for private health insurers to promote cost-efficiencies, and the inability of insurance funds to control the costs of health providers, may push up the fees charged for medical services (Hopkins and Frech 2001), thereby contributing to the growth in gap fees and out-of-pocket costs incurred by patients.

Even if private healthcare adds to total costs, it might be seen as economically valuable when it supports clinically worthwhile outcomes that the public system would not have provided. But why should other taxpayers subsidize these outcomes?

The most plausible argument is that subsidizing private health overcomes consumer myopia: Perhaps people systematically pay less for health services than is in their own interests. But, the evidence suggests that the increased spending results in inefficiency—more low-value care and longer stays—not improved outcomes. Further, the fact that the proportion of younger people who are privately insured is declining and the proportion of older people insured is increasing suggests that consumers are making accurate assessments of their relative actuarial risk profile and the likely expected value of insurance for them.

The argument for subsidizing private healthcare is weaker if it adversely affects public care. Subsidizing private healthcare may divert medical professionals from the public system, reducing its capacity to meet patient needs. Higher remuneration in the private sector encourages doctors to allocate more time to private patients and to offer preferential treatment to private patients in public hospitals (Cheng et al. Yong 2015). When doctors work more hours in the private sector, they are available to work fewer hours in the public sector (Cheng, Joyce, and Scott 2013; Cheng, Kalb, and Scott 2013).

In a tight labor market, if doctors are attracted away from the public system, public hospitals may have reduced capacity to meet patient needs. The higher remuneration for medical specialists in the private sector may give an incentive to doctors working in both sectors to maintain waiting lists in the public system to encourage patients to be treated privately, creating horizontal inequity. Although the direction of causality is unclear, longer waiting times for public care and higher private care proportions are associated (Duckett 2005, 2018).

Private hospitals may engage in "cream skimming"—the selection of patients whose treatment will yield higher profit margins (Cheng et al. 2015). Hospitals may engage in "vertical" cream skimming or patient selection by focusing on patients who yield the same revenue but are lower cost to serve because their conditions are less severe. Hospitals and doctors may engage in "horizontal" cream skimming by choosing to specialize in more profitable medical procedures.

Public hospitals must accept all patients, so they have little or no scope to cream skim. Consequently, cream skimming by private hospitals may leave public hospitals with higher-cost patients. This reduces the surplus on funded services that would otherwise be used in the public sector to support additional services.

It has been suggested that PHI has subsidized queue jumping, meaning some people get access to healthcare based on their insurance status rather than clinical needs (Hindle and McAuley 2004). If a subsidy provides people who can afford it with the opportunity to bypass public-sector waiting lists, which are based on the greatest clinical needs, a subsidy operates to undermine the universality of the system, reduces equity of access to healthcare, and also reduces efficiency by reducing the average net value of clinical care provided.

Bringing it all Together: The Adverse Impact of PHI on Equity, Efficiency, and Quality

The insured—who are more likely to be wealthy (see Figure 4.1)—receive faster and therefore inequitable access to care than the uninsured. But there is also horizontal inequity within the insured population. About three-quarters of the population is covered for all elective procedures, creating differential access compared to the other quarter without complete coverage. Even among those covered for all procedures, three-quarters have a financial excess or deductible. Despite recent rationalization of product descriptions, contributors to PHI may not know the details of their product coverage and the rules about how much they will be out of pocket if they use a private hospital. Because the rebate is paid as a percentage of product price, those contributors eligible for the rebate electing more generous cover—more procedures covered with lower deductibles—are doubly rewarded with both better coverage and a bigger subsidy, creating horizontal inequity among the insured.

This chapter has said little about quality differences, principally because coding practices differ between the two sectors—mostly in terms of extent or "depth" of coding—so it is difficult to standardize for case mix differences. What we do know is there is more low-value care in private hospitals, and when adverse events occur private hospital patients are transferred to public hospitals. But there are key elements of quality where private hospitals perform well: Quicker access, although inequitable, is a component of quality; a longer length of hospital stay, although inefficient, may be perceived by patients as a positive and becomes another dimension of quality; so too is generally better food and other aspects of environmental quality.

Overall, the performance of the Australian healthcare system is good—Australia spends less per head and as a share of gross domestic product on health spending than its peers and has better gross outcomes in terms of life expectancy, albeit there is inequity here as well because indigenous life expectancy is about a decade shorter than the average.

Private health insurance remains one of the key contested domains of public policy in Australia and health policy in Australia: There are significant differences in ideology between the Conservative Liberal-National coalition and the Labor Party. Although the modus vivendi is now that Labor does not attempt to reduce subsidies, Liberal-National governments continue to support and extend membership contribution levels of PHI through subsidies and coercive policies. Liberal-National coalition parties also attempt to narrow and undermine inviversality, with rhetoric about Medicare being a residual rather than a universalist policy.

The ideological contest continues unabated despite the declining membership of PHI—people are voting with their feet—the inequitable impact of a two-speed system, and the inefficiency created in the private sector.

This chapter has shown that the arguments for government subsidies for private health services are weak if private health services only complement public health services. The argument would be stronger if the private sector delivers health services more efficiently than the public sector, but the evidence of this is contested. It is reasonable to argue for private health subsidies if they reduce the cost of health services to government—but only if minimizing the size of government is seen as an important objective.

Australia's current health system is an unhappy mix in which private care not only complements the public system by offering additional services and dimensions otherwise not publicly available, but also to some extent competes with the public system by offering substitute services.

This chapter has described the dual role of private healthcare as a complement to and substitute for public care. The emphasis on each of these roles has varied over time, reflecting attitudes to the role and size of government at the time. What has been demonstrated here is that the various arguments for subsidizing PHI, whether it is a complement or a substitute, are on very weak ground indeed. This does not stop politicians and self-interested stakeholders asserting the benefits of subsidizing PHI, regardless of the evidence.

There is clearly an ideological divide in Australia's policy: Conservative governments strongly support PHI and promote subsidies and penalties to increase coverage. Labor, on the other hand, tolerates PHI possibly because, with 40% of the population insured, it fears an electoral backlash if it proposed withdrawing subsidies. Given many—maybe more than a third—of those with PHI only have it because of penalties if they do not, the size of the potential political backlash may be overrated, but it would be a brave Opposition that decided to test those waters.

The interaction between the public and private sectors in Australia is complex and not healthy—the private sector competes for resources, both staff and money, with the public sector and provides little benefit in terms of reducing public-sector demand. Unfortunately, unlike belief in the Easter bunny and Father Christmas, people tend not to grow out of the belief that supporting PHI benefits the public sector. The Australian muddled and contested PHI system provides one big lesson for other countries: Subsidies, once introduced, are hard to withdraw no matter how irrational they are.

References

Australian Bureau of Statistics. 2020. *Patient Experiences in Australia: Summary of Findings, 2019–20*. Canberra: ABS.

Australian Institute of Health and Welfare. 2020a. *Admitted Patients*. Canberra: AIHW.

Australian Institute of Health and Welfare. 2020b. *Elective Surgery Waiting Times 2019–20*. Canberra: AIHW.

Australian Institute of Health and Welfare. 2020c. *Emergency Department Care 2019–20*. Canberra: AIHW.

Australian Institute of Health and Welfare. 2020d. *Health Expenditure Australia 2018–19*. Catalog no. HWE 80. Canberra: AIHW.

Australian Institute of Health and Welfare. 2021. *Admitted Patients 2019–20*. Canberra: AIHW.

Badgery-Parker, Tim, Sallie-Anne Pearson, Kelsey Chalmers, Jonathan Brett, Ian A. Scott, Susan Dunn, Neville Onley, and Adam G. Elshaug. 2019. "Low-value care in Australian public hospitals: prevalence and trends over time." *BMJ Quality & Safety* 28(3): 205–214. doi: 10.1136/bmjqs-2018-008338.

Bartlett, Ben, and John Boffa. 2001. "Aboriginal Community Controlled Comprehensive Primary Health Care: The Central Australian Aboriginal Congress." *Australian Journal of Primary Health* 7(3): 74–82. doi: https://doi.org/10.1071/PY01050.

Bartlett, Ben, and John Boffa. 2005. "The impact of Aboriginal community controlled health service advocacy on Aboriginal health policy." *Australian Journal of Primary Health* 11(2): 53–62.

Bhargava, Saurabh, George Loewenstein, and Justin Sydnor. 2017. "Choose to lose: Health plan choices from a menu with dominated options." *Quarterly Journal of Economics* 132(3): 1319–1372.

Brameld, Kate, DArcy Holman, and Rachael Moorin. 2006. "Possession of health insurance in Australia--how does it affect hospital use and outcomes?" *Journal of Health Services & Research Policy* 11(2): 94–100.

Butler, J. R. G. 2002. "Policy change and private health insurance: Did the cheapest policy do the trick?" *Australian Health Review* 25(6): 33–41.

Chalmers, Kelsey, Sallie-Anne Pearson, Tim Badgery-Parker, Jonathan Brett, Ian A. Scott, and Adam G. Elshaug. 2019. "Measuring 21 low-value hospital procedures: claims analysis of Australian private health insurance data (2010–2014)." *BMJ open* 9(3): e024142.

Cheng, Terence Chai, John P. Haisken-DeNew, and Jongsay Yong. 2015. "Cream skimming and hospital transfers in a mixed public-private system." *Social Science & Medicine* 132: 156–164. doi: http://dx.doi.org/10.1016/j.socscimed.2015.03.035.

Cheng, Terence Chai, Catherine M. Joyce, and Anthony Scott. 2013. "An empirical analysis of public and private medical practice in Australia." *Health Policy* 111(1): 43–51. doi: http://dx.doi.org/10.1016/j.healthpol.2013.03.011.

Cheng, Terence Chai, Guyonne Kalb, and Anthony Scott. 2013. Public private or both?: analysing factors influencing the labour supply of medical specialists. In *Working Paper*. Melbourne: Melbourne Institute.

Doiron, Denise, Glenn Jones, and Elizabeth Savage. 2008. "Healthy, wealthy and insured? The role of self-assessed health in the demand for private health insurance." *Health economics* 17(3): 317–334.

Doiron, Denise, and Nathan Kettlewell. 2018. "The Effect of Health Insurance on the Substitution between Public and Private Hospital Care." *Economic Record* 94(305): 135–154. doi: 10.1111/1475-4932.12394.

Donabedian, Avedis. 2002. *An introduction to quality assurance in health care.* New York: Oxford University Press.

Duckett, Stephen. 2005. "Private care and public waiting." *Australian Health Review* 29(1): 87–93.

Duckett, Stephen. 2018. "Coercing, Subsidising and Encouraging: Two Decades of Support for Private Health Insurance." In *Wrong Way: How Privatisation and Economic Reform Backfired*, edited by Damien Cahill and Phillip Toner, 40–58. Melbourne: La Trobe University Press in conjunction with Black Inc.

Duckett, Stephen, and Matt Cowgill. 2019. *Saving private health 2: Making private health insurance viable.* Melbourne, Vic.: Grattan Institute.

Duckett, Stephen, and Terri Jackson. 2000. "The new health insurance rebate: An inefficient way of assisting public hospitals." *Medical Journal of Australia* 172(9): 439–444.

Duckett, Stephen, and Greg Moran. 2021. *Stopping the death spiral: creating a future for private health.* Melbourne, Vic.: Grattan Institute.

Duckett, Stephen, and Kristina Nemet. 2019a. *The history and purposes of private health insurance.* Melbourne, Vic.: Grattan Institute.

Duckett, Stephen, and Kristina Nemet. 2019b. *Saving private health 1: reining in hospital costs and specialist bills.* Melbourne, Vic.: Grattan Institute.

Dunlevy, Sue. 2012. "Tony Abbott to Axe Health Insurance Means Test 'as Soon as We Can.'" *The Australian* February 15. http://www.theaustralian.com.au/national-affairs/means-test-pledge-swells-tony-abbotts-budget-savings-task/news-story/9f79a8ffd42f81120e4b9fa8b99a5511

Dwyer, Judith, K. O'Donnell, E. Willis, and J. Kelly. 2016. "Equitable care for indigenous people: Every health service can do it." *Asia Pacific Journal of Health Management* 11(3): 11–17.

Eagar, Kathy. 2004. "The weakest link?" *Australian Health Review* 28(1): 7–12. doi: https://doi.org/10.1071/AH040007.

Einarsdóttir, Kristjana, Fatima Haggar, Gavin Pereira, Helen Leonard, Nick de Klerk, Fiona J. Stanley, and Sarah Stock. 2013. "Role of public and private funding in the rising cesarean section rate: a cohort study." *BMJ open* 3(5): e002789.

Eldridge, Damien S., Ilke Onur, and Malathi Velamuri. 2017. "The impact of private hospital insurance on the utilization of hospital care in Australia." *Applied Economics* 49(1): 78–95.

Ellis, Randall, and Elizabeth Savage. 2008. "Run for cover now or later? The impact of premiums, threats and deadlines on private health insurance in Australia." *International Journal of Health Care Finance and Economics* 8(4): 257–277. doi: 10.1007/s10754-008-9040-4.

Hall, Jane, Richard De Abreu Lourenco, and Rosalie Viney. 1999. "Carrots and sticks—the fall and fall of private health insurance in Australia." *Health Economics* 8(8): 653–660.

Hindle, Don, and Ian McAuley. 2004. "The effects of increased private health insurance: a review of the evidence." *Australian Health Review* 28(1): 119–138.

Hopkins, S., and H. E. Frech. 2001. "The rise of private health insurance in Australia: Early effects on insurance and hospital markets." *Economic and Labour Relations Review* 12(2): 225–238.

Judkins, Simon. 2021. "ED Overcrowding, Under-resourcing Worst in 30 Years." *MJA Insight*, April 16. https://insightplus.mja.com.au/2021/14/ed-overcrowding-under-resourcing-worst-in-30-years/

McLean, J., and M. K. Walsh. 2003. "Lessons from the Inquiry into Obstetrics and Gynaecology Services at King Edward Memorial Hospital 1990–2000." *Australian Health Review* 26(1): 12–23.

Peacock, Stuart J., and Jeffrey R. J. Richardson. 2007. "Supplier-induced demand: re-examining identification and misspecification in cross-sectional analysis." *The European Journal of Health Economics* 8(3): 267–277.

Productivity Commission. 2009. *Public and private hospitals: Research Report.* Canberra: Productivity Commission.

Productivity Commission. 2010. *Public and private hospitals—multivariate analysis: supplement to research report.* Melbourne: Productivity Commission.

Richardson, Jeffrey R. J. 2005. "Priorities of health policy: cost shifting or population health." *Australia and New Zealand Health Policy* 2(1): 1–19.

Richardson, Jeffrey R. J., and Stuart J. Peacock. 2006. "Supplier-Induced Demand: Reconsidering the Theories and New Australian Evidence." *Applied Health Economics and Health Policy* 5(2): 87–98. doi: 10.2165/00148365-200605020-00003.

Robson, Alex, and Francesco Paolucci. 2012. "Private Health Insurance incentives in Australia: The effects of recent changes to price carrots and income sticks." *The Geneva Papers on Risk and Insurance. Issues and Practice* 37(4): 725–744.

Schilling, Chris, Catherine Keating, Anna Barker, Stephen F. Wilson, and Dennis Petrie. 2018. "Predictors of inpatient rehabilitation after total knee replacement: An analysis of private hospital claims data." *Medical Journal of Australia* 209(5): 222–227.

Schram, Arthur, and Joep Sonnemans. 2011. "How individuals choose health insurance: An experimental analysis." *European Economic Review* 55(6): 799–819. doi: https://doi.org/10.1016/j.euroecorev.2011.01.001.

Selvaratnam, Roshan J., Mary-Ann A. Davey, Robyn M. Hudson, Tanya Farrell, and Euan M. Wallace. 2021. "Improving maternity care in Victoria: An accidental learning healthcare system." *Australian and New Zealand Journal of Obstetrics and Gynaecology* 61: 165–168.

Thompson, Geoff, Nicholas J. Talley, and Kelvin M. Kong. 2017. "The health of Indigenous Australians." *Medical Journal of Australia* 207(1): 19–20.

van der Weyden, M. B. 2005. "The Bundaberg Hospital scandal: the need for reform in Queensland and beyond." *MJA* 183(6): 284–285.

Willcox, Sharon, Mary Seddon, Stephen Dunn, Rhiannon Tudor Edwards, Jim Pearse, and Jack V. Tu. 2007. "Measuring and reducing waiting times: A cross-national comparison of strategies." *Health Affairs* 26(4): 1078–1087. doi: 10.1377/hlthaff.26.4.1078.

Wilson, R. McL., W. B. Runciman, R. W. Gibberd, B. T. Harrison, L. Newby, and J. D. Hamilton. 1995. "The quality in Australian health care study." *Medical Journal of Australia* 163(6 November): 458–471.

Yu, S., D. Fiebig, R. Viney, V. Scarf, and C. Homer. 2019. Private provider incentives in health care: the case of birth interventions. In *Working Paper*. Sydney: Centre for Health Economics Research and Evaluation.

Zweifel, Peter, and H. E. Frech. 2016. "Why 'Optimal' Payment for Healthcare Providers Can Never be Optimal Under Community Rating." *Applied Health Economics and Health Policy* 14(1): 9–20. doi: 10.1007/s40258-015-0207-0.

5

The Public/Private Healthcare Mix in France

Implications and Current Debates

Aurélie Pierre and Zeynep Or

Introduction

Three major values—solidarity, liberalism, and pluralism—define the foundations of the French health system and shape the care organization and its funding. Solidarity requires equal access to care by need and a financing system where the healthy and rich support the less wealthy and sick. Liberalism refers to the freedom for health professionals to be able to decide the type and place of their practice and for patients to choose their care providers and insurance levels. Pluralism relates to a wide range of healthcare providers and multiple private health insurers. The complex hybrid public/private organization and funding of the French health system reflects the weight of these values, as well as, in some respect, their contradictions. Solidarity is mainly provided by universal health insurance allowing the redistribution of resources for supporting the sick and low-income individuals, while plurality can be seen in the mix of public and private providers and private insurance schemes. Nevertheless, this plurality in care provision and funding, together with a high degree of freedom for care providers and patients, has been challenging the objectives of solidary and equal access to high-quality healthcare as well as system-wide efficiency for better health outcomes.

The public health insurance scheme is a noncompetitive statutory health insurance (SHI) model that covers all of the French population. It provides a comprehensive basket of care and funds about 77% of health expenditures but requires cost sharing for all services, including doctor visits and hospitalizations (Direction de la Recherche, des Études, de l'Évaluation

Aurélie Pierre and Zeynep Or, *The Public/Private Healthcare Mix in France* In: *The Public/Private Sector Mix in Healthcare Delivery*. Edited by: Howard A. Palley, Oxford University Press. © Oxford University Press 2023. DOI: 10.1093/oso/9780197571101.003.0005 et des Statistiques [DREES] 2019). About 96% of the French population hold a complementary private insurance (CHI), mainly to cover these copayments. Therefore, the French have one of the lowest average out-of-pocket expenditures (around 9%) among the Organization for Economic Cooperation and Development (OECD) countries. Private complementary insurance finances around 14% of the health expenditure, covering all or part of the costs left to patients by the SHI, and plays a key role in ensuring access to care (Buchmueller et al. 2004; Grignon et al. 2008), especially to services for which the costs are not well covered or regulated by the SHI, such as specialist and dental care. In other words, healthcare in France is funded by a mixture of public and private health insurance schemes reimbursing the same benefit package. Different from some other countries, private health insurance is not used for obtaining faster access to certain treatments or for jumping public-sector queues. Waiting times, which could be problematic in some areas due to the unequal distribution of doctors in the territory, are by no means as large an issue as in some other countries, such as Canada and England (Flood and Thomas 2020). No matter the level of their private insurance, patients have a large choice of public and private healthcare providers. Most health professionals work on a fee-for-service (FFS) basis and contract with the SHI fund. They usually respect the tariffs set by the SHI, with a possibility, for some of them, to charge extra fees. Private hospitals also contract with the SHI and are paid by regulated tariffs set at the national level. They play an essential role in care provision, especially in providing surgery. About 55% of all surgery and 25% of obstetric care is provided by private for-profit hospitals.

The health outcomes of the French population rank among the best in the OECD area, with high life expectancy (OECD 2019). Patients have a large choice of providers, and the health system's responsiveness is rated high. However, promoting a universal health system built on a mix of public and private funding and provision raises numerous challenges for ensuring the equity in access, solidarity, and efficiency of the system. The system is expensive, complex, and fragmented in its organization and funding. Large differences in health status between socioeconomic groups as well as social and geographical inequalities in access to care have been a persistent problem (Devaux 2015; Chevillard et al. 2018). A high concentration of out-of-pocket expenditures by the poorest and the sickest part of the population is a real concern (Franc and Pierre 2016b; Perronnin and Louvel 2018). Therefore, the equity principle that is rooted in law and reinforced in all health plans as a strategic objective requires continuous tuning of the health system (Ministère des solidarités et de la santé 2017, 2022).

In this chapter we present the unique mix of public/private healthcare funding and delivery in France and discuss the extent this mix contributes to achieving the overall health system goals of better health outcomes, quality, equity, and efficiency. The first section that follows explains the role of private insurance in healthcare funding and shows how public decision-makers regulate the private insurance market to reduce the issues for equity of access to care and efficiency. The next part focuses on the role of private providers in care delivery and implications of this plurality on care quality, efficiency, and access. We then summarize the most recent measures tackling the major issues with the organization and funding of the public/private mix in the French health system and suggest some avenues for improvement.

A Distinctive Hybrid Public/Private Health Insurance System

France stands out from other countries with similar public and private insurance organization (e.g., Switzerland, Germany, and South Korea) by the fact that public and private insurances reimburse jointly the same health services on almost all type of care. The unique place of private health insurance in France is reflected in the high complementary insurance coverage in the general population (96% in 2019) and the high share of private insurance (14% in 2018) in total health expenditure (Paris and Polton 2016). Funding for the public SHI comes mainly from income-based contributions from employers and employees, as well as, increasingly, through taxation. CHI is based on contractual freedom; while insurers are not allowed to select patients, premiums are mostly conditioned on age (i.e., on risk) without considering ability to pay, and the level of benefits varies mainly according to income.

The Public Health Insurance: Solidarity in the French Health System

Universal Coverage with Contributions on the Basis of Means
Since its creation in 1945, public health insurance in France has been based on two founding principles, namely, access to care depending on need, not

income (the principle of horizontal equity), and solidarity between high- and low-income classes for financing the system (vertical equity). The principle of horizontal equity is reflected by the SHI's reimbursements, which depend on health needs, resulting in solidarity between the healthy and the sick, and the principle of vertical equity is reflected in the progressive nature of financial contributions to SHI, which are proportional to income, with a higher contribution for wealthier individuals (Figure 5.1). Until the 1970s, the funding of SHI was based almost exclusively on payroll contributions. In the past few decades, to ensure financial sustainability, the sources of funding have been broadened to include a wider range of income. The most important change has been the introduction of the *Contribution Sociale Généralisée* (CSG)—taxes applied to a broader range of income, such as financial assets and investments, pensions, gambling, and so on—to finance SHI. A number of earmarked taxes on alcohol, tobacco, and pharmaceutical companies have also been introduced to support public health financing over time. In 2019, about 55% of revenues for SHI came from payroll contributions, 25% from the CSG, and 20% from other taxes (Commission*Comptes de la Sécurité Sociale* 2020).

Statutory health insurance is compulsory and universal for all individuals who work or reside regularly in France. It is provided under various insurance schemes, with mandatory enrollment determined by employment status (wage earners, self-employed, farmers and agricultural employees, students, etc.) or by previous employment status for the retired. Individuals

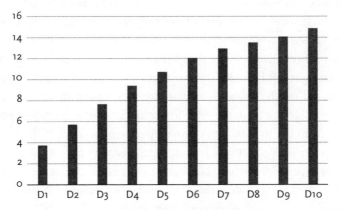

Figure 5.1 Contributions of households to SHI funding, by income deciles.

Note: D1 corresponds to 10% of the population with the lowest income and D10 to the top 10%.

Source: Jusot et al. 2016.

cannot choose their scheme or insurer or opt out. Thus, there are no competing health insurance markets for public health coverage in France. Three
main SHI schemes cover the entire French population. The first one, *le
Régime Général*, insures wage and salary earners, self-employed, and their
dependents and covers about 88% of the population. The second one, *la
Mutualité sociale Agricole*, for farmers and agricultural employees, covers
about 10% of the population. The last one, *les Régimes spéciaux*, includes
about 10 small schemes that cover specific professional categories (e.g.,
notaries, military, etc.), representing 1% of the population. All SHI insurers
provide the same basket of services and goods.

The SHI became universal in 2000 after the implementation of the
"Universal Health Insurance" law (*CMU*[1]), which allowed covering the 2%
of individuals who were not under any scheme given their employment
status. There is also a fully state-funded scheme, *l'Aide médicale d'Etat*, which
provides access to a specific standard benefit package for illegal immigrants
(which differs from the SHI benefit package). It is means tested, and
applicants must be resident for more than 3 months in the French territory.
In 2018, about 310,000 people benefitted from this scheme.

The Comprehensive Benefit Package

The standard benefit package under the SHI system covers a wide range of
goods and services, including inpatient hospital and rehabilitation care
(in both private and public facilities), home care, dental care, prescription
drugs, cost of transport, and care provided by paramedical professionals
(physiotherapists, speech therapists, etc.). Patients usually pay the cost of
ambulatory services at the point of delivery and then claim reimbursement
from their insurance funds. The SHI reimbursements are based on prede-
fined rates of regulated prices that vary according to the type of care, reflecting stronger solidarity for the most severe diseases. Patients' copayments
are calculated on the basis of regulated prices, called *tickets modérateurs*,
varying from 20% of regular fees for hospital care to 30% for physician
visits and from 0% to 85% for approved prescription drugs.[2] There are also
a number of small deductibles for physician visits, paramedical procedures,
drugs, and medical transport, cumulated with extra-billing fees from some
physicians. As a result, while the SHI covers, on average, about 78% of the
total cost of healthcare, this goes up to 92% for hospital care, 65% for ambulatory treatments, and 45% for drugs and medical goods, including optical and
dental devices (Table 5.1).

Table 5.1. Percentage of health expenditure funded by SHI from 2010 to 2019

	2010	2011	2012	2013	2014	2015	2016	2017	2018	2019
All	76.3	76.2	76.3	76.6	77.1	77.3	77.6	77.9	78	78.2
Hospital care	91.5	91.2	91.1	91.1	91.1	91.2	91.5	91.7	91.6	91.6
Public	92.2	91.9	91.9	91.8	91.9	91.9	92.3	92.5	92.4	92.6
Private	89	88.8	88.7	88.6	88.5	88.5	88.7	88.7	88.7	88.4
Outpatient care	63	63	63.3	63.7	64.3	64.8	64.9	65.2	65.8	66
Transport	93	92.9	92.9	92.7	92.8	92.9	93	93	93	93
Drugs	68	68.4	68.9	69.5	71	71.3	71.9	72.8	73.4	74.3
Medical goods	41.2	40.7	40.8	41.7	42.5	43	43.9	44.6	44.7	44.6
Optical	4.1	3.9	3.8	3.9	3.9	4.1	4.1	4.1	4.1	3.9
Other medical goods	73	71.8	71.7	71.8	71.5	71.2	71.1	71.1	71.3	72

Note: In 2019, of hospital expenditures, 91.6% were paid by SHI.
Source: DREES 2020.

There are some exemptions from copayments for individuals who suffer from specific chronic conditions. The *Affection Longue Durée* (ALD) scheme, which today covers 32 groups of diseases (cancer, tuberculosis, poliomyelitis, mental illness, etc.), allows patients to be exempt from the copayments concerning treatments associated with their ALD conditions, irrespective of their income status. However, they still have to pay copayments that concern other conditions, as well as, regardless of their condition, deductibles and extra-billing charges. In 2017, over 10 million individuals were covered by the ALD scheme, representing about 17% of SHI beneficiaries and accounting for roughly 60% of the health expenditure reimbursed by the SHI fund. The number of ALD beneficiaries has continuously increased in the last decade (10.7 billion in 2017 vs. 8 billion in 2005). Despite the increasing demand, the average share of SHI in total health expenditure has remained stable in the past 15 years (around 77%), mainly because of better control of a drug benefit basket and regulation of prices.

The Unique Place of Private Complementary Health Insurance

About 96% of the French population holds a private CHI policy that finances on average about 14% of healthcare expenditures. CHI is more

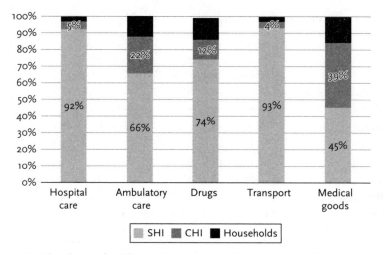

Figure 5.2 The share of public and private complementary health insurance and out-of-pocket payments in health expenditure.
Source: DREES 2020.

important than for hospital care (5%) for paying outpatient care (22% of health expenditures), drugs (12% of health expenditures), and "other medical goods," including optical devices (39%) (Figure 5.2).

Historically, private CHI providers have focused on reimbursing copayments left to patients. Most CHI plans also offer better coverage for medical goods and services that are poorly covered by the public scheme, especially dental and optical devices. Some CHI plans also pay for a part (or the totality) of extra-billing charges asked by some physicians, and some would offer an extended benefit basket, including goods and services that are not covered by the SHI, such as surgery for myopia, or access to an individual room in a hospital. Most of the CHI contracts are not allowed to reimburse deductibles, which are capped by SHI (maximum of €50 per year for medications and €50 for consultations).

Types of Private Insurance
The CHI policies can be purchased through either an employer, that is, a **collective contract**, for private-sector employees and their dependents; or individually, that is, an **individual contract**, for public-sector employees, self-employed individuals, and those unemployed. Collective CHI contracts, partly paid by the employer, have been subsidized since 1979 via tax and social contribution exemptions. CHI premiums vary depending on the age of the policyholder for those insured individually, or on the average age of

the pool of those insured for collective contracts, where the premiums are uniform for all persons insured under the same contract. Those enrolled in the individual CHI market—students, civil servants, self-employed, un-employed, retired—are free to buy (or not) a CHI and choose their level of coverage. Except in the case of specific exemptions, subscription to a col-lective CHI has been required by law for all private sector employees since 2016 (Franc and Pierre 2015). In general, collective CHI contracts are more advantageous than individual ones in terms of guarantees and premiums be-cause of the bargaining power of employers and the concentration of indi-viduals with good health risks (e.g., younger, of working age). Thus, at an equivalent coverage level, premiums for collective contracts are often lower than for individual contracts, even before the contribution made by the em-ployer. In addition, they reimburse more often all or part of the extra-billing charges (Barlet et al. 2020). In 2014, about 60% of CHI owners had an indi-vidual contract, while 40% were covered by collective contracts. The rate of collective contracts has slightly improved since the implementation of the ANI reform in 2016, but the exact rate is not known.

Mix of CHI Providers

The private CHI market is quite competitive. Around 500 providers offer different kinds of CHI policies. There are three distinctive categories of insurers. First, the *mutuelles*, which are nonprofit mutual insurance com-panies that have traditionally dominated the health insurance market and cover approximately 60% of the insured, mostly by individual contracts. Second are the *institutions de prévoyance*, which are nonprofit institutions jointly managed by representatives of employers and employees. They offer almost exclusively collective contracts (i.e., they cover mainly working-age individuals) and cover about 15% of the insured. Last, the *assurances*, private for-profit companies, which have entered into health market more recently, cover around 25% of the CHI beneficiaries, mostly with individual policies. These three types of providers operate under distinct regulatory schemes,[3] but the differences in their premium rates (prices) have diminished over time because of the high competition.

Regulation of the Complementary Health Insurance

In free and competitive markets, health insurers adjust their insurance premiums to the risk of the insured. This can be done directly, using health status and morbidity, or indirectly, using age as an indicator of health status. Access to private health insurance is therefore inequitable since older and sicker individuals, who need care the most, would pay higher premiums. Moreover, private insurers are not required to pursue the system-wide efficiency and cost-containment objectives that are pursued by the public payers. For all these reasons, the CHI market in France is highly regulated.

Tackling Risk Selection

As early as 1989, French authorities have required CHI providers to give a lifetime guarantee for anyone insured so that their premium cannot increase over time, on renewal of a contract, above the price set for others in the same pool of insured for that contract (as part of the *loi Évin*). This law also aims to protect young pensioners, benefiting from a collective contract, who may face higher insurance premiums in individual markets on retirement. Moreover, since 2002, a tax reduction was applied to contracts in which the health status of the insured is not used as a variable of risk adjustment (selection) when defining the price. These contracts, called *contrats solidaires*, prohibit private insurers from using a health questionnaire when setting the insurance plan.

Subsidies for Private CHI for Low-Income Groups and Wage Earners

Given the importance of copayments and the role of CHI in ensuring access to care in France, the expansion of CHI among the poorest, but also for other segments of the population, has been a constant objective of successive governments for decades.

Two schemes were introduced, in 2000 and 2005, for supporting low-income individuals to acquire CHI. The first, the *Couverture maladie universelle complémentaire* (CMU-C), a state-funded insurance scheme, allows people whose monthly income is about 20% below the poverty line to benefit, free of charge, from a CHI contract. The CMU-C covers 100% of negotiated prices of all drugs and services included in the benefit package of SHI (no copayment required). It further covers, albeit modestly, a number of dental and orthodontic treatments and eyeglasses. Moreover, patients are exempted from upfront payments, and physicians are not allowed to extra-bill CMU-C patients. The second measure, the *Aide à la complémentaire santé* (ACS), provides public subsidies in the form of vouchers for buying a private CHI contract. It targets individuals under the poverty line who are not eligible for the CMU-C. ACS provides cash support in the form of vouchers that can only be used to buy a CHI contract. Since 2013, the beneficiaries of ACS have also been exempted from extra-billing. These two schemes supporting CHI for the poorest are funded through specific taxes on private health insurance (*taxe de solidarité additionnelle*; TSA), which amounted to €2 billion in 2012, and, marginally, from taxes on tobacco. In 2019, CMU-C and ACS schemes covered, respectively, 8% (5.9 million individuals) and 1.9% (1.7 million individuals) of the population.[4] In November 2019, CMU-C and ACS were joined under a single scheme, called *la complémentaire santé solidaire* (CSS), to simplify the system and to reduce non-take-up issues.

There has also been continuous political support for ensuring that all workers can have access to CHI—first with tax incentives for private sector employees and employers (since 1979), for the self-employed (since 1994), then by a mandate for all the private sector employees. Indeed, with the *Accord national interprofessionnel* law, all private sector employers must, as of 2016, offer a private CHI to all their employees and pay at least 50% of their premium (they can choose to pay a higher share). Moreover, in case of unemployment, individuals can benefit, free of costs, from the collective contract of their previous employer for up to 12 months. These contracts have to provide a higher minimum coverage concerning dental and optical care.

Controlling Health Expenditure Growth

While supporting access to CHI, successive governments have been constantly looking to regulate, legitimize, and enlarge the responsibility of the private health insurers in containing health expenditure. Therefore, although there is no restriction on what insurers are allowed to cover on the private CHI market, CHI contracts have to respect certain conditions in order to benefit from tax advantages and public subsidies. These contracts, called "responsible," are required to respect certain restrictions in reimbursement in order to promote good consumption behavior. For example, they cannot reimburse out-of-pocket payments when patients visit an outpatient specialist directly without a referral from a general practitioner (GP) (to support the voluntary gatekeeping reform introduced in 2004) or refund certain deductibles (0;50€ for each drug and paramedical act, 1€ for each healthcare visit, and 2€ for transport). In 2016, new constraints were introduced to limit differences in coverage levels between individual and collective contracts in order to reduce the impact of too generous collective contracts on healthcare prices. These contracts must now respect some price/reimbursement ceilings for optical devices and extra-billing charges to control the price inflation for optical devices and cap excess fees in sector 2. Today, almost all CHI contracts subscribed by individuals are defined as "responsible" (*solidaires et responsables*).

Issues in Terms of Equity and Efficiency

While SHI is universal, offers a comprehensive basket of care, and on average, the French population has a very low level of out-of-pocket payment compared to other OECD countries, the combination of public/private health insurance does not fully protect the most socially vulnerable households against the risk of high health spending. Indeed, out-of-pocket payments are not capped, and the mix of funding raises a number of issues about the horizontal equity in access to care, redistribution of public resources, and efficiency in containing the health expenditure growth.

Concerns for Equity

The public/private mix of the French health insurance system challenges the objective of horizontal equity, which is equal access to care by equal need, with significant inequalities in coverage of the least-advantaged part of the population, and, ultimately, in access to care. While on average the out-of-pocket expenditure per capita is very low in France, a small group of low-income individuals with poor health status appear to concentrate a high share of this expenditure. In 2012, an average of almost €5,000 per year in out-of-pocket payments for healthcare was faced by 1% of the population before CHI reimbursements (Haut Conseil pour l'Avenir de l'Assurance Maladie [HCAAM] 2021). Thus, patients with multiple and complex conditions have higher out-of-pocket payments left by SHI despite the existence of the ALD scheme (Franc and Pierre 2016b; Geoffard and de Lagasnerie, 2012). Yet, there is still a small part of the population who do not own a CHI. While only 5% of the population lacked CHI in 2014, the rate was 16% for the unemployed and 12% for individuals in the lowest-income quintile, despite the existence of CMU-C and ACS (Perronnin and Louvel 2018). Moreover, even when they own a CHI, low-income and older groups have less-generous insurance contracts. This is mostly due to the basic functioning of the private insurance market, where premiums increase with risk (i.e., age), and the level of guarantees subscribed by the insured (i.e., services covered) is not associated with needs but with income. Therefore, individuals insured by individual contracts with lower income spend proportionally more of their income on private health insurance, up to 10% of household income, despite owning lower-quality or less-generous contracts (Kambia-Chopin et al. 2008; Jusot et al. 2012). Also, the CHI contracts, even when they are "responsible," adjust their premiums as a function of age, hence requiring higher payments from those with higher needs, against the horizontal equity principle. Moreover, group contracts, which, by design, are more advantageous than individual contracts, are not accessible for the most precarious and sickest individuals. As a result, good CHI contracts with lower prices and better coverage are more often subscribed by the wealthier.

To tackle the issues in equity in access to care, the solution proposed by successive governments has been to increase private CHI coverage for a larger part of the population, including with public subsidies. Nevertheless, this politique has also been a source of a two-tier treatment in the system. In fact, the public subsidies given to private companies and employees for supporting collective contracts is considerable compared to those dedicated to low-income individuals (Franc and Pierre 2015). Moreover, the fact that health professionals are not allowed to charge extra fees for the beneficiaries of the public CHI schemes (CMU-C, ACS) appears to create two-tier treatment. Patients who are part of these schemes may face discrimination and have difficulties in getting an appointment with some physicians (Desprès et al. 2009), although it is illegal to refuse a patient because of insurance status.

Efficiency Concerns

The hybrid public/private insurance system, where private insurance complements the public funding for almost all types of care, implies a multiplicity of payers for the same basket of care and is not forcibly the most optimal way of using resources. First, the generous coverage offered by some private CHI contracts can be inflationary. This is especially the case for collective CHI contracts since they often reimburse extra fees charged by some health professionals. Second, the reimbursement of copayments by the private CHI cancels the incentives initially sought to reduce moral hazard in the core public plan (Askenazy et al. 2013; Geoffard 2006). Third, this combination of public/private insurance comes with a high management cost: France has the second-highest administrative costs (6% of the health spending) in the OECD, just after the United States, and almost half of this expenditure is related to CHI (Figure 5.3).

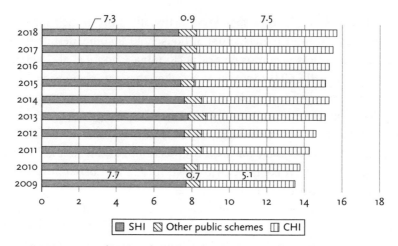

Figure 5.3 Amount of SHI and CHI management cost (in milliards of euros).
Source: DREES 2019.

Finally, even if the regulation of the CHI market is crucial to limit the most harmful effects of risk selection operated by insurers, the extent of this regulation may appear nonoptimal. Private insurers must adjust insurance premiums to the risk of the insured to face adverse selection. Thus, overly restrictive regulations push insurers to find new solutions to select risks, which can lead to a vicious circle that exacerbates market distortions without allowing policyholders to be fully protected from risk selection.

A Rich Mix of Public and Private Providers

Plurality in Care Delivery

With 3.2 physicians and 10.5 nurses per 1,000 population in 2019, health human resources in France is close to the OECD average (OECD 2019). This average, however, hides contrasting realities. Health professionals are free to practice in different settings (solo practice, medical centers, clinics, etc.) with different payment arrangements and obligations.

Ambulatory Care
Ambulatory care is mainly provided by private, self-employed health professionals—doctors, nurses, dentists, and medical auxiliaries—working

in their own individual practice, in health centers, or private clinics. In 2016, 47% of all doctors and 65% of the GPs were self-employed, while 42% were employed in a hospital or another healthcare facility, and 11% had mixed (public and private) activity (DREES 2017). Self-employed health professionals are paid according to a national FFS schedule. The official tariffs for reimbursement are set via a formal national negotiation process between the government, the union of SHI funds, the union of CHI schemes, and unions of health professionals. Doctors usually contract with SHI to define their practice mode and pricing. Those who charge the negotiated fee are known as "sector 1" contractors (Box 5.1). In return they receive their social contributions (including pension) paid by the SHI fund. Some doctors, known as "sector 2," contractors, are allowed to charge higher fees but must purchase their own pension and insurance coverage. The creation of sector 2 in the 1980s aimed to reduce the cost of social contributions for the SHI fund, but it did not have the expected impact, and the demand for the sector was much higher than predicted. Consequently, access to sector 2 has been limited since 1990 to a controlled number of doctors each year. In 2016, the average fees for physicians in sector 2 were about 52% higher than conventional tariffs, overbilling rates varying between 10% (for Cantal) and 115% (for Paris area).

Inpatient Care

Inpatient care is delivered by a large number of public, private for-profit, and nonprofit hospitals. Patients can freely choose between public and private hospitals without needing a referral. Doctors and other health professionals (nurses, etc.) working in public hospitals are usually paid by salary, while doctors working in private hospitals are paid by FFS. While the total number of hospital beds has decreased over the past decade, the French system remains highly hospital centric, with one of the highest hospitalization rates in the OECD area, and hospital care represents almost half of all health spending (OECD 2019).

Public hospitals have the legal obligation to provide a range of services, including 24-hour care, and have to take part in activities related to national/regional public health priorities. They represented 45% of all hospitals and 62% of all acute inpatient beds in 2018 (Drees 2021). The private for-profit sector represents 25% of all inpatient beds and specializes mostly in elective surgery. About 55% of all surgeries and 20% of obstetric care are provided by private for-profit hospitals. Their market share goes up to 65% for knee replacement,

---

Box 5.1. DIFFERENT SECTOR OF PRIVATE PRACTICE IN FRANCE

Sector 1: Health professionals are required to bill the conventional tariffs set out in the national agreements with the SHI. Extra-billings above these amounts are limited to a very few circumstances (out-of-hour visits, etc.). In return, health professionals get a part of their compulsory social contributions paid by SHI. In 2018, 52% of specialists and 95% of generalists were working in sector 1, adhering to the national tariffs.

Sector 2: Health professionals who have signed the medical convention with the SHI are permitted to extra-bill. They must purchase their own pension and insurance coverage. There is no official limit to how much care providers can charge extra, but the social security code and the medical code of ethics require that extra-billing be of a "reasonable amount"— without defining the term.[a] The entry to sector 2 has been restricted to a specific number of specialists since 1990. In 2018, 47% of specialists and 5% of generalists were working in sector 2, with a high degree of variation across specialties (37% of doctors in sector 2 among psychiatrists vs. 65% and 31% among gynecologists and ophthalmologists, respectively) and across regions (75% of ophthalmologists are in sector 2 in the Paris area vs. 40% in Bretagne).

Sector 3: Health professionals who do not have the convention with SHI have complete freedom to set their fees, but the reimbursement from SHI is lower than for sectors 1 and 2. Less than 1% of generalists and specialists work in sector 3.

[a] Section L162-1-14-1 of the social security code and section 53 of the medical code of ethics apply.

---

more than 80% for certain ambulatory surgery, such as cataracts and endoscopies. On the other hand, certain complex care/procedures (e.g., stroke care, burn treatment, or surgery for multiple traumas) are provided almost exclusively by public hospitals. Three-quarters of private nonprofit hospitals, which represent about 14% of acute care, have a special agreement with the state to provide "public services," such as emergency care, and are eligible for public subsidies. Private hospitals also contract with the SHI and respect the same quality and safety regulations as public hospitals in order to be funded.

Until 2004, public and private hospitals were paid under two different schemes. On the one hand, public and most private not-for-profit hospitals had global budgets mainly based on historical costs. On the other hand, private for-profit hospitals had an itemized billing system that was inflationary, with daily tariffs covering the cost of accommodation, nursing, and routine care and a separate payment based on the diagnostic and therapeutic procedures carried out (Or and Gandré 2021). The difference in payment between public and private hospitals has always been a subject of conflict: Public hospitals considered global budgets as an instrument of rationing, insensitive to changing demand, while private hospitals advocated that global budgets rewarded inefficiency of public hospitals. The introduction of activity-based payment, ABP (*tarification à l'activité*, or T2A in French) in 2005 to pay for acute hospital services was therefore very welcomed by all parties initially. The major objectives of ABP were to increase hospital efficiency and to create a "level playing field" for payments to public and private hospitals. While it achieved half of its objectives by increasing productivity in both sectors, ABP also created new problems regarding quality and appropriateness of care.

From the patients' point of view, while the competition between public and private hospitals improves choice and contribute to innovation in care (Or et al., 2020), the extra-billing for physician services, common in private for-profit hospitals, is a source of inequality in access. While some doctors are also allowed to extra-bill in public hospitals, this is much less common. Until recently, there was little information on the extra fees charged in hospitals, but some reports have shown that extra-billing charges can be up to four times higher than regulated prices in hospital settings (*France Assos Santé* 2015). However, according to the observation of tariffs, different measures introduced by the SHI in recent years have been successful in containing extra fees in hospitals; the fees were (on average) about 45% over the regulated fees in 2016, versus 80% in 2005.

Unsustainable Freedom in "Liberal Medicine"

Historically, liberal medicine in France has been organized around four principles delineated by law: confidentiality of medical information, office-based FFS practice in the ambulatory sector, freedom of practice for physicians, and the patient's free choice of provider. These principles have been challenged over time to limit the escalating healthcare costs and chronic problems, with unequal geographic distribution of doctor supply (Cour des comptes 2017), but they are still strongly rooted in the system.

Freedom of practice for physicians implies that doctors (and medical auxiliaries) are free to choose their place of practice as well as, their practice mode, and sometimes prices. While pricing rules have been strengthened over time, freedom to choose the place of practice remains a historic right for doctors to which medical unions are very attached (Hassenteufel 2008). Notwithstanding a relatively high density of doctors, the unequal geographical distribution of health workers, skewed to the well-off urban areas, has been a long-standing problem for access to care. The lack of specialists, such as not only gynecologists, ophthalmologists, and anesthetists, but also GPs in some areas, has become a serious policy concern in the past decade (Lucas and Chevillard 2018) (Figure 5.4). The average waiting time for an appointment was 44 days for gynecologists, 50 days for cardiologists, and 80 days for ophthalmologists (Millien et al. 2018). While 95% of the French population live a 15-minute drive from a GP (Coldefy et al. 2011) and 50% of GP appointments are obtained within 48 hours, there are wide variations across regions.

At the same time, most patients get an appointment within a week for an urgent problem, but rather wait, sometimes up to 3 to 4 months for regular

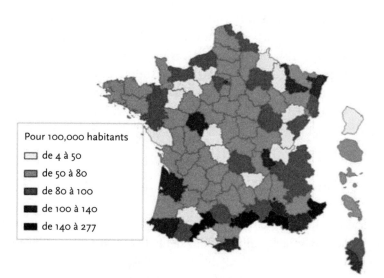

Figure 5.4 Density of specialists in France in 2016.

Source: "La médecine libérale de spécialité: contenir la dynamique des dépenses, améliorer l'accès aux soins" (Cour des comptes 2017).

check-ups or for a first visit to see a specialist, especially in rural territories (Millien et al. 2018). Also, in areas where there is a shortage of providers, access to specialists who do not extra-bill patients can be difficult (Cour des comptes 2017). The fact that patients are not systematically asked for a referral from a GP to visit a specialist (especially for gynecologists, ophthalmologists, and stomatologists) makes it difficult to orient patients' access to services as a function of their need (Figure 5.5). The gatekeeping reform, introduced in 2004, financially punishes patients (with lower reimbursement rates) when they do have a regular GP as a gatekeeper. However, this reform did not have a significant impact on improving care pathways (Naiditch and Dourgnon 2009; Bras 2020), since primary care physicians and specialists, mostly paid on a FFS basis and in competition for patients, have little incentive to invest in collaboration and care coordination.

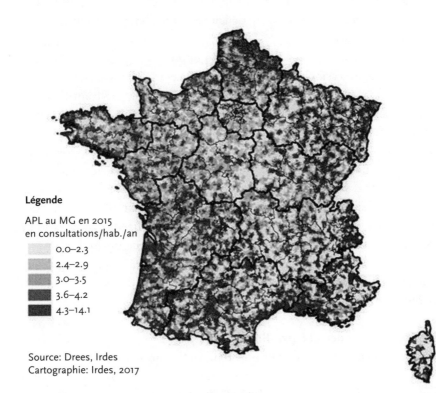

Légende

APL au MG en 2015
en consultations/hab./an

- 0.0–2.3
- 2.4–2.9
- 3.0–3.5
- 3.6–4.2
- 4.3–14.1

Source: Drees, Irdes
Cartographie: Irdes, 2017

Figure 5.5 Density of GPs in France in 2015.

Sources: "Le système de santé: enjeux et défis." Ouvrage collectif du Collège des Economistes de la santé (Chevillard et al. 2021).

Tackling Inequities in Access to Care

Incentives for Improving Geographical Access

Following the national ranking exams, medical students choose a specialty and a region in which they will do their internship. Since 2005, successive governments have been subsidizing medical students to choose certain underserved areas. Financial aid in the form of housing aid, study grants, and other related assistance have been offered to students who choose to study in these areas. Financial aid also targets health workers already in practice to encourage them to move in underserved areas. Doctors and nurses who settle in deficit areas benefit from subsidies from local authorities (installation bonuses, loan of premises, income guarantees). The government also encourages group practices in primary care by paying €50,000 over 2 years to GPs who settle, for at least 3 years, in health centers in underserved areas. Moreover, doctors who practice in deficit areas are exempted from some social and fiscal charges.

Nevertheless, these measures aiming to improve geographic distribution of healthcare professionals had only limited success. The measures targeting medical students are based on the assumption that physicians trained in a region will choose to exercise in that region. However, quality of life, expected income, and working conditions are also major factors that determine physicians' choice. Financial incentives are considered to be too low compared to the financial benefits expected from settling in a richer region. It is also shown that young doctors care more about the family life and working conditions than potential income when deciding their place of practice (Barriball and al. 2015; Munck et al. 2015). Group practice appears to be more attractive for young generalists than solo practice in rural or underserved areas (Chevillard and Mousquès 2020). Hence, encouraging group practice in primary care has been a lever for increasing the density of GPs in underserved areas.

Reducing the Burden of Extra-Billing

The question of extra-billing or how to limit the amount has been a public concern for several decades, even though the prices were poorly monitored by the public authorities. In 2007, the General Inspectorate of Social Affairs revealed that the average amount of extra-billing between 1995 and 2004 increased three times faster than average incomes in France (Igas 2007). Also, despite the restrictions on access to sector 2 for GPs,

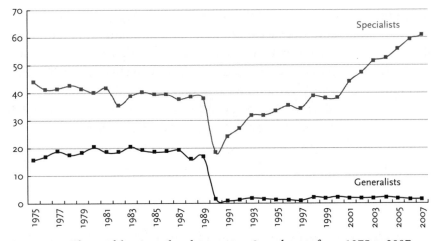

Figure 5.6 Share of doctors who chose sector 2, each year from 1975 to 2007.
Source: Les comptes de la santé 2010" (DREES 2011).

the proportion of specialists who settle in sector 2 each year is increasing (Figure 5.6).

The public health code requires physicians to inform their patients of all costs related to their visit, displaying prices inside their medical practices. Hence, the cost of a visit to a sector 2 physician is not known to patients before the appointment. There is also no platform allowing comparison of prices of providers. In 2012, SHI created an observatory of tariffs to follow up more closely the extra-fees charged by physicians. Moreover, since 2013, voluntary contracts (called contracts with Mastered tariffs[5]) have been introduced to encourage sector 2 physicians to freeze their fees and not charge more than the average price observed during the last 3 years. They are also asked to perform a share of their services at regulated SHI-tariff levels. In return, they receive a partial payment of social security contributions, usually reserved for sector 1 doctors (up to € 4,300 per year on average). In 2018, about 50% of doctors had signed this contract.

Despite all these attempts to regulate extra-billing, the financial burden of extra-billing for patients is still an issue, with a high concentration of extra-billing costs among the sickest and low-income individuals (Franc and Pierre 2016b; Perronnin 2016). In some regions and areas, patients have no other choice than to pay extra fees to see a specialist. While the implementation of new contracts in 2016 allowed a slight reduction of the average amount of extra-billing (about 3%), sector 2 physicians still have great latitude in fixing their prices. Moreover, the small reduction in fees should be put against the amount SHI devotes to subsidize social security contributions for these doctors, who can even benefit from a windfall effect: signing up to the contract to reduce social charges even if they did not intend to increase their fees (Bras 2015). Ultimately, extra-billing introduces strong disparities in remuneration between doctors that are not justified by their level of qualification or quality of care provided. They allow sector 2 doctors to reduce their level of activity compared to sector 1 doctors or simply to compensate for lower productivity. Hence, they contribute to accentuating the problems of territorial access to care.

Concerns for Efficiency and Quality of Care Delivery

Growing Health Expenditure

With about 11% of gross domestic product (GDP) dedicated to health, the rising cost of healthcare has been a major concern in France in the past decades. Traditionally, most of the cost containment efforts have concentrated on regulating prices of healthcare. While France had visible success in controlling prices of healthcare services and pharmaceuticals, low prices seem to have a limited impact on health expenditure growth. Healthcare providers, mostly paid by FFS or activity volumes, tend to compensate for reduced revenues by increasing the volume of services they provide. The system encourages more hospital utilization, medical tests and medications with high risk of duplication of services, and inefficient care processes. Ambulatory physicians and other healthcare providers, paid by FFS, have little interest or incentive to control the volume and the cost of their prescriptions or to invest in prevention, health promotion, and care coordination. In the hospital sector, while the introduction of ABP globally improved hospital productivity in both public and private hospitals, it has also created new problems for the quality and appropriateness of hospital care. Since 2005, both the number of beds per capita and the average length of stay fell significantly with an increase in ambulatory surgeries,[6] but avoidable hospital admissions, readmissions, and emergency visits also increased visibly over this period, especially for older people (Bricard et al. 2020).

The macro-level budgetary management of healthcare specific to France has exacerbated the some of the issues of quality and allocative efficiency in the system. Since 2010, the specification of an overall expenditure target for healthcare, known as the National Objective for Health Insurance Spending

(Objectif National de Dépenses de l'Assurance Maladie, ONDAM), has been the key strategy to contain health spending in France. There are different budget targets for ambulatory, hospital, and social care sectors. To control hospital expenditures, national-level expenditure targets for acute care (with separate targets for the public and private sectors) are set by the Parliament each year. If the actual growth in total hospital volume exceeds the target, the prices go down the following year. But the growth of activity is monitored only at an aggregate level (separately for the public and private sectors), and prices have been adjusted downward regularly since 2006 as the hospital volumes have been increasing faster than the targets set. This mechanism meant that the prices have become (progressively) unrelated to hospitals' costs (and quality) and created a financially unstable and opaque environment, which fostered frustration and resentment, especially in public hospitals (Or 2014). Contrary to private hospitals, public facilities have little flexibility in their management and cannot specialize in a few profitable services as they wish. In the absence of clear price and quality signals, public hospitals have been concerned with balancing their accounts by increasing their volume of activity. Moreover, there has been a gradual underinvestment in public hospital infrastructure since the hospital prices were to cover partly the cost of investment.

Regulating Volume Rather than Quality

Against a rapidly rising volume of activity in the hospital sector, several measures were introduced to ensure quality and appropriateness of care. One major regulatory tool has been to link authorizations to minimum activity thresholds. There are volume norms for cardiac surgery, obstetrics services, cancer care, and so on. Furthermore, at the regional level, hospital volumes are monitored to identify hospitals that have high levels of activity/growth within the region. A list of 32 interventions (including cholecystectomy, cataract surgery, hysterectomy, prostatectomy, etc.) are defined as priority based on three criteria: strong growth rate in the past 3 years, high variations between/within regions, and/or potentially harmful consequences for patients. Since 2014, for a number of high-volume/fast-growing surgeries (including knee prosthesis and cataract surgery), the Ministry of Health sets a national rate of activity growth. If a hospital's caseload (for a given surgery) grows faster than the threshold set, the corresponding tariff goes down by 20%. There is not enough information on the impact of this politic on the hospitals, but there is an increasing consensus now for concentrating on "appropriateness of care" and reducing interventions considered as "low-value" care.

Nevertheless, France has been backward in monitoring and reporting publicly the quality of care providers. While important progress has been made for collecting data on quality, in particular security, of care in hospitals, most indicators are focused on process. Major indicators, such as 30-day re-admission rates, mortality, and adverse events, are not monitored regularly across providers or across regions/territories. More recently, data on patient experience in hospitals were collected, but benchmarking of efficiency and care quality is discouraged even when data are available. In primary and long-term care sectors, there is almost no information available to the public on patient experience and quality of care of different providers. This reduces France's capacity to identify problem areas as well as good practices to push forward policies for improving care quality and efficiency.

Problems with Care Coordination

The lack of coordination between ambulatory, hospital, and social care has been recognized as a major drawback in terms of both cost-control and quality of care (Larcher 2007). The fact that most providers work as inde-pendent providers—and with little collaboration between hospital, primary, and social care/services—means that patient care is fragmented, and patients need to navigate a complicated system. Moreover, uncoordinated care and the high degree of independence and choice both for providers and patients have been identified as key drivers of healthcare cost. Increasingly, health-care providers are asked to account for the cost and quality of services they provide.

It is largely recognized that organizational changes that contribute to better service delivery, such as formal collaboration between different health professionals, are less likely to occur in solo practice. Therefore, the latest reforms encourage group practice in primary care settings and test alterna-tive payment models for improving care provision and efficiency. Finding an effective way of funding group practice that will give more emphasis on prevention and care coordination in primary care has been a strong policy objective.

Perspectives for Improving the Equity and Efficiency of the French Public/Private Model

The recent sanitary crisis provoked by Covid-19 has highlighted some of the major structural weaknesses of the French public/private model and accelerated ongoing reforms tackling long-standing issues. The segmented approach to the management and funding of primary, secondary, and long-term care is increasingly criticized. It is also recognized that the division between healthcare providers in different sectors are reinforced by the payment models based on volumes (FFS or ABP) at the local level. Moreover, the Covid-19 crisis revealed that the cost-sharing imposed by the SHI for all services, including hospitalizations without surgery, is problematic for fully protecting the population against financial risk associated with serious conditions.

Better Funding and Payment of Care Providers

In order to improve the efficiency and quality of healthcare provision, it is necessary to have a holistic approach to care provision and funding across different settings. While the implementation of macro-level ONDAM targets has been quite successful in containing overall expenditure in the past decade, this strict budgetary process has accentuated a segmented approach to healthcare. The division of budgets between providers ignores the fact that healthcare provided in one sector has consequences on the others: The care provision in the community determines the need for hospital care, home care services impact the need for long-term care facilities, and so on. This reinforces the division of healthcare supply at the local level and reduces the capacity to improve the coordination of service delivery across sectors in order to strengthen the resilience of the health system to effectively serve an aging population with chronic diseases.

In 2019, a new financing law with a dedicated budget (Article 51 of the 2018 Social Security Financing bill) was introduced to encourage new care models based on new funding modes. It waives regulatory barriers for testing innovations in care organization and payment, encouraging bottom-up proposals. All health professionals and healthcare organizations were given the possibility of experimenting new healthcare models, including alternative funding models, provided that pilots aimed to improve the quality of health and social care services and patient experience. This new bottom-up approach aims to remove financial barriers to innovation in order to promote efficiency, prevention, and care coordination. During the first wave of the pandemic, some of the initiatives born under this law were reactive and developed quick solutions locally to ensure continuity of care for their patients. The Ministry of Health has announced that this law will support the sustainability of innovations born during the Covid-19 crisis.

Less Competition and More Collaboration in Care Delivery

The fact that healthcare professionals are paid by FFS and patients are free to choose their care providers from a wide range of options, without almost no restriction, creates a highly competitive environment for care providers in France. Health professionals aiming to retain a certain income level need to maintain a certain level of activity (procedures, visits, etc.). This in turn creates an unfavorable environment for collaboration and task shifting since "sharing patients" and "delegating tasks" may present a financial risk. In the hospital sector, the competitive environment created by the ABP, while it contributed to some efficiency gains in hospitals, also raised questions on care quality and allocative efficiency of the system. The recent sanitary crisis highlighted the weaknesses of fragmented management of public health, primary, secondary, and social care (Ferrand 2020; Or and Gandré 2021) and revealed the need to cultivate a health prevention and promotion culture involving all healthcare providers.

Several recent policies have aimed at increasing local coordination between healthcare providers. These include the creation of local hospital groups (*Groupement hospitalier de territoire*) and the development of regional/local care networks (*Communautés professionnelles territoriales de santé*) incorporating hospital and primary care physicians, nurses, and other professionals (including social workers, administrative staff, etc.). In addition to the experiment with new payment models, including bundled payments, these reforms aim to improve the continuum of care throughout the entire patient care pathway and to reduce competition between local care providers. The local hospital groups encourage reorganization of hospital services around the local population, allowing hospitals to share their resources and activity by specializing on certain services. Currently, these groupings concern only public hospitals, but they are supposed to include private hospitals also in near future.

However, to support collaboration between care providers while preserving the benefits of a yardstick competition, France needs to refine and diffuse indicators for benchmarking the quality of care across settings, in particular to monitor patient experience in and out of hospitals, including readmissions, complication rates, inappropriate prescriptions, and other health-related items (for specific patient groups) across local areas and providers. There is also a need improve public information on prices of different care providers. While there has been a visible improvement in this area with the creation of observatories of prices, it is still very difficult for patients to compare prices of care providers in ambulatory and hospital settings.

Altering the Role of Private Insurance

The general policy of promoting private CHI as a means to achieve public system goals of equity of access and cost containment for avoiding more structural reforms may not be sustainable. The specific setup of public/private health insurance in France has perverse consequences for both patients and public and private insurers. On the one hand, the SHI operates in a market where incentives for pursuing public policy goals and reducing moral hazard can be counterbalanced by the private CHI, to which access depends on income rather than needs (Franc and Pierre 2016a). On the other hand, private insurers operate in a highly regulated market, with constraints that appear contradictory to deal with adverse selection issues. Today, there is a consensus in the public debate to call for a structural reform reorganizing the roles of public and private insurance in healthcare financing, but without any consensus concerning the model (HCAAM 2021; Cour des Comptes 2016; Askenazy et al. 2013). While many experts suggest separating public and private insurance benefit baskets and to provide higher SHI reimbursement for essential services, there is no agreement on the types of care that should be excluded from the public basket, the extent of SHI reimbursement, and the level of regulation in the CHI market.

Conclusion

The French healthcare system is founded on the main principles of solidarity, plurality, and liberalism. Equal access to quality healthcare is one of the major objectives of the system routed in public health law. The health status of the population ranks among the best in the world, French patients have a large choice of public and private providers, without the chronic waiting time problems observed in other OECD countries, and have generally high satisfaction rates. Nevertheless, the system is expensive, complex for users, fragmented in its organization, and characterized by many inequalities in access to care. The unsustainable growth of health spending has also been a long-standing concern.

Notwithstanding the high share of public funding of health expenditure, increasing reliance on private insurance to cover some of the costs of healthcare, raises concerns for solidarity, equity in access to care, and efficiency of the system. A mixture of regulatory measures and financial incentives are used to reduce the difficulties that the sickest and the poorest would otherwise face in a competitive health insurance market, but the cost and efficiency of this complex system is increasingly questioned. At the same time, the French system promotes plurality and choice for patients. The health insurance model operates with self-employed healthcare professionals and care facilities paid mainly based on volume. While this allows a variety of care options and choice for patients, it also creates problems of care coordination, access to care, and induced demand. The high level of freedom for care providers (in deciding where to practice) and the dominant FFS payment and extra-billing by most specialists result in persisting inequalities in access between socioeconomic groups and geographical regions. In the hospital sector, where a high number of public and private hospitals operate in the same market, the highly competitive environment created by the ABP not only allowed increasing productivity but also exacerbated the issues of care quality and appropriateness. In order to improve its sustainability while pursuing equity goals, the French system needs to ensure that care providers are working together with the same quality and efficiency objectives in a collaborative approach.

Several initiatives are currently being deployed to test and encourage new payment models and for improving organization of healthcare delivery. The Covid-19 pandemic in 2020 accelerated some of these initiatives by shifting the traditional divide between the public and private sectors and the traditional boundaries between medical professions. In the early days of the pandemic, while public hospitals were under stress, private clinics in the same region were underutilized and waiting for patients. In some regions, initially, instead of mobilizing local capacities, patients were transferred by medical trains and helicopters to public hospitals in less-affected regions, including in neighboring countries. Regional health authorities have gradually included private capacity in their planning and provided temporary authorizations for setting up intensive care units in private hospitals. Public/private collaborations have become more fluid in the second wave since the networks of public and private physicians, developed during the first wave, were mobilized quickly.

Overall, the French system has been torn between the pressures to curb the growth in health expenditure and to ensure equity of access and quality of care while maintaining a unique public/private mix that allows plurality and choice. The recent measures put in place suggest that there are opportunities for improvement that should be monitored over time, even if changing the public/private funding model risks becoming more complicated.

Acknowledgment

We are grateful to our colleagues Guillaume Chevillard, Marie-Caroline Clément, Véronique Lucas, Marc Perronnin, and Sylvain Pichetti for their guidance and helpful comments in preparing this chapter. All errors and omissions remain our responsibility alone.

Notes

1. This became the *Protection Universelle Maladie* (PUMA) in 2016.
2. The reimbursement level by SHI is determined by the effectiveness of a given drug and the gravity of the disease treated: 100% for rare, highly effective, or expensive drugs (e.g., for cancer); 65%, 35%, or 15% for diminishing therapeutic value, respectively. Drugs evaluated as ineffective are not reimbursed by the SHI.
3. Mutuelles are regulated by the *code de mutualité*, nonprofit provident institutions by the social security code, and private insurance companies by the commercial insurance code.
4. The number of people eligible for these schemes is estimated to be higher: About 30% of the individuals who are eligible to CMU-C and 60% of those eligible for the ACS are not exercising their rights.
5. Two contracts were introduced: CAS (*Contrat d'Accès aux Soins*) in 2013 and OPTAM (*OPtion TArifaire Maitrisée*) in 2016.
6. Between 2013 and 2018, the number of discharges increased by 8%, while the number of days in the hospital declined by 1% (DREES 2021).

References

Askenazy, Philippe, Brigitte Dormont, Pierre-Yves Geoffard, and Valérie Paris. 2013. "Pour un système de santé plus efficace. Les notes du Conseil d'Analyse." *Economique*, 8(8): 1–12.

Barlet, Muriel, Mathilde Gaini, Lucie Gonzalez, and Renaud Legal. 2020. *La complémentaire santé: Acteurs, bénéficiaires, garanties—Édition 2019*. Panoramas de la DREES.

Barriball, L., J. Bremner, J. Buchan, I. Craveiro, M. Dieleman, O. Dix, G. Dussault, C. Jansen, M. Kroezen, A.M. Rafferty, and W. Sermeus. 2015. *Recruitment and Retention of the Health Workforce in Europe*. Brussels: European Commission.

Bras, Pierre-Louis. 2015. "La liberté des tarifs médicaux: La victoire des médecins spécialistes." *Les Tribunes de la santé*, 3(48): 73–92.

Bras, Pierre-Louis. 2020. "La rémunération des médecins à la performance: Efficacité clinique ou efficacité symbolique?" *Les tribunes de la santé*. 2(64): 61–77.

Bricard, Damien, Zeynep Or, and Anne Penneau. 2020. "Évaluation d'impact de l'expérimentation Parcours santé des aînés (Paerpa)." Final Report. 575, 2020/11. IRDES.

Buchmueller, Thomas, Agnès Couffinhal, Michel Grignon, and Marc Perronnin. 2004. "Access to Physician Services: Does Supplemental Insurance Matter? Evidence from France. *Health Economics* 13(7): 669–687.

Chevillard, Guillaume, Véronique Lucas-Gabrielli, and Julien Mousquès. 2018. "Déserts médicaux en France: État des lieux et perspectives de recherches." *L'Espace géographique* 4(47): 362–380.

Chevillard, Guillaume, Véronique Lucas-Gabrielli, and Julien Mousquès. 2021. "Comment améliorer l'accès aux soins primaires selon les spécificités des territoires?" In *Le système de santé français aujourd'hui: enjeux et défis. Ouvrage collectif du Collège des Economistes de la santé (CES)*. Coordonné par Thomas Barnay, Anne-Laure Samson, and Bruno Ventelou. Paris: Editions Eska, chapitre 11, 2021/07.

Chevillard, Guillaume, and Julien Mousquès. 2020. "Les maisons de santé attirent-elles les jeunes médecins généralistes dans les zones sous-dotées en offre de soins?" n°247. In *Question d'Economie de la Santé*. IRDES.

Coldefy, Magali, Laure Com-Ruelle, Véronique Lucas-Gabrielli, and Lionel Marcoux. 2011. *Les distances d'accès aux soins en France métropolitaine au 1er janvier 2007*. Rapport Irdes n°550. IRDES.

Commission des Comptes de la Sécurité sociale. 2020. *Les comptes de la Sécurité sociale: Résultats 2019 et prévision 2020*. Rapport des comptes de la Sécurité Sociale.

Cour des comptes. 2009. "Les centres d'examen de santé. Rapport de la Cour des comptes." In *Rapport de la sécurité sociale de 2009*.

Cour des comptes. 2016. *La participation des assurés au financement de leurs dépenses de santé: une charge croissante, une protection maladie à redéfinir*. Rapport de la cour des comptes.

Cour des comptes. 2017. "La médecine libérale de spécialité: Contenir la dynamique des dépenses, améliorer l'accès aux soins." In *La sécurité sociale: Rapport sur l'application des lois de financement de la sécurité sociale* (Chapitre 5).

Desprès, Caroline Guillaume, Stéphanie Couralet, and Pierre-Emmanuel. 2009. *Le refus de soins à l'égard des bénéficiaires de la Couverture maladie universelle complémentaire à Paris*. Fonds de financement de la protection complémentaire de la couverture universelle du risque maladie, La documentation française, collection des rapports publics.

Devaux, Marion. 2015. "Income-Related Inequalities and Inequities in Health Care Services Utilisation in 18 Selected OECD Countries." *European Journal of Health Economics* 16(1): 21–33. doi:10.1007/s10198-013-0546-4

Direction Générale de l'Offre de Soins (DGOS). 2018. *Les chiffres clés de l'offre de soins.* 2018 ed. Ministère des solidarités et de la santé.

Direction de la Recherche, des Études, de l'Évaluation et des Statistiques (DREES). 2020. "Les dépenses de santé en 2019, résultat des comptes de la santé." https://drees.solidari tes-sante.gouv.fr/publications-documents-de-reference/panoramas-de-la-drees/les-depenses-de-sante-en-2019-resultats

Direction de la Recherche, des Études, de l'Évaluation et des Statistiques (DREES). 2021. *Panorama des établissements de santé.* 2020 ed.

Ferrand, Richard. 2020. *Rapport d'information sur l'impact, la gestion et les conséquences dans toutes ses dimensions de l'épidémie de Coronavirus-Covid-19.* National Assembly. N°3053.

Flood, Colleen, and Thomas Bryan. 2020. *Is Two-Tier Health Care the Future?* Ottawa, Canada: Press of Ottawa. https://press.uottawa.ca/is-two-tier-health-care-the-fut ure.html

Franc, Carine, and Aurélie Pierre. 2015. "Compulsory Private Complementary Health Insurance Offered by Employers in France: Implications and Current Debate." *Health Policy* 119(2): 111–116.

Franc, Carine, and Aurélie Pierre. 2016a. "Conséquences de l'assurance publique et complémentaire sur la redistribution et la concentration des restes à charge: Une étude de cas." *Economie et Statistique* 475–476, 31–49.

Franc, Carine, and Aurélie Pierre. 2016b. *Restes à charge élevés: Profils d'assurés et persistance dans le temps.* Questions d'économie de la santé n°217. IRDES.

France Assos Santé. 2015. "Dépassements d'honoraires: Le 'match' public-privé." France Assos Santé. https://www.france-assos-sante.org/2015/01/16/depassements-dhonorai res-le-match-public-prive/

Geoffard, Pierre-Yves. 2006. *L'AMO ne suffit plus à garantir un accès aux soins sans barrière financière.* Regards 2016/1 (N° 49). École nationale supérieure de Sécurité sociale.

Geoffard, Pierre-Yves, and Grégoire de Lagasnerie. 2012. "Réformer le système de remboursement pour les soins de ville, une analyse par microsimulation." *Economie et statistique* 455–456: 89–113.

Grignon, Michel, Marc Perronnin, and John N. Lavis. 2008. "Does Free Complementary Health Insurance Help the Poor to Access Health Care? Evidence from France. *Health Economics* 17(2): 203–219.

Hassenteufel, Patrick. 2008. "Syndicalisme et médecine libérale: le poids de l'histoire." *Les Tribunes de la santé* 18(1): 21–28.

Haut Conseil pour l'Avenir de l'Assurance Maladie (HCAAM). 2021. *La régulation du système de santé.* Rapport du Haut Conseil pour l'Avenir de l'Assurance Maladie.

Inspection Générale des Affaires Sociales (IGAS). 2007. *Les dépassements d'honoraires médicaux.* Rapport de l'Inspection Générale des Affaires Sociales.

Jusot, Florence, Clémence Perraudin, and Jérôme Wittwer. 2012. "L'accessibilité financière à la complémentaire santé en France: Les résultats de l'enquête Budget de Famille 2006." *Economie et Statistique* 450: 29–46.

Jusot, Florence, Renaud Legal, Alexis Louvel, Catherine Pollak, and Amir Shmueli. 2016. "A quoi tient la solidarité de l'assurance maladie entre les hauts revenus et les plus modestes en France?" *Revue française d'économie* 31(4): 15–62.

Kambia-Chopin, Bidénam, Marc Perronnin, Aurélie Pierre, and Thierry Rochereau. 2008. "Les contrats complémentaires individuels: Quel poids dans le budget des ménages?" In: *Enquête sur la Santé et la Protection Sociale 2006.*

Larcher, Gérard. 2007. *Les missions de l'hôpital.* Inventory Prepared by the Consultative Commission on Hospital Missions.

Millien, Christelle, Hélène Chaput, and Marie Cavillon. 2018. La moitié des rendez-vous sont obtenus en 2 jours chez le généraliste, en 52 jours chez l'ophtalmologiste. Etudes et Résultats n°1085. DREES.

Ministère des solidarités et de la santé. 2017. "La stratégie nationale de santé 2018–2022." Les dossiers du Ministère des solidarités et de la santé. https://solidarites-sante.gouv.fr/IMG/pdf/dossier_sns_2017_vdef.pdf

Ministère des solidarités et de la santé. 2022. "Ma santé 2022: Un engagement collectif." Les dossiers du Ministère des solidarités et de la santé. https://solidarites-sante.gouv.fr/systeme-de-sante-et-medico-social/masante2022/

Munck, Stéphane, Sophie Massin, Philippe Hofliger, and David Darmon. 2015. "Déterminants du projet d'installation en ambulatoire des internes de médecine générale." *Santé Publique* 27: 49–58. https://doi.org/10.3917/spub.151.0049

Naiditch, Michel, and Paul Dourgnon. 2009. *The Preferred Doctor Scheme: A Political Reading of a French Experiment of Gate-keeping.* IRDES Working Papers, no. 22, 2009/03.

Organization for Economic Cooperation and Development (OECD). 2019. "OECD Health Statistics, Health Expenditure and Financing." https://stats.oecd.org/

Organization for Economic Cooperation and Development countries (OECD). 2020. *Health at a Glance: Europe 2020. State of Health in the EU Cycle.* Paris: OECD.

Or, Zeynep. 2014. "Implementation of DRG Payment in France: Issues and Recent Developments." *Health Policy* 117(2): 146–150.

Or, Zeynep, and Coralie Gandré. 2021. *Sustainability and Resilience in the French Health System.* London: LSE.

Paris, Valérie, and Dominique Polton. 2016. *L'articulation entre assurance maladie obligatoire et complémentaire, une spécificité française?* Regards 2016/1 (N° 49). École nationale supérieure de Sécurité sociale.

Perronnin, Marc. 2016. *Out-of-Pocket Spending for Ambulatory and Hospital Care after Reimbursement by the French Public Health Insurance: Unequally Distributed Financial Burden.* Questions d'Economie de la santé n°218. Publications Irdes.

Perronnin, Marc, and Alexis Louvel. 2018. *La complémentaire santé en 2014: 5% de non-couverts et 12% parmi les 20% les plus pauvres.* Questions d'Economie de la santé n°229. Publications Irdes.

6

Sweden's Public/Private Sector Mix in the Financing and Delivery of Healthcare Services

How It Relates to Health Equity and the Quality of Healthcare Services

Anna Häger Glenngård

Development of the Current Healthcare System

The present structure of the Swedish healthcare system reflects a long history of public funding and ownership together with a strong tradition of local self-government (Anell, Glenngård, and Merkur 2012). Swedish healthcare rests on a strong tradition of quality healthcare for all. The 2017 Health and Medical Services Act, which is the most important law governing Swedish healthcare, emphasizes not only equal access to services on the basis of need but also a vision of equal health for all. Health and medical services are mainly tax financed, traditionally publicly provided, and primary care is regarded as the first point of entry to healthcare services. Healthcare expenditures as a proportion of gross domestic product amounted to 10.9%%in 2019 (Statistics Sweden 2021).

A relatively large proportion of the resources available for medical services has traditionally been allocated to the provision of care and treatment at the hospital level, and a relatively small share has been allocated to primary care. However, there has been a continuous decrease in the number of hospital beds since the 1970s. Structural changes continued in the 1990s, with a shift from hospital inpatient care toward outpatient care and primary care and, when the municipalities took over the responsibility, long-term care (Anell et al. 2012). National policies and reforms during the past

Anna Häger Glenngård, *Sweden's Public/Private Sector Mix in the Financing and Delivery of Healthcare Services* In: *The Public/Private Sector Mix in Healthcare Delivery*. Edited by: Howard A. Palley, Oxford University Press. © Oxford University Press 2023. DOI: 10.1093/oso/9780197571101.003.0006 decades have also focused on moving patients out of hospitals toward primary and municipality-based care in the pursuit of patient-focused care. Such reforms have transferred responsibilities from hospitals to primary care and from regions to municipalities in an effort to move care "closer to patients" (Lövtrup 2017; SOU [Statens offentliga utredningar] 2019, 29). Despite the structural changes during the past decades, primary care only accounted for approximately one-fifth of the total healthcare expenditures in 2019 (Swedish Association for Local Authorities and Regions [SALAR] 2021). Moreover, there are relatively few doctors in primary care compared to specialized care.

Similar to other Nordic countries, major changes and market-like structures have been implemented in the Swedish healthcare system since the 1980s. The traditional objective of distributive justice has been accompanied by objectives related to cost control, efficiency, value, and quality. Quality here refers to both patients' perceptions about quality and clinical quality (e.g., the provision of care according to evidence-based clinical guidelines). The Swedish development toward waiting list guarantees, patient rights to choose providers, and other market-oriented reforms can be viewed as a response to such objectives. Similar reforms, under the umbrella of New Public Management (NPM), are visible across publicly funded healthcare systems also in several other northern European countries (Martinussen and Magnussen 2009; Cutler 2002).

Organization and Financing of the Health System

Three Levels of Government

The Swedish healthcare system is highly decentralized. The responsibility for organizing and financing healthcare rests with the 21 regions and 290 municipalities. The 2017 Swedish Health and Medical Services Act (HSL 2017:30) is designed to give the local authorities considerable freedom in organizing healthcare services. Reforms are often introduced by individual regions and municipalities, leading to regional and local variation, although reforms in one area are often replicated in other areas. The central government, through the Ministry of Health and Social Affairs, is responsible for overall healthcare policy and legislation, working together with a number of government agencies. There are eight government agencies directly involved in the area of health, medical care, and public health:

National Board of Health and Welfare
Swedish Health Agency
Health and Social Care Inspectorate
Swedish Agency for Health and Care Services Analysis
Public Health Agency
Swedish Agency for Health Technology Assessment and Assessment of
    Social Services
Dental and the Pharmaceutical Benefits Agency
Medical Products Agency

The 21 regions have the overall responsibility for financing and provision of healthcare services in hospitals and primary care centers (PCCs). There are about 70 hospitals at the region level. Highly specialized care, often requiring the most advanced technical equipment, is concentrated at seven university hospitals to ensure high quality and greater efficiency and to create opportunities for development and research. Regions are grouped into six medical care regions to facilitate cooperation regarding tertiary medical care. Primary care forms the foundation of the healthcare system, and there are about 1,200 PCCs in the country. Team-based primary care is practiced, with a mix of different staff categories at each PCC (e.g., general practitioners [GPs], registered nurses, physiotherapists, and psychologists). Regions also have the responsibility to provide care by GPs in municipal healthcare in cooperation with staff in the municipalities. The 290 municipalities have the responsibility to meet the needs of older people and people with functional impairments in special and ordinary housing. Registered nurses, assistant nurses, occupational therapists, and physiotherapists are the most common staff categories involved in healthcare in the municipalities. There is no hierarchical relation between municipalities and regions. They all have their own self-governing local authorities with responsibility for different activities. Healthcare constitutes the most important responsibility for the regions, while the municipalities are responsible for several different tasks, such as social services, elderly care, childcare, primary and secondary school and sewage.

The local and regional authorities are guided in their decisions by local priorities as well as national regulation and guidelines. Each region and municipality has an elected assembly that makes decisions on municipal and regional matters. General elections at the regional and local levels, as well as the national level, are held every 4 years. In the elections, political parties are elected to represent the citizens in the three political assemblies (i.e., the municipal and regional assembly and the national parliament). Nationally, the municipalities and regions are represented by SALAR. SALAR strives to promote and strengthen local self-government and provide local authorities with expert assistance. It compiles and disseminates information about such things as quality and waiting times in both primary care and specialized care at hospitals. SALAR also works as the employers' central association for negotiating terms of employment and local wage bargaining for staff employed by the regions and municipalities. All categories of healthcare staff are normally salaried employees (Anell et al. 2012).

Healthcare Is Primarily Publicly Funded

Healthcare is primarily tax funded. In 2019, about 85 % of total healthcare expenditures was publicly financed, i.e., by the regions (58%), municipalities (25%), and the central government (2%). Regions and municipalities levy proportional income taxes on their populations to finance their activities. Healthcare expenditures constituted approximately 85% of the regions' total expenditures and almost 20% of the municipalities' total expenditures in 2019 (SALAR 2021; Statistics Sweden 2021). The regions and municipalities also receive subsidies and national government grants, financed by national indirect and income taxes. General government grants are designed to redistribute resources among municipalities and regions based on need. Targeted government grants finance specific initiatives, such as reducing waiting times and improving the care and care coordination for elderly with multiple diseases.

The role of private health insurance is marginal in Sweden. In 2019, private health insurance, in the form of supplementary coverage, accounted for less than 1% of total health expenditures (Statistics Sweden 2021). It is mainly purchased by employers and primarily used to ensure quick access to an ambulatory care specialist and to avoid waiting lists for elective treatment. Healthcare insurers are for profit. In 2017, there were 633,000 individuals with private insurance, representing roughly 13% of all employed individuals ages 16 to 64 years (Swedish Insurance Federation 2018).

Private Spending Is Mainly Out of Pocket

Copayments from patients also help finance healthcare services. In 2019, private spending amounted to 15% of total healthcare expenditures. Almost all private spending is out of pocket (14% of total healthcare expenditures in 2019) (Statistics Sweden 2021). Outpatient medicines, dental care, and medical products (corrective lenses, hearing aids, wheelchairs, etc.) account for the largest share of out-of-pocket payments, which is related to the absence of caps on user charges in these areas (Glenngård and Borg 2019). While there are caps on user-charges for healthcare services and prescribed pharmaceuticals, there is no cap on user charges for dental care or over-the-counter medicines.

The regions set copayment rates for care provided in PCCs and hospitals, which leads to some variation across the country. The caps for primary care and outpatient visits at hospitals (SEK [Swedish krona] 1,150 in 2021) is set at the national level. People under 20 years are exempt from user charges in primary and hospital care throughout the country. Moreover, certain preventive services targeted at high-risk groups (e.g., involving maternity care, vaccination programs, and screening program) are exempt from copayments.

Pharmaceutical and dental benefits are determined at the national government by the Dental and Pharmaceutical Benefits Agency. For outpatient prescribed medicines and outpatient medical devices, approved for national reimbursement, there is a separate cap (SEK 2,350 in 2021). Individuals pay the full cost for noncovered medicines and medical devices, including over-the-counter medicines. Contraceptives are free of charge for people under 20 years. People under 23 years have free access to all covered dental care. There are two types of subsidies for dental care for people aged 23 years and above. There is a fixed annual subsidy to help cover costs for preventive dental care, such as annual dental check-ups. For other dental services within a 12-month period, a high-cost protection scheme means that people pay the full cost of services up to SEK 3,000 (USD 360), and thereafter they are entitled to an increasing level of state subsidy, but there is no absolute cap on user charges for dental care.

Public/Private Mix of Services

While the vast majority of all healthcare is publicly funded in Sweden, there is a mix of publicly and privately owned and operated health facilities. All seven university hospitals are publicly owned and operated. Of the approximately 70 hospitals at the regional level, only 6 are private, 3 for profit and 3 not for profit (Anell et al. 2012). In 2019, of the regions' expenditures for specialized (psychiatric and somatic) care, 8% was allocated to private providers (SALAR 2021). Whereas hospitals are predominantly publicly owned and operated, Swedish primary care is a rather unique case in the European context, with a mix of public and private PCCs. Of the about 1,200 PCCs in the country, more than 40% are privately owned, predominantly for profit. In 2019, of the regions' expenditures for primary care, 40% was allocated to private providers (SALAR 2021). In this chapter, the example of primary care is used to illustrate issues of health equity and quality of care related to the public/private mix regarding services.

The Development of Swedish Primary Care

Swedish primary care has traditionally been provided in fairly large and predominantly publicly owned PCCs with a mix of staff categories. PCCs have been responsible for the needs of primary care in a population in a geographical area, and resources have been allocated based on the size of the catchment population. This way of organizing primary care can best be described as an integrated community model, which ideally performs well in regard to effectiveness, productivity, continuity, equity, and quality, but often displays problems with accessibility and responsiveness toward individual patients' needs and expectations (Lamarche et al. 2003). As part of the NPM-inspired reforms introduced in Swedish healthcare during the past decades, a regulated market was introduced in primary care in the late 2000s. Expanded patient choice in combination with privatization and competition among providers was gradually introduced by the regions during 2007–2010. Since January 1, 2010, freedom of choice of PCC for individuals and freedom of establishment for providers passing the requirements decided by each region is mandatory, following a change in the Health Care Act decided by Parliament (Anell 2011). The introduction of such freedoms in a regulated market constituted a major change in the way that primary care is organized and provided in Sweden. The idea behind expanded choice and competition is that market mechanisms should lead to improved efficiency, quality, and responsiveness of providers in relation to their patients (Le Grand 2007, 2009). In the Swedish case, the introduction of the market reform was particularly targeted at problems with poor accessibility, continuity, and responsiveness of primary care, ideally without negative consequences for objectives related to equity (Anell 2011; Glenngård 2016).

A persisting challenge in Swedish primary care, before as well as after the 2007–2010 market reform, is a shortage of GPs. This shortage has consequences for access to and continuity in GP visits. In connection with the reform, the number of PCCs increased by over 20% in Sweden. The increase in the number of PCCs was not accompanied by a corresponding increase in GPs or other healthcare staff. The existing primary care staff was rather spread out over more PCCs. Not only are there relatively few doctors in primary care, compared to other specialized care, but also Swedish GPs devote a relatively smaller share of their working time to patients compared to GPs in several other European countries (Swedish Agency for Health and Care Services Analysis 2020). The principle of team-based primary care implies that individuals register with a PCC rather than with an individual GP (Anell 2011; Glenngård 2016). The idea is that GPs should devote their time to patients with worse conditions as other staff categories attend to patients with less-severe problems (i.e., substitution of GP labor input for non-GP labor input). While this is one possible explanation why GPs devote less time to patients, evidence also showed that Swedish GPs devote more time to administrative work and experience more work-related stress compared to GPs in other European countries (Swedish Agency for Health and Care Services Analysis 2020). Also, other staff categories experience work-related stress and a high administrative burden (Holmgren et al. 2019; Hollman, Lennartsson, and Rosengren 2014). A number of policy initiatives to tackle persisting challenges with a shortage of GPs was initiated in 2020–2021 (e.g., targeted national grants to strengthen primary care and a new legislation targeting access, patient centeredness and continuity in primary care) (Ministry of Health and Social Affairs 2020).

Possible future developments in Swedish primary care include shifting some of the responsibilities from the regional to the national level (Anell 2020): To tackle the current and future needs and challenges, not least in regard to moving the care "closer to patients" (SOU 2019,29) and the persisting shortage of GPs, the central government needs to take more comprehensive responsibility for funding in order to secure greater health access and the quality of healthcare delivery of services, rather than using short-term targeted grants. Increased central government funding should have consequences for governance and leadership at this level, especially in the area of planning and managing human resources.

Differences between Public and Private PCCs

In connection with the 2007–2010 reform, 223 new PCCs were established, equal to a 23% increase throughout the country. The increase consisted predominantly of private for-profit providers, establishing in densely populated areas with a low level of socioeconomic deprivation (Swedish National Audit Office 2014; Isaksson et al. 2018; Burström et al. 2017). The proportion of private PCCs increased from 28% to 37% on a national level (Swedish Competition Authority 2010). The proportion of private PCCs did not correspond to market share in terms of the proportion of citizens, compared to the mainly public PCCs existing before the reform, as the new PCCs were smaller (Swedish National Audit Office 2014). Public PCCs were almost twice as large as private ones in 2010, as measured by the number of individuals on the PCC list (i.e., 8,800 compared to 4,600 individuals on average) (Swedish Competition Authority 2012). The characteristics of private and public PCCs differed also in regard to other factors than PCC list size (e.g., differences in the division of labor between GPs and other staff categories, with a larger proportion of GP visits and better continuity in GP visits at private PCCs) (Swedish Agency for Health and Care Services Analysis 2015b:9).

Comparing performance with regard to ownership of PCCs is challenging as there are limited data available about the content of care and outcomes for patients. Since 2009, an annual National Patient Survey (NPS) in primary care is used to collect information about patients' perceptions about different dimensions about the quality of care provided at public and private PCCs (e.g., respect and responsiveness, continuity, and coordination and accessibility. According to results from the NPS in the years immediately following the reform, patients were more satisfied with private PCCs than public ones, but when adjusting for patient mix, the division of labor, and PCC list size, such differences did not remain for most dimensions (Glenngård 2013; Glenngård and Anell 2017). This indicates that differences in patients' perception at the PCC level mirror structural characteristics of PCCs.

In more recent years, relatively few PCCs have entered the market each year, but the private PCCs that have been established are to a greater extent located in socioeconomically deprived (densely populated) areas, compared to those that established in connection with the reform. Moreover, the initial difference in size between public and private PCCs has decreased over time as more individuals have registered with private PCCs. Ten years after the market reform, the proportion of individuals at private PCCs corresponds fairly well to the proportion of private PCCs on the market. On a national level, the proportion of private PCCs was 44% in 2020, and the private PCCs accounted for 41% of all registered individuals (Dagens medicin 2021a). An analysis of registry data from Region Skåne, the southernmost region of Sweden, also indicated that differences in size, patient mix, and patients' perceptions about the quality of care between public and private PCCs either have decreased or do not persist at all one decade after the reform (Anna Häger Glenngård data on file covering the years 2018–2019). Differences in the division of labor between GPs and other staff across owner types have also decreased over time. Private PCCs seem to gradually have substituted GP visits for visits with other professional groups as more patients have listed without an accompanying increase in GPs (Anna Häger Glenngård data on file, covering the years 2018–2019), and public PCCs have been found to change their administrative practices when faced with competition from private PCCs (Dackehag and Ellegård 2019). Altogether, this suggests that private and public PCCs have become more similar over time.

Equity and Quality of Primary Care Services

For expanded choice and competition to lead to improved quality, accessibility, and responsiveness of providers in relation to their patients, it is vital that individuals have access to choose among alternative providers and that individuals are interested and informed enough to be able to make a choice of provider (Le Grand 2007, 2009). Hence, for such gains to be made without adverse consequences for equity in access to care and distribution of services, it is important that there are no major differences in the availability of alternative providers across population groups. This relates to both horizontal equity, defined as the principle in which people with similar needs should have similar access to the healthcare services, and vertical equity, which stipulates that individuals with greater needs should have access to healthcare services appropriate to these greater needs.

Proponents of the 2007–2010 market reform argued that choice and competition would increase the total number of PCCs, thereby improving the overall quality in and access to primary care. Opponents feared that the establishment of new private providers would have negative consequences for equity in access to primary care as they expected that new (private) providers would establish foremost in densely populated and privileged areas and that low-need patients would increase their utilization more than high-need patients (Fredriksson, Blomqvist, and Winblad 2013; Burström 2009; Kullberg, Blomqvist and Winblad 2018). One decade later, there is mixed evidence available, partly supporting both sides. On an overall level, Dietrichson et al. (2020) found that, despite the increase in PCCs, the effects of introducing choice and competition has been modest. Based on analysis of register data, they found small improvements of patients' overall satisfaction with care but no significant effects on quality as measured by avoidable hospitalization as a result of the reform. One possible reason is that the increase in PCCs was not followed by a corresponding increase in GPs.

Available evidence regarding horizontal and vertical equity in Swedish primary care is mixed. Next, issues of equity and quality of Swedish primary care is further elaborated based on available data and previous research on geographical accessibility, distribution of GP visits, and patients' perceptions about primary care. Results from available research regarding variation in geographical access to alternative providers and on socioeconomic distribution of GP visits are used to illustrate issues related to horizontal equity. Finally, findings from research about variation in patients' perceptions about the quality of care between socioeconomic groups are presented to illustrate equity in patient-reported outcomes.

Variation between Regions—Equity in Geographical Accessibility

Geographical accessibility can be defined as the distance, or travel time, between patients and healthcare providers and equity in geographical accessibility as all citizens having a similar, or minimum, travel distance to the nearest healthcare provider (Isaksson, Blomqvist, and Winblad 2016). There is some evidence that the access to alternative PCCs varies across regions, with better access in more densely populated areas.

First, there is geographical variation in the overall access to alternative providers. Individuals living in more densely populated areas have better access to alternative PCCs compared to individuals living in less densely populated areas. The providers entering the market in connection with the 2007–2010 reform mainly became established in densely populated areas. This led to variation in the overall availability of alternative PCCs to choose among for the population. The Swedish Competition Authority (2012, 2014) evaluated the extent individuals actually had access to alternative providers in 2011 and 2014. Throughout the country, around 80% of the population had less than a 5-minute car journey, while about 2% of the population—or 205,000 individuals—had more than a 20-minute car journey to an alternative PCC than the one closest to their home in both years investigated. Only 5% of the people living in the densely populated Stockholm region had more than a 5-minute car journey to an alternative PCC, while more than 30% of the populations in eight other—mainly less densely populated—regions had more than a 5-minute care journey to an alternative PCC. PCCs that have established in more recent years are also mainly located in densely populated areas (Dagens Medicin 2021a).

Second, there is geographical variation in the access to different types of PCCs. Individuals living in less densely populated areas have less access to private PCCs, compared to individuals living in more densely populated areas, who may choose among both public and private PCCs. In connection with the market reform, the proportion of private PCCs increased from 28% to 37% on a national level. The proportion varied widely between regions, however, from 3% in some of the northernmost and less densely populated regions to between 40% and 63% in the more densely populated regions in the southern parts of Sweden (Swedish Competition Authority 2010). Although private PCCs have increased in size and some private PCCs have established in more recent years, the variation between regions, with regard to proportion of private PCCs, remains one decade later. In 2020, the proportion of patients listed with a private PCC was 44% at the national level, with a variation between 11% in Region Västerbotten, one of the northernmost less densely populated regions, and 63% in Region Stockholm, the most densely populated region (Dagens medicin 2021b).

Variation between Socioeconomic Groups—Equity in Distribution of Services

The fact that most private PCCs entering the market in connection with the reform established in densely populated areas with a low level of socioeconomic deprivation have led to inequities in geographical accessibility and access to alternative PCCs between socioeconomic groups (Swedish National Audit Office 2014; Isaksson et al. 2018; Burström et al. 2017). Evidence about the socioeconomic distribution of visits following the reform is mixed. Studies from different parts of Sweden pointed in different directions. Beckman and Anell (2013) analyzed differences in GP visits before and after the market reform in Region Skåne (i.e., the southernmost and densely populated region in Sweden). They found that the reform led to improved access to GP visits on an overall level, but that individuals with a higher income benefited more from the reform than individuals with a lower income. Agerholm et al. (2015) also found that the total number of GP visits increased significantly, and that the reform had a negative impact on equity, based on an analysis of register data from Region Stockholm, the largest region in Sweden in terms of population. Sveréus et al. (2018) analyzed changes in socioeconomic distribution following the market reform, based on data from the three largest regions (in terms of population) in Sweden (i.e., Region Stockholm, Region Skåne, and Västra Götaland region). Similar to Beckman and Anell (2013) and Agerholm et al. (2015), they concluded that the number of visits increased for all population groups, that is, that the reform led to increased access to GP visits. Contrary to Beckman and Anell (2013) and Agerholm et al. 2015), they found that there were few or no changes in the socioeconomic distribution of visits. Their results indicated that the increase in visits were pro-poor in absolute terms but not in relative terms. A report by the Swedish Agency for Health and Care Services Analysis (2015a:6), based on analysis of three large regions, also concluded that the reform resulted in a significant increase in GP visits, most pronounced in Region Stockholm. The results in the report also showed that groups of individuals with low income and/or low education had more GP visits compared to other groups both before and after the reform. Finally, San Sebastián et al. (2017) analyzed the use of GP services in the four northernmost regions in Sweden—Region Jämtland-Härjedalen, Region Västernorrland, Region Västerbotten, and Region Norrbotten—before and after the market reform. They concluded that the reform led to higher use of GPs by individuals with higher income after adjusting for health needs. In summary, available studies showed that the reform led to improved access to GP visits, but there is uncertainty regarding consequences for horizontal equity. However, a limitation of all these studies is that none had access to information about length or content of visits. Such data, which are largely missing in the Swedish context, are needed to draw certain conclusions about the distribution of services and interventions across PCCs and population groups and to assess if an increased number of visits occurred at the expense of reduced quality (e.g., length and content of visits).

Variation between Socioeconomic Groups—Equity in Patient-Reported Outcomes

Available research suggests that patients' perceptions about primary care vary with respect to socioeconomic conditions in Sweden. Several studies, based on patient survey data at the PCC level, found a negative correlation between high socioeconomic deprivation and different dimensions of patients' experiences with care (Angelis, Glenngård, and Jordahl 2021; Dahlgren et al. 2014; Glenngård 2013; Glenngård and Anell 2017, 2018). The majority of the published studies were based on survey data from different regions during the years shortly after the reform. One possible explanation for the negative relationship between difficult socioeconomic circumstances and worse patient satisfaction is that the PCCs that entered the market in connection with the introduction of choice and competition primarily were located in more affluent areas.

If PCCs choose not to establish in areas with a high socioeconomic burden, the mechanism behind expanded patient choice and provider competition risks failing in such areas, with adverse consequences for equity. Previous research showed that individuals in lower socioeconomic groups often have lesser capabilities to exercise choice compared to people with higher income and/or education because they have lesser abilities to search for information, articulate demands, and travel to nonlocal providers (Fotaki et al. 2008; Barr, Fenton, and Blane 2008). However, a recent study based on 2019 NPS data from the southernmost region in Sweden, where several private PCCs have established in socioeconomically unfavorable areas in recent years, found a similar relationship (Glenngård 2021). This indicates that there is a variation in perceptions about the quality of care with regard to socioeconomic conditions, at least at the PCC level, even in areas with good access to different types of PCCs. However, variation in patients' perceptions about the quality of care does not necessarily mirror differences in the content of visits. As mentioned, a challenge when assessing the distribution of services and interventions in Swedish primary care is a lack of data about the content and length of visits.

Governance Mechanisms to Ensure Health Equity and Health Quality

The 2007–2010 market reform had major consequences for governance and leadership in the Swedish regions because payment was separated from provision, and private providers become involved in the delivery of primary care. In this chapter, the definition of governance and leadership in publicly funded healthcare systems as a continuous process consisting of three parts—priority setting, monitoring, and accountability—is used (Smith et al. 2012). In general terms, this implies that governments set priorities based on population needs and political decisions, with respect to available resources, and then allocate resources and tasks to healthcare providers based on such priorities. Next, they collect information to be able to assess provider activities. Finally, they evaluate providers against their expectations and consequently hold providers to account for their conduct. In Swedish primary care, this means allocating resources and tasks to the public and private PCCs through agreements, monitoring, and assessing PCCs in regard to such agreements and deciding whether to allow providers to continue practice primary care with public funding. The underlying assumption in welfare markets is that choice and competition may suffice to achieve increased accessibility and responsiveness toward individuals' needs and preferences, but not to achieve important goals from a population perspective. Governments need to compensate for differences in the ability to make informed choices in different groups of the population to ensure that accessibility and responsiveness toward some groups is not improved at the expense of worse accessibility and responsiveness in other groups in the population.

The fact that the market reform in Swedish primary care was initiated by individual regions, rather at the national level, reflect the strong tradition of decentralization in this setting. This has led to rather flexible legislation. By law it is stipulated that individuals have the right to choose a

PCC, that providers cannot deny an individual from enrolling at the PCC list, that payment to providers should follow people's choice, and that the same requirements apply to public and private PCCs (Health and Medical Services Act 2017,30). However, it is up to each region to decide on the specific compliance requirements for PCCs to be allowed to practice care with public funding, in accordance with local priorities and identified needs in the population. This has led to some variation, for example, in the organization of care for elderly with complex needs and coordination of such services between regions and municipalities. It is also up to each region to decide on the principles for allocating resources to PCCs and how to monitor and hold providers to account for adherence to stipulated requirements. Next, a description of how the regions use principles for resource allocation and monitoring of providers to ensure equity and quality in primary care follows.

Principles for Resource Allocation

In connection with the introduction of patient choice and provider competition, the 21 regions introduced different systems for allocating financial resources and financial responsibility to PCCs. There was a variation in the proportion of fixed and variable payment and in principles for risk adjustment of the fixed payment with regard to patient mix and location of PCCs (Anell 2011). The proportion of fixed payment varied between 40% and 100% across the regions. Provider payment models have become more similar over the decade since the reform was introduced. All regions now allocate resources to PCCs based on fixed capitation, risk adjusted with regard to expected greater demands for primary care in accordance with the level of socioeconomic deprivation, age, and/or the level of morbidity and among individuals on the PCC list (Isaksson et al. 2016; Glenngård 2019). The proportion of fixed payment varies between 60% in Region Stockholm and 80% and almost 100% in most other regions. Morbidity is usually measured by average adjusted clinical groups (ACGs), and socioeconomic deprivation is usually measured by care need index (CNI) among individuals on the PCC list. ACG is a measure that quantifies morbidity in a group of individuals based on their age, gender, and the constellation of diagnoses over a defined time period (Reid et al. 1999). CNI is a measure that quantifies the level of social deprivation based on seven factors (e.g., composition of the household, country of birth, education, and unemployment) (Sundquist et al. 2003).

Risks associated with fixed payment to providers include cream skimming, cost shifting (referrals), and skimping on quality (Anell 2011). The idea behind risk adjustment of the fixed payment is to prevent cream skimming, that is, that providers avoid individuals with expected great needs of primary care services. As mentioned, providers cannot deny anyone from enrolling at the PCC list by law. However, providers can choose in what area to establish a PCC, which has a somewhat similar result since people tend to register with a PCC close to their home.

Observed differences in patient mix and patient satisfaction between public and private PCCs during the period following the market reform, together with evidence that patients' experiences varied with regard to socioeconomic conditions, raised concerns that increased choice and provider competition is difficult to achieve without adverse consequences for equity (Fredriksson et al. 2013; Swedish National Audit Office 2014; Burström et al. 2017). While the PCCs that established in connection with the reform mainly located in favorable areas, PCCs that have established in more recent years are to a higher extent located in socioeconomically deprived areas. In this respect, the use of risk adjustment of fixed capitation based on CNI appear to be a successful governance mechanism. Anell, Dackehag, and Dietrichson (2018) concluded that risk-adjusted capitation affects private providers' establishment decisions. They found that risk-adjusted capitation based on CNI increases the supply of private PCCs in areas with unfavorable socioeconomic and demographic characteristics in Sweden.

Risk adjustment of the fixed payment does not prevent skimping on quality or an appropriate volume or a certain distribution of services. Other governance mechanisms are needed to prevent such risks. In regard to principles for resource allocation, this includes variable payment for visits and certain services and performance-based payment based on fulfilment of goals related to different aspects of quality. Most regions use a small proportion of variable payment, primarily for visits. In connection with the market reform, most regions also included performance-based payment for reaching targets related to continuity in GP visits, waiting times, results in patient surveys, participating in national quality registries, and adherence to clinical guidelines. While the use of pay-for-performance schemes created strong financial incentives to reach stipulated targets in certain areas (e.g., related to prescription guidelines), in some regions it led to crowding-out effects in other areas. Several regions have abandoned performance-based payment altogether, and in regions where this is still used, the number of performance targets have been substantially reduced (Glenngård 2019).

In summary, differences in the models for allocating resources to PCCs have decreased over time, with a trend toward more fixed payments and less reliance on detailed pay-for-performance schemes. Regions use principles for allocating resources to public and private PCCs to prevent cream-skimming (risk-adjustment fixed payment) and skimping on some aspects of quality (pay for performance related to adherence to clinical guidelines). Other governance mechanisms, related to monitoring of providers, are used to prevent skimping on other aspects of (primarily clinical) quality and possible underprovision of services.

Principles for Monitoring Providers

There is a long and strong tradition of performance measurement in Swedish healthcare, especially in specialized care, driven by intraprofessional use of measures for quality improvement work. For example, there are more than 100 national quality registries, managed by specialist organizations, with voluntary participation by provider. Registries store individualized data on diagnosis, treatment, and treatment outcomes in inpatient and outpatient care, including primary care. There are also national data registries covering services in healthcare and social services, administered by the National Board of Health and Welfare, that are mandatory for providers to report to, and databases administered by SALAR, where data are collected from administrative systems in regions and municipalities. There has been a shift in the use of performance measurement—from intraprofessional quality improvement work toward external control and in support of accountability. Examples of external control by regions include the use of performance targets in agreements between regions and providers, sometimes included in pay-for-performance schemes, to improve quality and ensure accountability for the use of allocated resources. At the national level, such external control includes monitoring the adherence to Swedish national guidelines in different disease areas by the National Board of Health and Welfare and transparent presentation of results to enhance quality and equity in healthcare. While the early NPM-inspired reforms largely focused on increased efficiency, where output concerned the volume of care, a shift in focus toward health outcomes and quality of care and a more general trend toward increased transparency can be noted during the past two decades (Anell et al. 2012). Since 2006, the government, together with SALAR, published annual performance comparisons and rankings, called "regional comparisons" of PCCs and hospitals, using data from national quality registries, health data registries, and patient and waiting time surveys. The regional comparisons included over 350 measures organized into various categories, such as prevention, patient satisfaction, waiting times, trust, and access. Many indictors are presented at an aggregated level for each region or municipality, and some are presented for individual hospitals and PCCs. Statistics on patients' experiences and waiting times for each PCC are also made publicly available by SALAR to help guide people in their choice of PCC.

Criticism about the shift toward the use of performance measurement for external control has increased in Sweden as elsewhere. It has been argued that assessment of providers has come to focus on performance measures that are easy to collect and that external control ultimately undermines intrinsic motivation among professionals. There is regional variation in specific measures used to assess PCC performance and hold providers to account for their conduct, related to variation in the specific requirements that PCCs have to comply with to be allowed to practice care with public funding in each region. Most regions, as well as government agencies, use a framework called "good healthcare and social services" to identify appropriate areas and indicators to use in their assessment of PCCs. The framework was developed by the Swedish National Board of Health and Welfare in 2006, inspired by the Institute of Medicine in the United States (National Board of Health and Welfare 2009; Institute of Medicine 2001). It contains six domains: The care provided should be patient centered, knowledge based, safe, accessible, efficient, and equitable. The regions and national agencies, such as the National Board of Health and Welfare, monitor and assess provider quality with regard to the six domains by the use of proxy measures, such as adherence to evidence-based guidelines as proxy measures for knowledge based and safe care, results from waiting time surveys to monitor accessibility, and results from patient surveys to monitor patient-centeredness.

Another critique in the Swedish healthcare system is that providers are subject to a heavy administrative burden and coercive controls, as they are supposed to act in accordance with targets and clinical performance indicators based on national guidelines and local priorities (Fredriksson, Blomqvist, and Winblad 2014; Glenngård and Anell 2017). More recently, policy interest has turned toward governance approaches allowing for a higher degree of professional autonomy and a more enabling use of performance measurement systems. As noted above, there has been a trend in most regions in recent years toward more fixed payments and less reliance on detailed pay-for-performance schemes. Moreover, most regions combine performance measurement with some kind of dialogue or feedback to support quality improvements and continuous learning (SALAR 2013). However, all regions also use a variety of measures to monitor and assess PCCs and to hold providers to account for their adherence to requirements stipulated in agreements. Hence, the regions' use of performance measurement serves the two purposes of forcing compliance with agreements to ensure external accountability for the use of allocated resources and to offer providers support for learning and quality improvement (Glenngård 2019). The importance of maintaining and further developing governance mechanisms to take both these perspectives into account together with a need to involve healthcare professionals in the processes of governance were also emphasized in a recent report on the future governance of Swedish healthcare (Anell 2020).

Concluding Remarks

There is a saying that every system is perfectly designed to get the results it gets. This is certainly the case in Swedish primary care. A system based on the idea of free choice of PCC for individuals and competition among (public and private) providers combined with a strong tradition of local self-government have resulted in variation in several areas. Different principles for allocating resources to PCCs and use of performance measurement to ensure equity and quality of services were introduced in the regions when implementing the 2007–2010 market reform. The establishment patterns among private PCCs entering the market in connection with the reform led to inequities in geographical accessibility and access to alternative providers between socioeconomic groups and variation in characteristics between public and private PCCs. The evidence on how this affected the socioeconomic distribution of visits is mixed, while several studies have demonstrated that groups of individuals with worse socioeconomic conditions are less satisfied with the primary care services they receive. However, data about the length and content of visits in primary care are largely missing in the Swedish context, which makes it difficult to draw certain conclusions about the distribution of services and interventions across PCCs and population groups.

Ten years after the introduction of the market reform, there are tendencies that some differences have decreased. More private PCCs have established in less favorable areas, and public and private PCCs have become more similar in regard to patient mix, the division of labor, and patients' perceptions of quality of care. These changes can be related to several factors. The principle of risk adjusting the fixed payment to PCCs in relation to socioeconomic deprivation among individuals on the PCC list has encouraged private PCCs to establish in less favorable areas. The shortage of GPs has led to changes in the division of labor among private PCCs as more individuals have listed without an accompanying increase in GPs. As the characteristics of public and private PCCs have become more similar, it is perhaps not surprising that variation in patients' perceptions in regard to ownership have decreased. Such perceptions tend to mirror structural characteristics of PCCs, including patient mix.

Mechanisms for governance to ensure health equity and quality have also become more similar across the 21 regions. There is a trend toward more enabling—rather than coercive—governance mechanisms, allowing for a higher degree of professional autonomy and support to continuous learning and quality improvements. However, it is important to stress that regions strive to include two overall components in their current governance models; to ensure external accountability for the use of allocated resources by control of compliance with agreements and support to learning and quality improvement. This dual purpose of governance is important to maintain and further develop to balance current and future needs and challenges in Swedish primary care. Moreover, it is important to tackle the situation with a shortage of GPs in order to improve taccess to as well as continuity in GP visits. Possible solutions involve a more comprehensive responsibility for funding and governance at the national level.

References

Agerholm, Janne, Daniel Bruce, Antonio Ponce de Leon, and Bo Burström. 2015. "Equity Impact of a Choice Reform and Change in Reimbursement System in Primary Care in Stockholm County Council." *BMC Health Services Research* 15: 420.

Anell, Anders. 2011. "Choice and Privatisation in Swedish Primary Care." *Health Economics, Policy and Law* 6: 549–569.

Anell, Anders. 2020. *Vården är värd en bättre styrning* [In Swedish]. Stockholm: SNS Förlag.

Anell, Anders, Margareta Dackehag, and Jens Dietrichson. 2018. "Does Risk-Adjusted Payment Influence Primary Care Providers' Decision on Where to Set Up Practices?" *BMC Health Services Research* 18: 179.

Anell, Anders, Anna Häger Glenngård, and Sherry Merkur. 2012. "Sweden: Health System Review." *Health Systems in Transition* 14(5): 1–159.

Angelis, Jannis, Anna Häger Glenngård, and Henrik Jordahl. 2021 "Management Practices and the Quality of Primary Care." *Public Money and Management* 41(3): 264–271.

Barr, David A., Laura Fenton, and David Blane. 2008. "The Claim for Patient Choice and Equity." *Journal of Medical Ethics* 34: 271–274.

Beckman, Anders, and Anders Anell. 2013. "Changes in Health Care Utilisation Following a Reform Involving Choice and Privatisation in Swedish Primary Care: A Five-Year Follow-Up of GP-Visits." *BMC Health Services Research* 13: article 452.

Burström, Bo. 2009. "Market-Oriented, Demand-Driven Health Care Reforms and Equity in Health and Health Care Utilization in Sweden." *International Journal of Health Services* 39: 271–285.

Burström, Bo, Kristina Burström, Gunnar Nilsson, Göran Tomson, Margareth Whitehead, and Ulrika Winblad. 2017. "Equity Aspects of the Primary Healthcare Choice Reform in Sweden—A Scoping Review." *International Journal for Equity in Health* 16(1): article 29.

Cutler, David. 2002. "Equality, Efficiency and Market Fundamentals: The Dynamics of International Medical-Care Reform." *Journal of Economic Literature* 40(3): 881–906.

Dackehag, Margareta, and Lina Maria Ellegård. 2019. "Competition, Capitation and Coding: Do Public Primary Care Providers Respond to Increased Competition?" *CESifo Economic Studies* 5: 402–423.

Dagens Medicin. 2021a. "Privata vårdcentraler listade 400 000 fler på fem år—offentlig vård ligger stilla" [In Swedish]. March 31.

Dagens Medicin. 2021b. "Så stor andel är privat listade i olika regioner" [In Swedish]. March 31.

Dahlgren, Cecilia, Hilja Brorsson, Sofia Sveréus, Fanny Goude, and Clas Rehnberg. 2014. *Fem år med husläkarsystemet inom Vårdval Stockholm* [In Swedish]. Stockholm: Karolinska Institutet.

Dietrichson J, Ellegård LM, and Kjellsson G. 2020. "Patient choice, entry and quality of primary care: Evidence from Swedish reforms." *Health Economics* 29(6): 716–730.

Fotaki, Marianna, Martin Roland, Alan Boyd, Ruth McDonald, Rod Sheaff, and Liz Smith. 2008. "What Benefits Will Choice Bring to Patients? Literature Review and Assessment of Implications." *Journal of Health Services Research & Policy* 13(3): 178–184.

Fredriksson, Mio, Paula Blomqvist, and Ulrika Winblad. 2013. "The Trade-off between Choice and Equity: Swedish Policymakers' Arguments When Introducing Patient Choice." *Journal of European Social Policy* 23(2): 192–209.

Fredriksson, Mio, Paula Blomqvist, and Ulrika Winblad. 2014. "Recentralizing Healthcare through Evidence-Based Guidelines—Striving for National Equity in Sweden." *BMC Health Services Research* 14: 509.

Glenngård, Anna Häger. 2013. "Is Patient Satisfaction in Primary Care Dependent on Structural and Organizational Characteristics among Providers? Findings Based on Data from the National Patient Survey in Sweden." *Health Economics Policy and Law* 8(3): 317–333.

Glenngård, Anna Häger. 2016. "Experiences of Introducing a Quasi-Market in Swedish Primary Care: Fulfilment of Overall Objectives and Assessment of Provider Activities." *Scandinavian Journal of Public Administration* 20(1): 72–86.

Glenngård, Anna Häger. 2019. "Pursuing the Objectives of Support to Providers and External Accountability through Enabling Controls—A Study of Governance Models in Swedish Primary Care." *BMC Health Services Research* 19: 114.

Glenngård, Anna Häger. 2021. "What Matters for Patients' Experiences with primary Care? A Study of Variation in Patient Reported Experience Measures with Regard to Structural and Organisational Characteristics of Primary Care Centres in a Swedish Region." *Nordic Journal of Health Economics.* https://doi.org/10.5617/njhe.8fc

Glenngård, Anna Häger, and Anders Anell. 2017. "Does Increased Standardisation in Health Care Mean Less Responsiveness towards Individual Patients' Expectations? A Register-Based Study in Swedish Primary Care." *Sage Open Medicine* 25(5): 1–8.

Glenngård, Anna Häger, and Anders Anell. 2018. "Process Measures or Patient Reported Experience Measures (PREM) for Comparing Performance across Providers? A Study of Measures Related to Access and Continuity in Swedish Primary Care." *Primary Health Care Research & Development* 19: 23–32.

Glenngård, Anna Häger, and Sixtem Borg. 2019. *Can People Afford to Pay for Health Care? New Evidence on Financial Protection in Sweden.* Copenhagen: WHO Regional Office for Europe.

Health and Medical Services Act. 2017. (Hälso—och sjukvårdslagen [2017:30], HSL).

Hollman, Djana, Sandra Lennartsson, and Kristina Rosengren. 2014. "District Nurses' Experiences with the Free-Choice System in Swedish Primary Care." *British Journal of Community Nursing* 19: 30–35.

Holmgren, Kristina, Gunnel Hensing, Ute Bültmann, Emina Hadzibajramovic, and Maria E. H. Larsson. 2019. "Does Early Identification of Work-Related Stress, Combined with Feedback at GP-Consultation, Prevent Sick Leave in the Following 12 Months? A Randomized Controlled Trial in Primary Health Care." *BMC Public Health* 19(1): 1110.

Institute of Medicine. 2001. *Crossing the Quality Chasm: A New Health System for the 21st Century.* Washington, DC: National Academies Press.

Isaksson, David, Paula Blomqvist, Ronnie Pingel, and Ulrika Winblad. 2018. "Risk Selection in Primary Care: A Cross-Sectional Fixed Effect Analysis of Swedish Individual Data." *BMJ Open* 8(10): e020402.

Isaksson, David, Paula Blomqvist, and Ulrika Winblad. 2016. "Free Establishment of Primary Healthcare Providers: Effects on Geographical Equity." *BMC Health Services Research* 16: 28.

Kullberg, Linn, Paula Blomqvist, and Ulrika Winblad. 2018. "Market-Orienting Reforms in Rural Health Care in Sweden: How Can Equity in Access Be Preserved?" *International Journal for Equity in Health* 17(1): 123.

Lamarche, Paul A., Marie-Dominique Beaulieu, Raynald Pineault, Damien Contandriopoulos, Jean-Louis Denis, and Neannie L. Haggerty. 2003. *Choices for Change: The Path for Restructuring Primary Healthcare Services in Canada.* Canadian Health Services Research Foundation, New Brunswick Department of Health and Wellness, Saskatchewan Department of Health, Ministère de la santé et des services sociaux du Québec and Health Canada.

Le Grand, Julian. 2007. *Delivering Public Services through Choice and Competition—The Other Invisible Hand.* Princeton, NJ: Princeton University Press.

Le Grand, Julian. 2009. "Choice and Competition in Publicly Funded Health Care." *Health Economics Policy and Law* 4: 479–488.

Le Grand, Julian, and William Bartlett. 1993. *Quasi-Markets and Social Policy*. London: Macmillan.

Lövtrup, Michael. 2017. "Rekordstor minskning av vårdplatserna 2016" [In Swedish]. *Läkartidningen* 114, EP9T.

Martinussen, Pål E., and Jon Magnussen. 2009. "Health Care Reform: The Nordic Experience." In *Nordic Health Care Systems—Recent Reforms and Current Policy Challenges*, European Observatory on Health Systems and Policies Series, edited by Jon Magnussen, Kaersten Vrangbaek, and Richard B. Saltman. Maidenhead, Berkshire, UK: Open University Press.

Ministry of Health and Social Affairs. 2020. *Lagrådsremiss—Inriktningen för en nära och tillgänglig vård—en primärvårdsreform* [In Swedish]. Stockholm: Ministry of Health and Social Affairs.

Reid, Robert J., Leonard MacWilliam, Noralou P. Roos, Bogdan Bogdanovic, and Charlyn Black. 1999. *Measuring Morbidity in Populations: Performance of the Johns Hopkins Adjusted Clinical Group (ACG) Case-Mix Adjustment System in Manitoba*. Manitoba Centre for Health Policy and Evaluation Department of Community Health Sciences Faculty of Medicine, University of Manitoba.

San Sebastián, Miguel, Paola A. Mosquera, Nawi Ng, and Per E. Gustafsson. 2017. "Health Care on Equal Terms? Assessing Horizontal Equity in Health Care Use in Northern Sweden." *European Journal of Public Health* 7(4): 637–643.

Smith, Peter, Anders Anell, Reinhard Busse, Luca Crivelli, Judith Healy, Anne Karin Lindahl, Gert Westert, and Tobechukwy Kene. 2012. "Leadership and Governance in Seven Developed Health Systems." *Health Policy* 106(1): 37–49.

SOU (Statens offentliga utredningar). 2019. *God och nära vård—Vård i samverkan* [In Swedish]. Stockholm: Statens offentliga utredningar.

Statistics Sweden. 2021. "Systems of Health Accounts (SHA) 2001–2019." https://www.sta tistikdatabasen.scb.se

Sundquist, Kristina, Marianne Malmström, Sven-Erik Johansson, and Jan Sundquist. 2003. "Care Need Index, a Useful Tool for the Distribution of Primary Health Care Resources." *Journal of Epidemiolgical Community Health* 57: 347–352.

Sveréus, Sofia, Gustav Kjellsson, and Clas Rehnberg. 2018. "Socioeconomic Distribution of GP Visits Following Patient Choice Reform and Differences in Reimbursement Models: Evidence from Sweden." *Health Policy* 122(9): 949–956.

Swedish Agency for Health and Care Services Analysis. 2015a. *En jämförande studie mellan tre landsting före och efter vårdvalets införande* [In Swedish]. Stockholm: Myndigheten för vårdanalys, report 2015:6.

Swedish Agency for Health and Care Services Analysis. 2015b. *Vården ur primärvårdsläkarnas perspektiv—en jämförelse mellan Sverige och nio andra länder* [In Swedish]. Stockholm: Myndigheten för vårdanalys, report 2015:9.

Swedish Agency for Health and Care Services Analysis. 2020. *Vården ur primärvårdsläkarnas perspektiv 2019* [In Swedish]. Stockholm: Myndigheten för vårdanalys, report 2020:5.

Swedish Association of Local Authorities and Regions (SALAR). 2013. *Landstingens arbete med uppföljning och kontroll av primärvårdsverksamhet—en översiktlig kartläggning* [In Swedish]. Stockholm: Swedish Association of Local Authorities and Regions.

Swedish Association of Local Authorities and Regions (SALAR). 2021. https://skr.se/skr/ ekonomijuridik/ekonomi/sektornisiffror.1821.html

Swedish Competition Authority. 2010. *Uppföljning av vårdval i primärvården—Valfrihet, mångfald och etableringsförutsättningar. Slutrapport* [In Swedish]. Stockholm: Swedish Competition Authority.

Swedish Competition Authority. 2012. *Val av vårdcentral—Förutsättningar för kvalitetskonkurrens i vårdvalssystemem* [In Swedish]. Stockholm: Swedish Competition Authority.

Swedish Competition Authority. 2014. *Etablering och konkurrens bland vårdcentraler— om kvalitetsdriven konkurrens och ekonomiska villkor* [In Swedish]. Stockholm: Swedish Competition Authority.

Swedish National Audit Office. 2014. *Riksrevisionen granskar: staten och vården. Primärvårdens styrning—efter behov eller efterfrågan* [In Swedish]. Stockholm: Riksrevisionen.

Swedish Insurance Federation. 2018. http://www.svenskforsakring.se

7

The Changing Private Sector Role in the Netherlands' Public/Private Sector Healthcare System

Some Considerations of Health Equity and Quality of Care

Florien M. Kruse and Patrick Jeurissen

Introduction

The Dutch welfare state emerged from the realization that collective effort was needed against widespread poverty among the working population. In 1901, the first social insurance scheme was born, although the church and other charities still provided most of the social safety net (van Oorschot 2006). Introduction of universal mandatory healthcare insurance took much longer. In 1941, the legal foundations for the Dutch contemporary healthcare system were laid, imitating the German Bismarck model (Wammes, Stadhouders, and Westert 2020). Over the years a patchwork of regulations came close to near-universal coverage for curative healthcare, while long-term care was steered by universal social insurance as early as 1968 (Companje 2014).

In the 1980s, the expansion of the Dutch welfare state came to a halt. Spiraling governmental expenditures, perceived inefficiencies, and lack of incentive for innovation in the delivery of public services contributed to this shift. As in other Western countries, the remedy offered was to "rethink" the relationship of the government with the private sector. This vogue later materialized into policy theory, so-called New Public Management, which argues that public organizations should be run like a business (Hood 1990, 1991); promoting ideas such as competition, privatization, decentralization, and entrepreneurship (Gruening 2001). These ideas also found momentum

Florien M. Kruse and Patrick Jeurissen, *The Changing Private Sector Role in the Netherlands' Public/Private Sector Healthcare System* In: *The Public/Private Sector Mix in Healthcare Delivery.* Edited by: Howard A. Palley, Oxford University Press. © Oxford University Press 2023. DOI: 10.1093/oso/9780197571101.003.0007 within the Dutch healthcare system, and the managed competition model as suggested by Alain C. Enthoven (Enthoven and van de Ven 2007) inspired various healthcare reforms. The aims: to make the healthcare system more responsive to the needs of patients and payers, to improve efficiency, and to foster innovation (Commissie Structuur en Financiering van de Gezondheidszorg 1987; Raad voor de Volksgezondheid en Zorgautoriteit 2000). Managed competition was tied to solidarity, and thus the aim was also to preserve affordability of care for patients and to create universal access.

In contrast to market-oriented healthcare reforms in various other countries, the shift toward (commercial) privatization did not take place in the Netherlands (Maarse 2006), and the number of for-profit healthcare insurers and providers is still limited today (Jeurissen et al. 2021).

This chapter examines how Dutch healthcare addresses horizontal equity, equal access to those with equal need and those with equal resources pay the same; and vertical equity, variation in access according to need and those with more resources pay more. We also address how the public/private mix works in Dutch healthcare, and how this system scores on equity and quality of care. This chapter follows the definition of quality of care of the Institute of Medicine in the United States: Quality of care is safe, effective, patient centered, timely, efficient, and equitable (Institute of Medicine 2001). The focus of this chapter is on the medical care and the long-term care sectors (primarily elderly long-term care).

This chapter is organized as follows: First, we give some background information about the Dutch healthcare system; second, we explain the public/private mix of finance and delivery in the medical and long-term care sectors. Third, we explore the possible impact of the public/private mix on equity and quality of care. Last, we reflect on our assessments and provide some lessons learned and policy recommendations.

Background

Dutch Healthcare System

To gain universal access to care, three healthcare systems/laws orchestrate the delivery of these services: (1) Health Insurance Act (HIA); (2) Long-Term Care Act (LTCA); (3) Social Support Act (SSA) (see Table 7.1).

Table 7.1. Healthcare systems in the Netherlands

	Health Insurance Act (HIA)	Long-Term Care Act (LTCA)	Social Support Act (SSA)
Scope	Medical care, pharmaceuticals, mental health, and nursing at home	Institutional long-term care	Social support at home
Eligibility	General practitioner is gatekeeper; some preauthorization by healthcare insurers	Needs-based assessment by a central office at the national level	Needs-based assessments by municipalities
Funding	Social and flat-rate premiums and some tax supplements	Social insurance	Taxes fund municipal block grants
Purchaser	Private healthcare insurance companies	Public care offices (executed by healthcare insurance companies)	Municipalities
Competition	Multiple payer	Single payer	Single payer
Copayments/deductible	€385 deductible, voluntary add-ons up to €885	Means-tested copayments	Fixed copayments
Introduction year	2006	2015	2007/2015

The HIA was implemented in 2006. It rests on three competitive managed markets: (1) insurance market; (2) purchasing market; and (3) provision market. Healthcare insurers act as third payers, representing their clientele. Subscribers are allowed to annually switch from their healthcare insurer (open enrollment), and each year about 7% actually do (Nederlandse Zorgautoriteit [NZa] 2019a). Healthcare providers then "compete" for insurer contracts and negotiate with them on price, volume, and quality (Maarse, Jeurissen, and Ruwaard 2016).

The reform of the Dutch long-term care system took place in 2007 and 2015. In contrast to the HIA reform, its aim was much more to control spiraling costs and to make long-term care services more client oriented (Maarse and Jeurissen 2016). Municipalities became responsible for all social care (SSA), while long-term care services (LTCA) on a continuing (24/7) bas were delegated to so-called regional care offices [Zorgkantoren]. These offices became responsible for purchasing all long-term care services in their respective regions. The largest regional healthcare insurer runs the regional

care office as a monopsony (Maarse and Jeurissen 2016). With regard to social care, the assumption was that decentralization toward the municipalities
should make care delivery more efficient, and therefore budgets were cut severely (Kroneman et al. 2016). In addition, the reform initiated a shift toward
nonresidential care—that people should receive care in their own homes for
as long as possible (Maarse and Jeurissen 2016).

Financing Medical Care—Public/Private Mix

Financing of medical care in the Netherlands under the HIA consists of a
mix of public and private funding. Public financing consists of a mix of social premiums and government grants (Wammes, Stadhouders, and Westert
2020). Private funding consists of nominal community-rated premiums,
a deductible, and certain copayments as well as complementary insurance
for those who seek such additional coverage. These resources are managed
and allocated by private healthcare insurers (active purchasing). In general,
copayments in the Netherlands are relatively low: 11% of the total healthcare
expenditure, compared to the 22% European average in 2018 (Organization
for Economic Cooperation and Development [OECD] 2020).

Before the 2006 reform, the sickness funds covered around 60% of the
population and were the main actors that purchased and financed healthcare (Walschots 2004). Although sickness funds were nominally private
(nonprofit) entities, they operated under public law, and market incentives
were minimal. The government stiffly regulated prices, volumes, contracts
with providers, and issues such as wages and internal reserves and claim
ratios. A parallel private restitution insurance scheme was also available for
the people over a certain income threshold (similar to the current German
system). This was provided by private companies or private subsidiaries
from the sickness funds. One of the main elements of the reform was that the
new insurance scheme became fully private: sickness funds transformed toward private companies. This holds important legal consequences because it
constrains the power of the government over healthcare insurers.

Under the new reform, private healthcare insurers were positioned to
be responsible to purchase healthcare and make contracts with healthcare
providers (Maarse, Jeurissen, and Ruwaard 2016). In a way, the reform
embodies a compromise between the publicly oriented sickness funds and
the private healthcare insurers. For example, the sickness funds received

from the reform a risk-adjustment scheme, social premiums, and purchasing agreements with providers, while the private insurers got a nominal premium, a deductible, and, most importantly, the regulation of the new health insurance scheme under private law rather than public law. Formally, healthcare insurers could operate for a profit. However, since they were not allowed to distribute profits, most decided to operate as nonprofit entities. Consult Box 7.1,for more information about the for-profit ban.

The Netherlands upholds a statutory medical care package. All residents and nonresidents are obliged to purchase healthcare insurance that covers for this package. Children, up to 18 years, are automatically covered (Wammes, Stadhouders, and Westert 2020). However, there exists a substantial variety among the different policies and add-ons that people can opt for, resulting in a large range of options. One can roughly divide these options into three main clusters. First, there is the option to opt for a benefits-in-kind plan, which limits the insured to the providers in the network (around 75% of the population), or a restitution plan, which guarantees full choice of providers (around 20% of the population) (NZa 2019a); 5% of the insured have a mix.

Box 7.1. For-Profit Ban in the Netherlands

Since 1977, the Netherlands has imposed a ban on distributing profits to third parties for healthcare providers. The ban applies to those healthcare providers that offer intramural reimbursable care (i.e., hospitals, independent treatment centers, and nursing homes) and provide reimbursable care (Plomp 2011). This implies that most outpatient care (domically care services) does not need to comply to this ban, although it appears that here nonprofits dominate the provider landscape.

The idea after the reforms was to lift this ban at some point in the future since for-profit ownership seemed a logical element in a private healthcare system that is (partly) steered by competition. However, the for-profit ban became a contested political issue, and a tug of war over a legal proposition to end the ban on profit distributions followed between political parties and between Parliament and the Senate. The law became too politically sensitive after two investor-owned hospital sites defaulted on their payments and after outcries sparked by media reports that revealed that certain commercial domiciliary care providers made excessive profits. As a result, the minister of health withdrew the law altogether (Bruins 2019).

Benefit-in-kind plans only partially reimburse out-of-network providers and have become stricter on who to include in their networks. Partly as a consequence of this, premium differences between benefit-in-kind plans and restitution plans have widened. The other reason is that people with chronic diseases tend to favor more lavish restitution plans over stricter versions of the in-kind benefit plans, most notably the so-called budget policies. The differences in premiums between the lowest and highest are currently €499 (NZa 2020c).

Second, people can opt for voluntary comprehensive healthcare packages. This package is an add-on to the statutory minimum medical care package, typically including physiotherapy and dentistry and the coverage of certain copayments. In 2020, this kind of comprehensive healthcare package was bought by 14.4 million (83.3%) of the insured (NZa 2020c). Last, the insured can reduce their premiums by increasing their deductible by up to €500, on top of the mandatory deductible of €385. The number of people who increased their deductible has increased substantially over the past 10 years and now totals almost 15% of all insured. The rebate of insurers for those that take up a voluntary deductible differs, but typically fluctuates around 45% of the chosen deductible (NZa 2020c). On average an adult person pays via earmarked payroll taxes €1.784 and €1.414 (plus deductibles) via their flat rate premiums per year (NZa 2020c).

Impact on Equity

The Netherlands scoresvery good on equity and access compared to other countries (Doty et al. 2021). Thus, accessibility is not deemed a pressing issue in the Netherlands. The system provides for high levels of solidarity (Jeurissen 2016). Solidarity is safeguarded by five main instruments. First, healthcare insurers are obliged to accept all applicants; in other words, they cannot deny or select enrollees (open enrollment). Second, healthcare insurers are not allowed to differentiate premiums based on the health risks of the insured (community rating). The government compensates the healthcare insurers based on the risk profiles of their clientele by means of collective risk adjustments. Third, a statutory obligation ensures coverage of a minimum package of medical care services, which means that, in principle, patients have access to the fundamental care they need. Fourth, people with lower incomes receive a healthcare allowance to be able to bear the

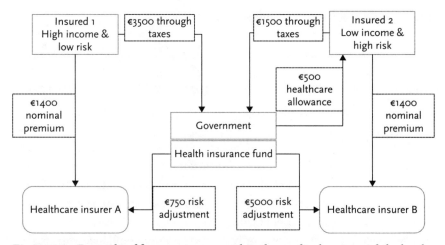

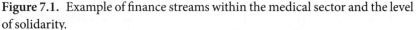

Figure 7.1. Example of finance streams within the medical sector and the level of solidarity.

Source: Inspired by (Nederlandse Zorgautoriteit (NZa 2016).

flat-rate premium of the statutory package (see Figure 7.1). Fifth, if people fail to pay premiums (defaulters), a law has been imposed that supports those people and ensures that they are still insured (*Wet structurele maatregelen wanbetalers zorgverzekering; Wet verbetering wanbetalersmaatregelen*) (Ministerie van Volksgezondheid Welzijn en Sport 2020).

As shown above, the insurance market is designed to minimize equity issues. However, several aspects still hamper equity and accessibility.

First, since 2012, the government has economized on the healthcare allowance by reducing the eligibility threshold. Since 2006, the number of people eligible has declined, reaching 300,000 in 2018 (Ministerie van Financiën/ Inspectie der Rijksfinanciën 2020). In practice this means that the working population with low incomes is less well compensated for their health expenses.

Second, the number of people who are uninsured is low. In 2018, these accounted for no more than 25,000 inhabitants, often undocumented immigrants (see Table 7.2). However, after a period of decline, these numbers are on the rise again. The number of people who fail to pay for their health insurance (defaulters), however, remains a bigger issue. On the upside, the number of defaulters have been in decline since 2014.

Third, one political contested issue is whether the mandatory deductible of €385 hinders people to seek (specialist) medical care. The deductible does

Table 7.2. Number of people uninsured in the Netherlands

	2014	2015	2016	2017	2018
Number of people uninsured	29,454	24,269	22,960	17,424	24,205
Number of people who fail to pay their healthcare insurance	325,810	312,037	277,023	249,044	224,714

Source: NZa 2019 (Nederlandse Zorgautoriteit (NZa 2019a).

not apply to primary care services, but it does apply for specialist medical care, mental health, allied health services, and pharmaceuticals. In 2019, a survey found that 5% of the respondents did not seek medical care because of healthcare costs (Meijer et al. 2020). In earlier surveys, researchers found that socioeconomic status was only related to noncompliance with regard to use of medicines (van Esch et al. 2015), and they also did not find a relationship between the increase of the deductible over the years and noncompliance effects (van Esch et al. 2017). Furthermore, the Netherlands scores compared well to other countries with respect the number of respondents who were said to have skipped doctor visits, tests, treatments, follow-up, or prescription medicines because of private cost (Doty et al. 2021). In 2020, of the respondents in the Netherlands, 9% said that they skipped care because of costs, and this is very low compared to other countries, such as Australia, New Zealand, and the United States, which scored above 20%. Only Norway scored better, with 8% (Doty et al. 2021). One study, however, did find that copayments of €200 for a specialist treatment have severely hindered access to mental care services (Ravesteijn et al. 2017; van der Lee, de Haan, and Beekman 2019). As a result, in 2013, the copayments specific for mental health were abolished.

Fourth, the possibility to choose a voluntary deductible may reduce risk solidarity between the healthy and those with existing health conditions; therefore, it may also introduce additional equity concerns that relate to the affordability of these deductibles across patient groups. Individuals with a low socioeconomic status who opt for a high deductible would be more at risk to high, possibly catastrophic, out-of-pocket costs. This is one reason that many municipalities offer their residents on welfare a collective plan that covers for the statutory deductible and is paid from local appropriations.

Evidence shows that persons who opted to increase the voluntary deductible have generally lower healthcare costs than those who stick to the mandatory deductible (Remmerswaal, Boone, and Douven 2019). In other words, those that choose to increase their deductible are aware of their health risks and, in turn, benefit from a premium discount (Remmerswaal, Boone, and Douven 2019). In addition, persons with a low income are more receptive then high-income people to shun care if they face a voluntary deductible (Remmerswaal et al. 2019).

Fifth, purchasing complementary voluntary insurance is another issue that holds potential consequences for equity. Complementary voluntary insurance might be quite expensive, and this might hinder access for people with lower socioeconomic status. Indeed, individuals who opt for a basic healthcare package are more often younger (≤35 years old) and healthier, but no clear relationship with income was found (NZa 2017b). In contrast, research showed that oral health (a service that falls under the complementary voluntary insurance scheme) for Dutch low-income people over 55 years old is worse compared to other European countries (Shen and Listl 2018).

Sixth, even though healthcare insurers are not allowed to deny any applicant (open enrollment) and are compensated for the risk profile of their clientele, the Dutch Healthcare Authority (NZa) raised concerns that healthcare insurers target their marketing at a low-risk population (NZa 2020c). For example, people who are young and who opt for a voluntary deductible and a strict (and cheap) network plan are most likely more profitable than people with chronic diseases and who enroll in plans with more choice and better coverage for complementary services. Even with a collective risk adjustment system, targeting a large low-risk clientele seems to be financially profitable—a worrying sign of adverse risk selection, which even in a sophisticated risk adjustment system as the Dutch have raises equity issues.

Seventh, healthcare insurers are obliged by law to ensure access to timely, spatially accessible, and sufficient quality of healthcare (NZa 2020a). This refers to all care covered by the basic medical package. The Dutch Healthcare Authority monitors whether healthcare insurers fulfill these obligations. However, this obligation is somewhat ambiguous and far from clearly defined. Although norms do exist for waiting times, these are not always enforced that strictly, and currently many areas of specialist mental health exceed these thresholds. Other elements are even less clear; for example, what is the maximum travel distance for the respective treatments? The obligation for healthcare insurance companies to ensure suitable and accessible care is essentially an open norm and is highly context dependent (NZa 2020a).

In light of this argument, it is also important to highlight the clause in the HIA that grants patients the freedom to choose their healthcare provider, also if a patient goes to an out-of-network provider. In such cases, healthcare insurers have to compensate approximately 75% of the average costs of that treatment (NZa 2018). While this clause improves the accessibility of care, it undermines the purchasing power of healthcare insurers, reducing their ability to select healthcare services that offer high-value care for their clientele (Rijksoverheid 2020b).

Impact on Quality

Medical services in the Netherlands are generally of good quality: Compared to other European countries, the Netherlands has low preventable and treatable causes of mortality (OECD 2020). Healthcare insurers and healthcare providers are supposed to negotiate with regard to price, volume, and quality. However, negotiating on quality has been proven to be less extensive than for price and volume. One study stated that insurers are in principle willing to fulfill this expectation but are hindered by the insensitivity of patients to be advised by their healthcare insurer, the lack of transparency of quality of care, consumer indifference, and reputation risks (Stolper et al. 2019). Empirical studies also showed that Dutch healthcare insurers still selectively contract healthcare providers based on quality of care (Heijink, Mosca, and Westert 2013). To tackle this, a few healthcare insurers and hospitals have been able to establish multiannual contracts with the aim of improving value of care—reducing costs and enhancing quality of care (van Dulmen et al. 2020). These multiannual contracts try to break the cycle of fee-for-service incentives. The idea is that such global budgets create the leeway toward providing only appropriate and necessary care required. Hospitals are also compensated for possible initial investments to reorganize their volume-maximization business models. Up to now, such contracts are not tied to explicit quality benchmarks, such as in accountable care organizations in the United States. However, hospitals and their doctors in a more qualitative way need to be accountable toward their payers by explaining how they are reforming their models of care (van Dulmen et al. 2020).

Delivery of Medical Care—Nonprofit Dominant

Private, nonprofit, hospitals have always been the dominant ownership form in the Dutch hospital sector (Jeurissen 2010). In the early 1900s, some of the hospitals were also owned by the government, but these were the minority (Jeurissen 2010). Currently, Dutch hospitals are nonprofit hospitals, owing mainly to the for-profit ban (see Box 7.1). However, since the reform of the medical care sector, three hospitals have been acquired by private investors (Jeurissen et al. 2021). Two of these hospitals—belonging to the same chain—defaulted on their payments (van Manen, Meurs, and van Twist 2020). One had to close its doors. The other hospital site merged with a local nonprofit hospital (Bruins 2018). In contrast to these two hospitals, the third investor-owned hospital is financially stable (BDO 2018) and currently the only surviving investor-owned hospital in the Netherlands; however, it is limited with respect to allocating profits to their investors.

In contrast to the hospital sector, independent treatment centers (ITCs) (in the United States called ambulatory surgical centers) tend to be more commercially oriented (Kruse 2021). The for-profit ban also applies to those ITCs that provide reimbursable care under the statutory benefit basket, but ITCs tend to share their rewards with their owners and employees via crafty accounting practices or high salaries (Kruse 2021; Baeten et al. 2019). ITCs have been on the rise in the Dutch healthcare sector (Kruse, Spierings, et al. 2018). Possible reasons for the growth of the ITC sector are various. One of these factors is that ITCs have carved out a niche market, distinguishing themselves from hospitals by organizing in "focus clinics" for elective, non-emergency, care. Another reason is that ITCs are typically more efficient and offer lower contracted prices (Kruse et al. 2019; NZa 2012). However, the out-of-network prices do not seem to differ between ITCs and general hospitals (Tulp et al. 2020). ITCs seem to be able to survive under the favorable patient freedom-of-choice clause in the HIA. Finally, the Covid-19 pandemic illustrated that ITCs could fulfill a crucial role in the Dutch healthcare system by offering spare capacity (Zelfstandige Klinieken Nederland [ZKN] 2020).

Impact on Equity

Access to medical care services is generally very good compared to other Western countries (Doty et al. 2021; van de Ven et al. 2013). However, several weaknesses are worth noting.

First, the pre-reform medical care system already showed signs that the migrant population had difficulties accessing healthcare providers, especially specialized medical care, infringing horizontal equity (Stronks, Ravelli, and Reijneveld 2001). Currently, almost 25% of the Dutch population has a migration background (2021), and this share has increased over the years (Centraal Bureau voor de Statistiek [CBS] 2021a, 2021 b). The five largest migration groups come from Turkey, Morocco, Surinam, Indonesia, Germany, and Poland (CBS 2021b). It remains unclear whether the reform eased these concerns or actually worsened them. Some studies found no prominent differences between ethnic groups (Klaufus, Fassaert, and de Wit 2014; Dahrouge et al. 2018), also not with respect to adverse events after treatments (van Rosse et al. 2013). However, other studies found unequal utilization patterns of care among the migrant population compared to the indigenous population (Uiters et al. 2006; Posthumus et al. 2016) (see Box 7.2).

Not only horizontal equity is important, but also vertical equity concerns can be raised for the migrant population, which require efforts to target these social groups in their healthcare needs (Dorgelo, Pos, and Kosec 2013). The non-Western population, and sometimes in particular the refugee group, shows different risk profiles compared to the Western population (e.g., for chronic diseases), implying that they require a different health provision approach (Oosterberg et al. 2013; Lamkaddem et al. 2013). Another aspect that relates to vertical equity is a language barrier between the healthcare professional and patient. This barrier can increase patient safety risks (van Rosse et al. 2016). Healthcare professionals could receive financial compensation for the use of an interpreter, but this compensation scheme, however, was abolished in 2012 for most healthcare sectors (Pharos et al. 2014). The majority of the hospitals neverthelessfound ways to finance the interpreter within their organization (van Rosse et al. 2013). Primary care services can

---

Box 7.2. Evidence on the Accessibility of Healthcare Services of the Non-Western Population in the Netherlands

One study showed that the Netherlands scores worse with respect to how immigrants experience access to healthcare services compared to other European countries (Hanssens et al. 2016). One study found that general practitioners (GPs) play a vital role for the migrant population: GPs support matter with respect to how well immigrants are able to access medical care (Uiters et al. 2006). Furthermore, the migrant population pays the GP a visit more often than the indigenous population does (van der Gaag et al. 2017). One possible explanation is that the migrant population has a higher health illiteracy, especially among the Turkish population (van der Gaag et al. 2017). The migrant population is however diverse, and utilization patterns differ between migrant groups (Uiters et al. 2006).

opt for financial support when they are located in deprived areas to compensate for additional costs, such as an interpreter. Yet, the removal of the financial compensation for an interpreter within the healthcare system remains a contested and political issue (van Ark 2021).

Second, waiting times have increased more recently. Professional norms exist with regard to a maximum acceptable waiting time for patients in need of nonacute and elective care, referred to as *Treeknormen*. Since 2015, waiting times have increased and noncompliance to the Treeknormen has increased sharply (Figure 7.2). A possible explanation for these increasing waiting times is that for several years pseudoglobal budgets have curbed the growth in healthcare costs in the Netherlands (Visser et al. 2017). These budgets apply to all healthcare providers that provide reimbursable medical care in the Netherlands. The percentage growth that hospitals were allowed by these global budgets has become tighter over the years. This has sharply slowed the growth in volumes, which probably has worsened the waiting times for care.

The impact of waiting times on the quality of care is unclear. On the one hand, this mainly relates to less-complex elective care. On the other hand, for most patients waiting longer for nonurgent care may reduce their quality of life. In certain subsectors, most notably care for severe mental disorders, waiting times might be so long that it could harm patients (Louwes and

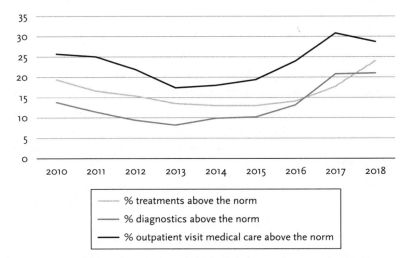

Figure 7.2. The share of treatments and diagnostics that are above the maximum acceptable waiting time (in %).

Source: Volksgezondheidenzorg.info 2021.

Raaijmakers 2020). The suspension of non–Covid-19 care during the pandemic has sharpened the discussion about the negative impact of long waiting times, for not only urgent care, but also elective care (Bulstra 2020; Rijksinstituut voor Volksgezondheid en Milieu 2020). For example, suspending a hip operation can impose restrictions on the patients' mobility and, therefore, on quality of life (Bulstra 2020).

Third, both the hospital sector and ITC sector have strongly consolidated over the years (Kruse Spierings, et al. 2018). Increasing one's market power against healthcare insurers is one explanation for this trend (Nederlandse Vereniging van Ziekenhuizen [NVZ] 2016). Regions with a few hospitals raised concerns about decreasing choice and accessibility (Maarse, Jeurissen, and Ruwaard 2016), which might affect quality of care. Furthermore, the professional associations and insurance companies imposed volume thresholds for complex care, only allowing those hospitals to perform complex treatments if they reach a specific threshold. This further fosters market concentration (den Engelsen, Hatenboer, and Hoff 2019).

Accessibility and Quality of ITCs

One of the concerns raised about ITCs is that they treat a different case mix compared to hospitals. There are indeed indications that this is applicable for the Dutch ITCs, and this is also in line with international studies (Street et al. 2010; Winter 2003). However, case mix differences between ITCs and general hospitals might be less stark in the Netherlands than in the United Kingdom or Greece (Kruse et al. 2019; Kruse, Stadhouders et al. 2018). Nevertheless, on average ITCs do seem to treat patients with high socioeconomic status (Kruse et al. 2019). One of the reasons could be that people with a high socioeconomic status more often have a restitution insurance package, while ITCs have not been contracted as much by healthcare insurers than by hospitals (Tulp et al. 2020).

The ITCs can reduce hospital waiting lists and free expensive and demanding hospital beds for complex patients. The specialties with the longest waiting times are those that involve allergology, ophthalmology, gastrointestinal services, and liver diseases (NZa 2017a). Most of these specialties are also offered by ITCs, who profile themselves as having short waiting times. During the Covid-19 pandemic, ITCs presented themselves as a solution to reduce the backlog of elective care (ZKN 2021).

Quality Differences of ITCs Compared to Hospitals

The rise of ITCs spark the question: Do ITCs provide better quality of care compared to general hospitals? In line with international studies (Trybou et al. 2014), studies that analyzed the Dutch context also painted a mixed picture: No clear quality differences between ITCs and general hospitals existed (Kruse et al. 2019; Tulp et al. 2020). This was measured in terms of outcome measures such as patient-reported outcome measures (i.e., PROMs) and share of revision within 1 year after a total hip or knee operation. However, ITCs do have better patient satisfaction scores than general hospitals (Kruse et al. 2019). And since contracted prices are on average lower for ITCs than general hospitals (Kruse et al. 2019), ITCs have the potential to be value-adding entities to the general healthcare system (Kruse 2021).

Financing Long-Term Care—Public/Private Mix

The long-term care system is mainly publicly funded, and private payments consist of approximately 9% of total long-term care costs (2018–2020) (based on our calculation) (CBS 2021c, 2021d).

Long-term care in the Netherlands is both needs and means tested. In the LTCA, the Central Administration Office defines eligibility and need for those that seek 24/7 care and support. For the SSA, municipalities are in charge to assess both eligibility and need, also referred to as the "kitchen table dialogues" (*keukentafelgesprek*). Those eligible for 24/7 care under the LTCA can opt for three healthcare packages to finance and organize their long-term care provision. The first package is an in-kind intramural care package—often, but not always, a package that is used in a nursing home setting. Alternative intramural packages might apply for disabled persons and for people who need continuous support for their mental disorder. For these in-kind packages, the care office purchases long-term care on behalf of the applicant. How much a care recipient has to pay out of pocket depends on their income level (see Figure 7.3). The vast majority of care—over 80%—is delivered through these in-kind packages (Post et al. 2019).

The second package is an in-kind extramural package, a home care package, also referred to as a total home care package or modular care package. The two other packages are designed for clients who seek more tailored solutions, creating more opportunities for a living environment

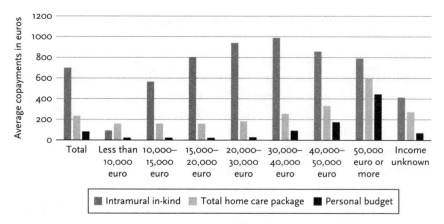

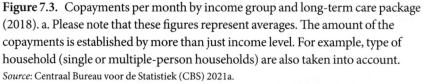

Figure 7.3. Copayments per month by income group and long-term care package (2018). a. Please note that these figures represent averages. The amount of the copayments is established by more than just income level. For example, type of household (single or multiple-person households) are also taken into account.
Source: Centraal Bureau voor de Statistiek (CBS) 2021a.

that fits with personal preferences. The use of these packages do increase more rapidly than the in-kind benefits (den Besten, Kiziltekin, and van der Lee 2019). For these packages, care offices only purchase the provision of care; the care recipient has to organize and finance their own housing. This could be either their own home or a private apartment that is operated by a nursing home. Copayments apply; however, these are significantly less than for the in-kind intramural care package (see Figure 7.3). The third and last option is a personal budget. This gives clients the strongest instrument for personal empowerment. Recipients of a personal budget have to purchase and organize their own care; a care office does not act like a third party in this regard. Housing is also a private responsibility. Copayments are the lowest for this option (see Figure 7.3), but for similar caseload, the financial compensation for personal budgets is also substantially lower than for in-kind care.

Equity

The Dutch long-term care system provides comprehensive coverage of costs, and every Dutch citizens has access to long-term care (Muir 2017). However, there are a few obstacles that hinder equity and access. First, as explained above, the benefits from the long-term care packages are means tested, and copayments' size differ per long-term care package. As a result, the selection of long-term care packages relates to socioeconomic status. This introduces equity and access issues in the long-term care system because people with high socioeconomic status are able to use certain delivery models of the long-term care system to their benefit and opt for an extramural care package instead of an intramural in-kind package and pay for housing privately, circumventing public copayments. Second, significant variation exists between municipalities with respect to the provision and use of social care (Pommer and Boelhouwer 2016). Social care has been decentralized, and municipalities have significant freedom to decide how to organize social care in their region and how much they want to spend (Kroneman et al. 2016). The fact that the central government has set the local copayments nationwide at a flat €19 per 4 weeks have made social services such as housekeeping much more attractive for a high-income clientele, who previously paid for such services themselves (Rijksoverheid 2020a). All in all, this could lead to inequal access to social care services across the Netherlands. Third, the long-term care reform in 2015 introduced different financing streams and organized the care in different silos. This made the long-term care system a complex web of institutions and laws that many care seekers found hard to maneuver (Kromhout 2018; Kromhout, van Echtelt, and Feijten 2020). This has implications for equal access to long-term care services, especially those with low "health literacy" (Heijmans et al. 2016).

Quality

The Netherlands is the biggest spender on long-term care as a share of economic output (gross domestic product) compared to other countries (OECD 2019). The question is however, if this also translates into better quality of care, such as patient-centered care. OECD statistics show that the Netherlands scores just about OECD average on quality in the long-term care sector (OECD 2019). This is measured in terms of percentage of long-term care facility residents with at least one healthcare-associated infection; antimicrobial-resistant bacterial isolates from healthcare-associated infections in long-term care; percentage of long-term care facility residents with at least one pressure ulcer. However, staff levels are probably at least as important for quality of care, and the Netherlands scores well in terms of the share of long-term care workers per 100 people aged 65 and over compared to other OECD countries (OECD 2019). The education of nurses can be categorized into three levels: intermediate, higher, and academic (Huisman-de Waal et al. 2019). Around 15% of the nurses in the LTCA (2019) have a bachelor (academic) degree (HBO) (based on our calculations, specialist nurses were a separate category) (CIBG 2021).

Competition on quality of care among long-term care providers is limited to the fact that they can earn small bonuses if they comply with certain quality standards or have conducted quality-increasing projects. This also applies for social care: Municipalities only apply a minimum quality threshold to contract providers.

The healthcare reform in 2015 came with additional cost-containment measures in the long-term care sector. However, this was short-lived. Shortly after the budget cuts, critical voices were aired that these measures jeopardize the quality of long-term care. The political attitude shifted along with the public mood, and (much) more money was invested to improve the quality of care. In 2017, an overarching quality norm for all nursing homes was introduced (*Kwaliteitskader Verpleeghuiszorg*) (Zorginstituut Nederland [ZiN] 2017), with also a much higher soft staff/client ratio norm. Additional public funds were allocated to the long-term care system to improve quality of care, so-called quality budgets (NZa 2019b). Long-term care providers can apply for these budgets at their care offices. Of the budget, 85% is earmarked for personnel (e.g., to increase the staff/client ratio), and the remaining 15% can be used more widely to improve the quality of care (Zorgverzekeraars Nederland 2019). In total these additional resources amounted to about 3% of the budget of the LTCA (2019) (NZa 2020b). This stands in sharp contrast to social care as social care budgets were significantly reduced with the long-term care reform (Maarse and Jeurissen 2016), and municipalities experienced substantial losses on their block grants (BDO 2021).

Delivery of Long-Term Care—Nonprofit Dominant

Similar to the hospital sector, the nonprofit sector dominates, primarily because of the for-profit ban (see Box 7.1). However, the for-profit nursing home sector has grown rapidly over recent years (Bos, Kruse, and Jeurissen 2020). In 2019, around 12% of the nursing home locations were for-profit organizations (Bos, Kruse, and Jeurissen 2020). The number of for-profit nursing homes' clients are however substantially under 12% because for-profit entities are generally much smaller (Kruse 2021). The for-profit nursing home sector has found a way to circumvent the for-profit ban by providing extramural care packages (i.e., extramural in-kind and personal budgets) and privately charge for rent and extra services (Plaisier and den Draak 2019).

Impact on Equity and Access

The Dutch long-term care system faces serious challenges to organize sufficient supply of appropriate services (Hinkema, van Heumen, and Egter van Wissekerke 2019). In the aftermath of the substantial budget appropriations, waiting times have been increasing in the long-term care sector. In 2019, the number of people on the waiting list was 16,164. This number was 16% higher than in 2018 (NZa 2019c). The number of people on the waiting list differs strongly by region (NZa 2019c). This regional variation sparks the question about equity and access: Where someone lives matters in so far as how long someone has to wait to receive suitable long-term care.

For-profit nursing home are mainly accessible for an affluent social group because of substantial private payments for rent and additional services. It is also financially beneficial for those of higher socioeconomic groups to opt for a for-profit home because of the substantial income-dependent copayments for intramural in-kind packages (see Figure 7.3). This enables those with deep pockets to skip the queue to access long-term care and to gain access to small-scale, often more person-oriented, care (Kruse 2021). To support this argument, a study also found that for-profit homes are mainly located in more affluent areas (Bos. Kruse, and Jeurissen 2020).

Impact on Quality

The for-profit nursing home sector offers small-scale, more person-oriented, care than the "traditional" nonprofit sector. Evidence has shown that small-scale homes—largely for-profit entities—relate to better quality of care compared to their counterparts (Pot and de Lange 2010). This relationship is more indirect, for example, because small-scale nursing homes tend to have higher average hours of care per client (Pot and de Lange 2010). However, direct comparisons between for-profit and nonprofit providers are difficult to make because of the large variation in case mix and organizational form.

From an ethical perspective, findings suggest that the market logic (e.g., the drive to maximize profits) and the logic of care (e.g., emotional and social values behind caregiving) can be largely reconciled in the Dutch for-profit nursing home sector, unlike the theory of the moral limits of markets would predict (Kruse et al. 2020). One explanation for this finding is that the provision of nursing home care should be considered as separate units. The nursing home setting has been strongly commodified in the Dutch for-profit sector, whereas the care relationship has been much less affected (Kruse et al. 2020).

Discussion

Accessibility and quality within the Dutch healthcare system are still among the best in the world, despite concerns raised when the healthcare system transformed toward a more market-oriented system. This may be due to the approach of reaping the benefits of the private sector, but taming its risks by applying strict regulations on how to finance and provide healthcare and keeping the market incentives on a strict leash. The for-profit ban for healthcare insurers and intramural care providers (i.e., ITCs, hospitals, and nursing homes) stands out in this regard. However, the high levels of horizontal and vertical equity in the Netherlands have witnessed some pressures in recent years. Within this chapter, two developments stand out.

First, commercially oriented providers have been increasingly able to carve out a parallel sector for services whereby a for-profit ban applies: ITCs and for-profit nursing homes. These providers have been able to grow because of the increasing reliance on market incentives and lack of public funding in a capital-intensive sector to accommodate growing wishes and demands. This parallel sector has introduced additional (horizontal) equity issues in the Netherlands because they tend to predominantly cater to residents with high socioeconomic status, especially in the nursing home sector.

Second, high-income people might have reaped more consumer surplus from the benefits of choice among increasingly diversified insurance plans under the HIA and more tailored packages in the LTCA that fit their needs as well as a nationwide flat rate, but low copayments, for all social support services. The high socioeconomic groups are better equipped to maneuver and use the complex healthcare system to their advantage. The different healthcare reforms introduced a web of separate laws, rules, systems, and institutions, making the system very complex. The complexity of the Dutch healthcare system makes it less accessible for people with low education, weaker social support system, and low health literacy. Groups such as some immigrant communities may face the need for additional support to address their higher needs. However, in a system dominated by insurance logic, the room for initiatives that improve vertical equity is limited to flanking policies, for example, to fund for native interpreters. As in other countries, people with high socioeconomic background live on average longer than people with a low socioeconomic background, and the gap has slightly increased over the years and currently stands at about 5 years (Broeders et al. 2018). The increasingly complex healthcare system and reliance on patient choice has created some equity challenges in a still very egalitarian system. It shows that healthcare delivery systems alone do not seem to be capable of narrowing this gap, which suggests that targeted policies are also needed to improve both public health and the social determinants of health.

References

Baeten, Steef, Pim Diepstraten, Jan-Peter Heida, Jori Hoendervanger, Luuk Willems, and Leslev Zanen. 2019. *Uitkering van dividend door zorgaanbieders. Praktijkanalyse en effectanalyse.* Utrecht: Finance Ideas and SiRM.

BDO. 2018. "BDO-Benchmark ziekenhuizen 2018. Zorginfarct dreigt. Sector vereist radicaal nieuw businessmodel." https://www.bdo.nl/nl-nl/perspectieven/benchmark-ziekenhuizen-2018-sector-vereist-radicaal-nieuw-businessmodel-bmz18

BDO. 2021. *BDO-benchmark Nederlandse Gemeenten 2021. Financiële situatie onhoudbaar. Tekorten groeien verder, uitvoering openbaar bestuur verschraalt.* Amsterdam: BDO.

Bos, Aline, Florien Kruse, and Patrick Jeurissen. 2020. "For-Profit Nursing Homes in the Netherlands: What Factors Explain Their Rise?" *International Journal of Health Services* 50(5): 431–443. https://doi.org/10.1177/0020731420915658

Broeders, Dennis, Djurre Das, Roel Jennissen, Will Tiemeijer, and Marianne de Visser. 2018. *WRR-Policy Brief 7. Van verschil naar potentieel. Een realistisch perspectief op sociaaleconomische gezondheidsverschillen.* Den Haag: Wetenschappelijke Raad voor het Regeringsbeleid (WRR).

Bruins, Bruno Johannes. 2018. *Faillissement MC Slotervaart en MC IJsselmeerziekenhuizen.* Den Haag: Ministerie van Volksgezondheid Welzijn en Sport.

Bruins, Bruno Johannes. 2019. *Wijziging van de Wet toelating zorginstellingen en enkele andere wetten teneinde investeringsmogelijkheden in medisch-specialistische zorg te bevorderen (Wet vergroten investeringsmogelijkheden in medisch-specialistische zorg).* Den Haag: Eerste Kamer der Staten-Generaal.

Bulstra, Sjoerd. 2020. "Afschalen electieve zorg niet zo onschuldig als het lijkt." https://www.skipr.nl/blog/afschalen-electieve-zorg-niet-zo-onschuldig-als-het-lijkt/

Centraal Bureau voor de Statistiek (CBS). 2021a. *Gefactureerde eigen bijdrage Wlz op MLZ-peildatum in maand.*

Centraal Bureau voor de Statistiek (CBS). 2021b. "Hoeveel mensen met een migratieachtergrond wonen in Nederland?" CBS. https://www.cbs.nl/nl-nl/dossier/dossier-asiel-migratie-en-integratie/hoeveel-mensen-met-een-migratieachtergrond-wonen-in-nederland-.

Centraal Bureau voor de Statistiek (CBS). 2021c. *Opgelegde eigen bijdrage voor AWBZ/ Wlz—en Wmo-zorg.*

Centraal Bureau voor de Statistiek (CBS). 2021d. *Wlz-zorg in natura; uitgaven/volume op basis van declaraties; leveringsvorm.*

CIBG. 2021. *DigiMV 2019* [Dataset]. The Haag: Ministerie van Volksgezondheid, Welzijn en Sport.

Commissie Structuur en Financiering van de Gezondheidszorg. 1987. *Bereidheid tot verandering.* The Haag: Distributiecentrum overheidspublicaties.

Companje, Karel-Peter. 2014. "Financing High Medical Risks in the Netherlands: Healthcare, Social Insurance and Political Compromises." In *Financing High Medical Risks*, edited by Karel-Peter Companje. Amsterdam: Amsterdam University Press.

Dahrouge, Simone, William Hogg, Elizabeth Muggah, and Ted Schrecker. 2018. "Equity of Primary Care Service Delivery for Low Income "Sicker" Adults across 10 OECD Countries." *International Journal for Equity in Health* 17(1): article 182. https://doi.org/10.1186/s12939-018-0892-z.

den Besten, Michiel, Tufan Kiziltekin, and Marcel van der Lee. 2019. *ZorgCijfers Monitor. Zorgverzekeringswet en Wet langdurige zorg 2e kwartaal 2019.* Diemen, Netherlands: Zorginstituut Nederland (ZiN).

den Engelsen, Bram, Douwe Hatenboer, and Jan-Luuk Hoff. 2019. *Invloed van kwaliteitsstandaarden op toegankelijkheid van medisch specialistische zorg.* Amersfoort, Netherlands: Twynstra Gudde & Zorginstituut Nederland.

Dorgelo, Annemiek, Sarah Pos, and Helena Kosec. 2013. *Handreiking Patiëntenparticipatie van migranten in Onderzoek, Kwaliteit en Beleid.* Utrecht: Pharos. https://www.pharos.nl/wp-content/uploads/2019/05/Handreiking_patientenparticipatie-Pharos.pdf

Doty, Michelle, Roosa Tikkanen, Molly FitzGerald, Katherine Fields, and Reginald Williams II. 2021. "Income-Related Inequality in Affordability and Access to Primary Care in Eleven High-Income Countries." *Health Affairs* 40(1): 113–120. https://doi.org/10.1377/hlthaff.2020.01566

Enthoven, Alain, and Wynand van de Ven. 2007. "Going Dutch—Managed-Competition Health Insurance in the Netherlands." *New England Journal of Medicine* 357(24): 2421–2423. https://doi.org/10.1056/NEJMp078199

Gruening, Gernod. 2001. "Origin and Theoretical Basis of New Public Management." *International Public Management Journal* 4(1): 1–25. https://doi.org/10.1016/S1096-7494(01)00041-1

Hanssens, Lise, Jens Detollenaere, Wim Hardyns, and Sara Willems. 2016. "Access, Treatment and Outcomes of Care: A Study of Ethnic Minorities in Europe." *International Journal of Public Health* 61(4): 443–454. https://doi.org/10.1007/s00038-016-0810-3

Heijink, Richard, Ilaria Mosca, and Gert Westert. 2013. "Effects of Regulated Competition on Key Outcomes of Care: Cataract Surgeries in the Netherlands." *Health Policy* 113(1–2): 142–150. https://doi.org/10.1016/j.healthpol.2013.06.003

Heijmans, Monique, Hanneke Zwikker, Iris van der Heide, and Jany Rademakers. 2016. *Hoe kunnen we de zorg beter laten aansluiten bij mensen met lage gezondheidsvaardigheden?* Utrecht: NIVEL.

Hinkema, Menno, Stefan van Heumen, and Norman Egter van Wissekerke. 2019. *Prognose capaciteitsontwikkeling verpleeghuiszorg.* Delft, Netherlands: TNO.

Hood, Christopher. 1990. "De-Sir Humphreyfying the Westminster Model of Bureaucracy: A New Style of Governance?" *Governance. An International Journal of Policy, Administration, and Institutions* 3(2): 205–214.

Hood, Christopher. 1991. "A Public Management for All Seasons?" *Public Administration* 69(1): 3–19. https://doi.org/10.1111/j.1467-9299.1991.tb00779.x

Huisman-de Waal, Getty, Theo Achterberg, Lisette Schoonhoven, and Maud Heinen. 2019. "The Netherlands." In *Strengthening Health Systems through Nursing: Evidence from 14 European Countries*, edited by Anne Marie Rafferty, Reinhard Busse, Britta Zander-Jentsch, Walter Sermeus, and Luk Bruyneel. Brussels: European Observatory on Health Systems and Policies.

Institute of Medicine. 2001. *Crossing the Quality Chasm: A New Health System for the 21st Century.* Washington, DC: National Academy Press.

Jeurissen, Patrick. 2010. "For Profit-Hospitals. A Comparative and Longitudinal Study of the For-Profit Hospital Sector in Four Western Countries." Doctoral thesis, Erasmus University Rotterdam.

Jeurissen, Patrick. 2016. *Steeds meer zorg, een betaalbare oplossing.* Oratie. Nijmegen, Netherlands: RadboudumcNijmegen.

Jeurissen, Patrick, Florien Kruse, Reinhard Busse, David Himmelstein, Elias Mossialos, and Steffie Woolhandler. 2021. "For-Profit Hospitals Have Thrived Because of Generous Public Reimbursement Schemes, Not Greater Efficiency: A Multi-Country Case Study." *International Journal of Health Services* 51(1): 67–89. https://doi.org/10.1177/0020731420966976

Klaufus, Leonie, Thijs Fassaert, and Matty de Wit. 2014. "Equity of Access to Mental Health Care for Anxiety and Depression among Different Ethnic Groups in Four Large Cities in the Netherlands." *Social Psychiatry and Psychiatric Epidemiology* 49(7): 1139–1149 https://doi.org/10.1007/s00127-014-0837-9.

Kromhout, Mariska. 2018. "Bedoelingen van de Hervorming Langdurige Zorg: het algemene kader." In *Veranderde zorg en ondersteuning voor mensen met een beperking*, edited by Mariska Kromhout, Nora Kornalijnslijper, and Mirjam de Klerk. Den Haag: Sociaal en Cultureel Planbureau (SCP).

Kromhout, Mariska, Patricia van Echtelt, and Peteke Feijten. 2020. *Sociaal domein op koers? Verwachtingen en resultaten van vijf jaar decentraal beleid.* Den Haag: Sociaal en Cultureel Planbureau (SCP).

Kroneman, Madelon, Wienke Boerma, Michael van den Berg, Peter Groenwegen, Judith de Jong, and Ewout van Ginneken. 2016. *Netherlands. Health System Review. 2016. European Observatory on Health Systems and Policies* 18(2): 1–240.

Kruse, Florien. 2021. "Healthcare Provision: Open for Business? Market Dynamics, Performance and Ethics of Commercially-Oriented Healthcare Providers, Using the Netherlands as a Case Study." PhD dissertation, Radboudumc.

Kruse, Florien, Stef Groenewoud, Femke Atsma, Onno van der Galiën, Eddy Adang, and Patrick Jeurissen. 2019. "Do Independent Treatment Centers Offer More Value than General Hospitals? The Case of Cataract Care." *Health Services Research* 54(6): 1357–1365. https://doi.org/10.1111/1475-6773.13201

Kruse, Florien, Wieke Ligtenberg, Anke Oerlemans, Stef Groenewoud, and Patrick Jeurissen. 2020. "How the Logics of the Market, Bureaucracy, Professionalism and Care Are Reconciled in Practice: An Empirical Ethics Approach." *BMC Health Services Research* 20(1): article 1024. https://doi.org/10.1186/s12913-020-05870-7

Kruse, Florien, Else Spierings, Eddy Adang, and Patrick Jeurissen. 2018. "Marktconcentratie is ook een punt van zorg bij zelfstandige behandelcentra." *Economisch Statistische Berichten (ESB)* 103(4766): 453–455.

Kruse, Florien, Niek Stadhouders, Eddy Adang, Stef Groenewoud, and Patrick Jeurissen. 2018. "Do Private Hospitals Outperform Public Hospitals Regarding Efficiency, Accessibility, and Quality of Care in the European Union? A Literature Review." *International Journal of Health Planning and Management* 33(2): e434–e453. https://doi.org/10.1002/hpm.2502

Lamkaddem, Majda, Karien Stronks, Annette Gerritsen, Walter Devillé, and Marie-Louise Essink-Bot. 2013. "Gezondheid en zorggebruik van vluchtelingen: Vervolgonderzoek onder mensen met een verblijfsvergunning in Nederland." *Nederlands Tijdschrift voor Geneeskunde (NTvG)* 157.

Louwes, Korrie, and Karina Raaijmakers. 2020. *Toezicht IGJ/NZa op aanpak wachttijden ggz.* Utrecht: IGJ & NZaUtrecht.

Maarse, Hans. 2006. "The Privatization of Health Care in Europe: An Eight-Country Analysis." *Journal of Health Politics Policy and Law* 31(5): 981–1014. https://doi.org/10.1215/03616878-2006-014

Maarse, Hans, and Patrick Jeurissen. 2016. "The Policy and Politics of the 2015 Long-Term Care Reform in the Netherlands." *Health Policy* 120(3): 241–245. https://doi.org/10.1016/j.healthpol.2016.01.014

Maarse, Hans, and Patrick Jeurissen. 2020. "Private Health Insurance in the Netherlands." In *Private Health Insurance. History, Politics and Performance*, edited by Sarah Thomson, Aanna Sagan, and Elias Mossialos. Cambridge: Cambridge University Press.

Maarse, Hans, Patrick Jeurissen, and Dirk Ruwaard. 2016. "Results of the Market-Oriented Reform in the Netherlands: A Review." *Health Economics, Policy and Law* 11(2): 161–178. https://doi.org/10.1017/S1744133115000353

Meijer, Marloes, Anne Brabers, Aafke Victoor, and Judith De Jong. 2020. *Negen procent van de mensen ziet af van zorg vanwege de kosten. Er is sprake van een daling in de periode 2016-2019.* Utrecht: NIVEL.

Ministerie van Financiën/Inspectie der Rijksfinanciën. 2020. *Eenvoud of maatwerk: Alternatieven voor bestaande toeslagenstelsel. IBO toeslagen deelonderzoek 2.* The Haag: Ministerie van Financiën/Inspectie der Rijksfinanciën.

Ministerie van Volksgezondheid Welzijn en Sport (VWS). 2020. *VWS—Verzekerdenmonitor 2020.* The Haag: Ministerie van Volksgezondheid Welzijn en Sport (VWS).

Muir, Tim. 2017. *Measuring Social Protection for Long-Term Care.* Paris: OECD

Nederlandse Vereniging van Ziekenhuizen (NVZ). 2016. *25 jaar patiënt in beeld. Brancherapport algemene ziekenhuizen 2016.* Utrecht: NVZ.

Nederlandse Zorgautoriteit (NZa). 2012. "Monitor zelfstandige behandelcentra—Een kwalitatieve en kwantitatieve analyse." Utrecht: NZa. https://www.zorgkennis.net/downloads/kennisbank/F4C-kennisbank-Monitor-zelfstandige-behandelcentra-817.pdf

Nederlandse Zorgautoriteit (NZa). 2016. *Monitor Zorgverzekeringen 2016*. Utrecht: NZa.

Nederlandse Zorgautoriteit (NZa). 2017a. *Actieplan wachttijden in de zorg*. The Haag: Ministerie van Volksgezondheid, Welzijn en Sport.

Nederlandse Zorgautoriteit (NZa). 2017b. "Monitor Zorgverzekeringen 2017." Utrecht: NZa. https://puc.overheid.nl/nza/doc/PUC_3656_22/1/

Nederlandse Zorgautoriteit (NZa). 2018. "Monitor Zorgverzekeringen 2018." Utrecht: NZa. https://puc.overheid.nl/nza/doc/PUC_3656_22/1/

Nederlandse Zorgautoriteit (NZa). 2019a. "Monitor Zorgverzekeringen 2019." Utrecht: NZa.

Nederlandse Zorgautoriteit (NZa). 2019b. *Onderzoeksrapport Sturing op kwaliteitsverbetering verpleeghuiszorg door zorgkantoren (Onderzoeksrapport toezicht op de langdurige zorg 2019*. Utrecht: NZa.

Nederlandse Zorgautoriteit (NZa). 2019c. *Samenvattend rapport. Uitvoering Wet langdurige zorg door zorgkantoren 2018/2019*. Utrecht: NZa.

Nederlandse Zorgautoriteit (NZa). 2020a. "De zorgplicht: handvatten voor zorgverzekeraars." Utrecht: NZa. https://puc.overheid.nl/doc/PUC_323566_22

Nederlandse Zorgautoriteit (NZa). 2020b. "Kerncijfers langdurige zorg." https://www.nza.nl/zorgsectoren/langdurige-zorg/kerncijfers-langdurige-zorg

Nederlandse Zorgautoriteit (NZa). 2020c. "Monitor Zorgverzekeringen 2020." Utrecht: NZa. https://magazines.nza.nl/nza-specials/2020/03/monitor-zorgverzekeringen-2020

OECD. 2019. *Health at a Glance 2019*. Paris: OECD.

OECD. 2020. *Health at a Glance: Europe 2020: A State of Health in the EU Cycle*. Paris: OECD.

Oosterberg, Eldine, Devillé Walter, Lizzy Brewster, Charles Agyemang, and Maria van den Muijsenbergh. 2013. "Chronische ziekten bij allochtonen. Handvatten voor patiëntgerichte zorg bij diabetes, hypertensie en COPD." *Nederlandse Tijdschrift voor Geneeskunde (NTvG)* 157: A5669.

Pharos, Nederlands Huisartsen Genootschap (NHG), Landelijke Huisartsen Vereniging (LHV), Koninklijke Nederlandse Organisatie van Verloskundigen (KNOV), Koninklijke Nederlandsche Maatschappij tot bevordering der Geneeskunst (KNMG), Nederlands Instituut van Psychologen (NIP), Nederlandse Patiënten Consumenten Federatie (NPCF), and Nederlandse Vereniging van Psychiatrie (NVvP). 2014. *Kwaliteitsnorm tolkgebruik bij anderstaligen in de zorg*. Utrecht: Pharos, NHG, LHV, KNOV, KNMG, NIP, NPCF, NVvP.

Plaisier, Inger, and Maaike den Draak. 2019. *Wonen met Zorg. Verkenning van particuliere woonzorg voor ouderen*. The Haag: Sociaal en Cultureel Planbureau (SCP).

Plomp, Emke. 2011. "Winst in de zorg. Juridische aspecten van winstuitkering door zorginstellingen." Doctoral thesis, UvA.

Pommer, Evert, and Jeroen Boelhouwer. 2016. *Overall rapportage sociaal domein 2015. Rondom de transitie*. The Haag: Sociaal en Cultureel Planbureau (SCP).

Post, Harry, Kees Huijsmans, Ronald Luijk, and Lisette Gusdorf. 2019. *Zorgthermometer ouderenzorg. Inzicht in de ouderenzorg*. Zeist, Netherlands: Vektis.

Posthumus, Anke, Gerard Borsboom, Jashvant Poeran, Eric Steegers, and Gouke Bonsel. 2016. "Geographical, Ethnic and Socio-Economic Differences in Utilization of Obstetric Care in the Netherlands." *PloS One* 11(6). https://doi.org/10.1371/journal.pone.0156621.

Pot, Anne Margriet, and Jacomine de Lange. 2010. *Monitor Woonvormen Dementie. Een studie naar verpleeghuiszorg voor mensen met dementie*. Utrecht: Trimbos Instituut.

Raad voor de Volksgezondheid en Zorgautoriteit (RVZ). 2000. *De rollen verdeeld.* The Haag: RVZ.

Ravesteijn, Bastian, Eli Schachar, Aartjan Beekman, Richard Janssen, and Patrick Jeurissen. 2017. "Association of Cost Sharing with Mental Health Care Use, Involuntary Commitment, and Acute Care." *JAMA Psychiatry* 74(9): 932–939. https://doi.org/10.1001/jamapsychiatry.2017.1847

Remmerswaal, Minke, Jan Boone, Michiel Bijlsma, and Rudy Douven. 2019. "Cost-Sharing Design Matters: A Comparison of the Rebate and Deductible in Healthcare." *Journal of Public Economics* 170: 83–97. https://doi.org/10.1016/j.jpubeco.2019.01.008

Remmerswaal, Minke, Jan Boone, and Rudy Douven. 2019. *Selection and Moral Hazard Effects in Healthcare.* The Haag: CPB Netherlands Bureau for Economic Policy Analysis. https://www.cpb.nl/sites/default/files/omnidownload/CPB-Discussion-paper-393-Selection-and-moral-hazard-effects-in-healthcare.pdf

Rijksinstituut voor Volksgezondheid en Milieu (RIVM). 2020. *Impact van de eerste COVID-19 golf op de reguliere zorg en gezondheid. Inventarisatie van de omvang van het probleem en eerste schatting van gezondheidseffecten.* The Haag: RIVM.

Rijksoverheid. 2020a. "Betaal ik een eigen bijdrage voor ondersteuning uit de Wmo?" https://www.rijksoverheid.nl/onderwerpen/zorg-en-ondersteuning-thuis/vraag-en-antwoord/eigen-bijdrage-wmo-2015#:~:text=Vanaf%202020%20betaalt%20u%20voor,is%20van%20een%20duurzame%20hulpverleningsrelatie

Rijksoverheid. 2020b. *Naar een toekomstbestendig zorgstelsel. Brede maatschappelijke heroverweging.* The Haag: Rijksoverheid.

Shen, Jing, and Stefan Listl. 2018. "Investigating Social Inequalities in Older Adults' Dentition and the Role of Dental Service Use in 14 European Countries." *European Journal of Health Economics* 19(1): 45–57. https://doi.org/10.1007/s10198-016-0866-2

Stolper, Karel, Lieke Boonen, Frederik Schut, and Marco Varkevisser. 2019. "Managed Competition in the Netherlands: Do Insurers Have Incentives to Steer on Quality?" *Health Policy* 123(3): 293–299. https://doi.org/10.1016/j.healthpol.2018.08.018

Street, Andrew, Peter Sivey, Anne Mason, Marisa Miraldo, and Luigi Siciliani. 2010. "Are English Treatment Centres Treating Less Complex Patients?" *Health Policy* 94(2): 150–157. https://doi.org/10.1016/j.healthpol.2009.09.013

Stronks, Karien, Anita Ravelli, and Sijmen Reijneveld. 2001. "Immigrants in the Netherlands: Equal Access for Equal Needs?" *Journal of Epidemiology and Community Health* 55(10): 701–707. https://doi.org/10.1136/jech.55.10.701

Trybou, Jeroen, Melissa De Regge, Paul Gemmel, Philippe Duyck, and Lieven Annemans. 2014. "Effects of Physician-Owned Specialized Facilities in Health Care: A Systematic Review." *Health Policy* 118(3): 316–340. https://doi.org/10.1016/j.healthpol.2014.09.012

Tulp, Anouk, Florien Kruse, Niek Stadhouders, and Patrick Jeurissen. 2020. "Independent Treatment Centres Are Not a Guarantee for High Quality and Low Healthcare Prices in The Netherlands—A Study of 5 Elective Surgeries." *International Journal of Health Policy and Management* 9(9): 380–389. https://doi.org/10.15171/ijhpm.2019.144

Uiters, Ellen, Walter Deville, Marleen Foets, and Peter Groenewegen. 2006. "Use of Health Care Services by Ethnic Minorities in The Netherlands: Do Patterns Differ?" *European Journal of Public Health* 16(4): 388–393 https://doi.org/10.1093/eurpub/ckl040

van Ark, Tamara. 2021. *Antwoorden op Kamervragen van het Kamerlid Dik-Faber (CU) over het belang van professionele tolken in de zorg.* The Haag: Ministerie van Volksgezondheid, Welzijn en Sport.

van der Gaag, Marieke, Iris van der Heide, Peter Spreeuwenberg, Anne Brabers, and Jany Rademakers. 2017. "Health Literacy and Primary Health Care Use of Ethnic Minorities in the Netherlands." *BMC Health Services Research* 17(1): 1–9. https://doi.org/10.1186/s12913-017-2276-2

van der Lee, Arnold, Lieuwe de Haan, and Aartjan Beekman. 2019. "Rising Co-payments Coincide with Unwanted Effects on Continuity of Healthcare for Patients with Schizophrenia in the Netherlands." *PloS One* 14(9). https://doi.org/10.1371/journal.pone.0222046

van de Ven, Wynand, Konstantin Beck, Florian Buchner, Erik Schokkaert, Frederik Schut, Amir Shmueli, and Juergen Wasem. 2013. "Preconditions for Efficiency and Affordability in Competitive Healthcare Markets: Are They Fulfilled in Belgium, Germany, Israel, the Netherlands and Switzerland?" *Health Policy* 109(3): 226–245. https://doi.org/10.1016/j.healthpol.2013.01.002

van Dulmen, Simone, Niek Stadhouders, Gert Westert, Erik Wackers, and Patrick Jeurissen. 2020. *Op weg naar hoge kwaliteit en lage kosten in de medisch specialistische zorg. Evaluatie veranderprogramma's Rivas Zorggroep en Bernhoven*. Nijmegen, Netherlands: IQ healthcare.

van Esch, Thamar, Anne Brabers, Christel van Dijk, Peter Groenewegen, and Judith de Jong. 2015. *Inzicht in zorgmijden. Aard, omvang, redenen en achtergrondkenmerken*. Utrecht: NIVEL.

van Esch, Thamar, Anne Brabers, Christel van Dijk, Lisette Gusdorf, Peter Groenewegen, and Judith de Jong. 2017. "Increased Cost Sharing and Changes in Noncompliance with Specialty Referrals in The Netherlands." *Health Policy* 121(2): 180–188. https://doi.org/10.1016/j.healthpol.2016.12.001

van Manen, Jaap, Pauline Meurs, and Marcus van Twist. 2020. *De aangekondigde ondergang. Onderzoek naar de faillissementen van het MC Slotervaart en de MC IJsselmeerziekenhuizen*. The Haag: Commissie onderzoek faillissementen ziekenhuizen.

van Oorschot, Wim. 2006. "The Dutch Welfare State: Recent Trends and Challenges in Historical Perspective." *European Journal of Social Security* 8(1): 57–76. https://doi.org/10.1177/138826270600800104

van Rosse, Floor, Martine de Bruijne, Maren Broekens, Karien Stronks, Marie-Louise Essink-Bot, and Cordula Wagner. 2013. *Etnische herkomst en zorggerelateerde schade. Monitor zorggerelateerde schade in Nederlandse ziekenhuizen*. Utrecht: NIVEL.

van Rosse, Floor, Martine de Bruijne, Jeanine Suurmond, Marie-Louise Essink-Bot, and Cordula Wagner. 2016. "Language Barriers and Patient Safety Risks in Hospital Care. A Mixed Methods Study." *International Journal of Nursing Studies* 54:45–53. https://doi.org/10.1016/j.ijnurstu.2015.03.012

Visser, Johan, Lydia van 't Veer, Jori Hoendervanger, Katlin Gaspar, Niek Stadhouders, Xander Koolman, and Jan-Peter Heida. 2017. *Eerste verkenning effecten hoofdlijnenakkoorden. In opdracht van het Ministerie voor Volksgezondheid, Welzijn en Sport*. Utrecht: SiRM, Celsus Academie & Talma Institute.

Walschots, Jan. 2004. *De prijsindexcijfers van zorg—en ziektekosten en de wijzigingen in de Ziekenfondswet en AWBZ per januari 2004*. Voorburg, Netherlands: Centraal Bureau voor de Statistiek.

Wammes, Joost, Niek Stadhouders, and Gert Westert. 2020. "International Health Care System Profiles. Netherlands." In *International Health Care System Profiles*, edited by R. Tikkanen, R. Osborn, E. Mossialos, A. Djordjevic, and G.A. Wharton. Washington, DC: Common Wealth Fund.

Winter, Ariel. 2003. "Comparing the Mix of Patients in Various Outpatient Surgery Settings." *Health Affairs* 22(6): 68–75. https://doi.org/10.1377/hlthaff.22.6.68

Zelfstandige Klinieken Nederland (ZKN). 2020. "Mediaoverzicht: Klinieken leveren hulp bij corona epidemie." ZKN. Last Modified March 27, 2020. https://www.zkn.nl/nie uws/mediaoverzicht-klinieken-leveren-hulp-bij-corona-epidemie/1080

Zelfstandige Klinieken Nederland (ZKN). 2021. "Klinieken kunnen helpen wachtlijsten ziekenhuizen weg te werken." ZKN. https://www.zkn.nl/nieuws/klinieken-kunnen-hel pen-wachtlijsten-ziekenhuizen-weg-te-werken/1432

Zorginstituut Nederland (ZiN). 2017. *Kwaliteitskader Verpleeghuiszorg. Samen leren en verbeteren.* Diemen, Netherlands: ZiN.

Zorgverzekeraars Nederland. 2019. *Toelichting model begroting verantwoording kwaliteitsbudget 2020 verpleeghuiszorg. Versie 2019-1.1.* Zeist, Netherlands: ZN.

8

The Public/Private Sector Mix in the Italian Healthcare System

Some Issues of Equity and Quality of Care

Federico Toth

Introduction

Since 1978, Italy has had a National Health Service (NHS), financed mainly through general taxation. The Italian NHS is committed to providing a wide range of healthcare services to all residents. The NHS absorbs approximately 6.6% of Italian gross domestic product (GDP) and employs over 650,000 people (including nurses, doctors, administrative staff, technicians, auxiliary personnel, managers, social workers, etc.). Approximately two-thirds of the healthcare financed by the NHS is provided by public providers (staff and facilities belonging to the NHS itself), and one-third is provided by freelancers and private facilities affiliated with the public service (Mapelli 2012; Toth 2014b). The NHS assists the entire population, and there is no possibility of opting out. Albeit the fact that the Italian NHS resolves to be universal and comprehensive, it fails to finance all the healthcare needed by Italians, who bear out-of-pocket costs for part of their pharmaceutical treatments, dental, and other specialist care. The private component corresponds to 26% of the total healthcare expenditure and is largely out of pocket (Organization for Economic Cooperation and Development [OECD] 2020).

As in the other contributions in this volume, special attention is paid in this chapter to the mix of public and private in the healthcare system (at the level of both financing and service provision) and the consequences in terms of the equity and quality of healthcare.

In the health field, the concept of equity can be attributed to various meanings (Mooney 1983; Le Grand 1987; Culyer and Wagstaff 1993; Culyer

Federico Toth, *The Public/Private Sector Mix in the Italian Healthcare System* In: *The Public/Private Sector Mix in Healthcare Delivery*. Edited by: Howard A. Palley, Oxford University Press. © Oxford University Press 2023.
DOI: 10.1093/oso/9780197571101.003.0008

2001; Braveman 2006). To avoid misunderstandings, it is then appropriate to define right away the conceptual categories that used in the next sections. The concept of equity can be applied to multiple dimensions of the healthcare system (Mooney 1983; Wagstaff and Van Doorslaer 2000). In this chapter, we specifically address: (1) equity in financing; (2) equity in resource allocation; (3) equity in access to healthcare; and (4) equity in healthcare utilization. Thus, it is crucial to look at these four forms of equity in more detail.

When it comes to equity in *healthcare finance,* we refer to the ways in which residents contribute to the financing of healthcare. In this regard, it is useful to make a distinction between *vertical* equity and *horizontal* equity (Wagstaff and van Doorslaer 2000; Culyer 2001). By vertical equity, we mean the principle according to which one must contribute in relation to one's ability to pay: Those who are richer must pay more than those who are poorer. The goal of vertical equity is therefore achieved through a system of healthcare contribution that is proportional or, even better, progressive with respect to income earned (Hussey and Anderson 2003). The principle of horizontal equity is instead achieved to the extent that individuals with an equal ability to pay actually end up making equal contributions, regardless of other conditions such as gender, occupation, place of residence, marital status, and so on.

It is interesting to reason in terms of equity in relation to the criteria of *allocation of health resources* (Culyer and Wagstaff 1993). As far as the Italian case is concerned, the reference is, specifically, to the criteria through which the national government allocates the health budget among the regions. Also, on this front, the principle of equity can be presented in two versions: assigning the same identical quota for each resident (regardless of the actual needs) or, on the contrary, allocating resources according to need (assigning to the regions a differentiated budget in proportion to the health needs of their respective populations).

The third dimension to which the principle of equity can be applied concerns *access to care* (Mooney 1983; Le Grand 1987; Goddard and Smith 2001). In this sense, equity corresponds to the formula "equal access to available care for equal need" (Whitehead 1992). This definition implies the requirement that individuals should face the same personal costs of receiving medical treatment (Le Grand 1987). The most common barriers to accessing healthcare are waiting times, user charges, distance between place of residence and place of care, language differences, and so on (Le Grand 1987; Goddard and Smith 2001).

Finally, we come to equity in healthcare utilization (Mooney 1983; Wagstaff and Van Doorslaer 2000). Here, again, a distinction can be made between vertical and horizontal equity (Culyer and Wagstaff 1993; Culyer 2001). Horizontal equity corresponds to the principle that persons in equal need should be treated the same (Le Grand 1987; Culyer and Wagstaff 1993). This implies that the delivery of medical care is independent of variables such as income, educational level, personal connections, gender, ethnicity, occupation, sexual orientation, and so on. Vertical equity corresponds to a separate goal, which can be summarized in the principle that people with different needs are appropriately treated differently. In other words, people with greater medical needs should receive more attention and resources than those with lesser needs (Culyer and Wagstaff 1993; Culyer 2001). Health equity is also related to the idea that patients are receiving a satisfactory quality of health care. Italy's NHS seeks to achieve quality of healthcare services through an accreditation process. Accreditation hinges on extensive quality criteria, including the appropriateness and timeliness of interventions, health status factors, and patient satisfaction. It encompasses management of human and technical resources, the consistency of the provider's activity with regional health planning, and the evaluation of the activities conducted and the results achieved (Donatini 2020).

We utilize and analyze various meanings of the concept of equity in the following sections. We try to understand the extent to which the architecture and actual functioning of the Italian healthcare system promote equity in its various forms.

The Regionalized Structure of the Italian Nhs

The NHS is structured into three levels: national, regional, and local.

Starting from the *national* level, despite the fact that the reforms of the last 30 years have aimed at promoting an accentuated decentralization, the Italian Ministry of Health still plays a central role in the planning of the healthcare system. First of all, the Ministry of Health is responsible for determining the overall budget to be allocated to the public health service. A second strategic task assigned to the Ministry of Health concerns the definition of the so-called essential levels of assistance (*Livelli Essenziali di Assistenza*, LEAs), a discussion of which follows. It is the responsibility of the national government and parliament to regulate the health professions, whereas the governance of pharmaceuticals rests with the Italian Medicines Agency (*Agenzia Italiana del Farmaco*, AIFA).

Turning to the *regional* level, since the reform of 1992–1993, regional governments have acquired great importance in the health field. The Italian Constitution places health protection among the matters of concurrent legislation between the state and the regions. This means, in essence, that the national government must limit itself to determining the principles of a general nature, whereas the regions and autonomous provinces are given wide discretion in planning and organizing healthcare in their territory. This discretion leads to the possibility for regional governments to configure their health service in the way they deem most appropriate, adopting organizational models that can be very different from each other (Toth 2014b; Cinelli et al. 2020). Some regional healthcare systems, including those of Lombardy and Lazio, outsource a greater volume of care to private providers. It is up to the individual regional government to establish the criteria for the accreditation and remuneration of providers, both public and private, and how to allocate resources among the different care areas (primary care, hospital care, prevention, etc.). Some regional systems, including those of Tuscany, Emilia-Romagna, and Veneto, have invested more in territorial care in recent years, whereas other regions, including Lazio and Lombardy, have traditionally devoted more resources to hospital care.

The regionalized structure of the Italian NHS is justified by the principle through which individual regions must be given the flexibility to adapt their services to the particular needs of their respective populations. In fact, as discussed below, regional autonomy poses a problem of horizontal inequity and disparity in the quality of care offered.

The autonomy recognized to the regions in health matters is such that there are those who argue that it no longer makes sense to speak of a unitary NHS in Italy: The Italian health system should rather be conceived as the federation of about 20 regional systems (Mapelli 2012). In fact, significant differences emerge between one region and another, in terms of both the organizational structures adopted and the quality of the services provided (Mapelli 2012; Toth 2014b). The gap between the north and the south of the country also appears to be particularly worrying (Toth 2014a). The differentiated ways in which Italian regions have coped with the Covid-19 pandemic (Toth 2021b) constitute further confirmation of the differences between one regional health system and another.

The regionalized structure of the Italian NHS is generating continuous friction between the national and regional governments: The former is called on to guarantee the uniformity of services throughout the country and must also check that the regions do not exceed the budget allocated to them; the regions, for their part, accuse the central government of not allocating sufficient resources to the funding of the NHS.

Finally, we come to the third level: the *local* one. In the majority of regions, with the exception of Lombardy,[1] the health authorities operate on the local level and are divided into two categories: population-based local health authorities (*Aziende Sanitarie Locali,* ASLs) and public hospital enterprises (*Aziende Ospedaliere,* AOs). The territorial authorities (ASLs) have the task of guaranteeing their patients all the services included in LEAs. Stating that the local health authorities must guarantee certain services does not mean they must necessarily provide them themselves: The local health authorities are free to outsource part of the services for which they are responsible to external suppliers. Each region can determine, at its own discretion, how many ASLs to set up in its territory and the relative size.[2]

The local health authorities, therefore, function with regard to the direct supply and commissioning of services. AOs, on the contrary, perform only production functions, having the primary task of providing specialized care. Only part of Italian public hospitals have been transformed into autonomous public enterprises; there are currently about 50 AOs in the entire national territory (Cinelli et al. 2020). Public hospitals that do not constitute autonomous public enterprises remain productive facilities within their respective local health authorities: They enjoy limited autonomy with respect to AOs. To underline the different nature of ASLs and AOs, it is established that the former are financed on the basis of the number of patients residing in their respective territories, whereas AOs are remunerated on the basis of the volume of specialist services actually provided.

It should be noted that, compared to the NHS in the United Kingdom and Nordic countries, the Italian NHS is less public and more open to private providers (Toth 2021a). About one-third of hospital beds are in privately owned facilities (OECD 2020). More than 90% of private hospitals are contracted with the NHS; this means that they provide part of their services on behalf of the public service. Private providers are funded in part by the NHS and, in part, directly by users.

Who Is Covered by the NHS?

The NHS can be assessed by the degree of *prevalence* and *generosity* of insurance coverage (Toth 2019). Prevalence refers to the breadth of insurance coverage (who is covered), whereas generosity refers to the depth (what services are guaranteed) and height (what proportion of cost is covered) of insurance coverage (WHO 2010; Stuckler et al. 2010; Lagomarsino et al. 2012). A high degree of prevalence should be a guarantee of horizontal equity in the access to healthcare. A low level of generosity usually results in low equity in healthcare finance, whereas a high degree of generosity should promote equity (both vertical and horizontal) in access to care.

Law No. 833 of 1978, which established the Italian NHS, stipulates that the latter be universal and comprehensive (Mapelli 2012; Toth 2014b). A system is considered universal to the extent that the right to healthcare is guaranteed to the entire resident population. The *comprehensiveness* of the system, on the other hand, concerns the generosity of the care provided: The public service is required to offer a generous package of health services, which takes charge of all the healthcare needs of the population. Healthcare that is deemed essential should be provided free of charge or, at most, with a copayment by users.

We first analyze the dimension of the prevalence of health coverage. One may ask whether the Italian NHS actually guarantees health coverage to the entire population or whether some categories remain to some extent excluded.

The Italian NHS provides assistance not only to all Italian citizens but also to foreigners who are, for various reasons, in the national territory. In case of emergency care, citizens of European Union (EU) member countries are entitled to care in all public facilities in Italy. Even non-EU citizens with a regular residence permit enjoy the assistance of the public health service; they can register, free of charge, with the NHS and choose their own family doctor (thus ensuring equal treatment with Italian citizens). Some non-EU countries (including Switzerland, Norway, Argentina, Brazil, and Australia) have signed specific agreements with the Italian government, under which the citizens of these states—by exhibiting a certificate issued in their country of origin—are entitled to urgent healthcare provided by the Italian NHS. They are therefore granted coverage in reference to urgent and non-postponable care.

Finally, we come to non-EU citizens without residence permits; they are also guaranteed medical care in Italy. In theory, this assistance should not be free of charge: Foreigners without a regular residence permit cannot register with the NHS and should pay for the medical treatments they receive. There is, however, a way to avoid payment: It is sufficient for the assisted person to fill in a self-certification in which the person declares to being indigent and therefore unable to meet medical expenses. In doing so, the foreigner without a stay permit is assigned an STP card—that is, a Temporarily Present Foreigner code that entitles one to not only free emergency care but also other treatments that are deemed indispensable and urgent.[3] The STP code does not grant the possibility to register with a family doctor, thus excluding access to most primary and preventive healthcare.

We can therefore conclude that, in Italy, at least on paper, urgent health-care is not denied to anyone. The situation is different with regard to visits, examinations, and procedures that are not deemed urgent. In fact, there are certain categories of persons who encounter difficulties in accessing the NHS for nonurgent care. Those who have difficulty in accessing nonurgent healthcare services are, above all, homeless persons, individuals without a regular residence permit, migrants hosted in collective facilities, and part of the Roma and Sinti populations. Individuals belonging to these categories are called, in jargon, "invisibles," as they are not formally registered with the NHS. The invisibles usually have peculiar healthcare needs compared to the rest of the population. With respect to these categories of disadvantaged, there is clearly a problem of equity, both horizontal and vertical, in access to care.

From a social and healthcare perspective, homeless people are especially at risk for merely bureaucratic issues—that is, individuals without a permanent place of residence are not registered with any ASL and therefore cannot select a family doctor. This problem is often bypassed by giving the homeless a fictitious domicile, but this is not always the case. Therefore, many homeless individuals and undocumented foreigners have access to emergency care (especially via the emergency ward) but do not receive a significant portion of primary and preventive care services (Toth 2016).

Usually a problem concerning foreigners more than Italians, some categories of individuals, despite having the right to the services of the NHS, do not access them (or access them only partially) because they are unable to follow the required administrative procedures or because they are unaware of their rights.

As explained further in this chapter, all of the categories just mentioned (undocumented immigrants, the poor, the homeless, other marginalized individuals, etc.) are not completely abandoned, as they can count locally on a varied network of public programs, charities, and nonprofit organizations.

The Comprehensiveness of the Services Provided by the NHS

In addition to universality, the second objective that the NHS must pursue concerns the comprehensiveness of the services provided. The public service is required to offer a vast array of healthcare services covering all of the population's healthcare requirements. So, it is important to next assess how generous the package of care offered by the Italian NHS is.

One can start by saying that, in Italy, the public health service provides a wide range of health-related services. The NHS's sphere of competence is not limited to the diagnosis and treatment of diseases or illnesses but spans healthcare from prevention to rehabilitation, from food hygiene to veterinary services, from protection of motherhood to workplace safety, from school health to mental health, and from assistance for the handicapped to the fight against drug addiction (Toth 2016). In Italy, the tasks assigned to the public health service are very broad indeed: The NHS would therefore seem to have adopted a comprehensive approach to health promotion.

However, some healthcare treatments are not financed by the NHS, at least not to all patients. Since the 1990s, it has been concluded that, in the health field, the formula of "giving everything to everyone," although desirable, is not financially sustainable. It was then preferred to draw up a list of services that the public health service is required to guarantee, in a uniform manner, to all its patients; these are the so-called LEAs. LEAs therefore constitute the package of services that Italians are entitled to receive from the NHS free of charge or, at the most, by making a copayment.

The definition of the list of LEAs constitutes a crucial junction in the relations between the central government and the regions, insofar as it is precisely from the determination of the essential levels that the amount of resources that the state undertakes to allocate to the financing of the NHS should descend. The Ministry of Health is responsible for defining and updating the list of LEAs, as already mentioned. The list of LEAs was drawn up for the first time in 2001 and then subsequently updated in 2017.

The list of treatments considered essential is very long and includes several thousand healthcare services, divided into three categories: prevention and public health; territorial assistance; and hospital care. To avoid misunderstandings, alongside the list of services considered essential, the Ministry of Health prepared two further lists: that of services *partially* excluded and that of treatments *totally* excluded from LEAs.

Services that are partially excluded (as they can only be provided under certain conditions or to certain categories of patients) include, for example, outpatient physiotherapy and dental care. The NHS is committed to providing dental care only to children up to 14 years of age and to some specific categories of adults in particularly vulnerable health conditions (i.e., those affected by serious illness) or those requiring social aid (social vulnerability criteria are established by the individual regions). For the rest of the population, the public service only guarantees dental emergency coverage (i.e., in the presence of acute infections) and diagnostic examinations in cases of cancer of the oral cavity (Toth 2014b). In all other cases, dental care is the responsibility of the individual citizen.

Totally excluded from LEAs are (1) procedures whose direct purpose is not the protection of health (like most cosmetic surgery); (2) treatments whose effectiveness is not considered sufficiently proven by scientific evidence, including nonconventional treatments such as phytotherapy, homeopathy, and chiropractic; and (3) procedures that provide parity of benefits for the patient but are more expensive than others available.

This is the situation on paper. In practice, the situation is somewhat different.

The Ministry of Health monitors each year to which extent individual regions actually provide LEAs. From this monitoring (Ministero della Salute 2020), it emerged that, in recent years, the regions of the center-north (e.g., Emilia-Romagna, Tuscany, Piedmont, Veneto) have usually been able to provide the majority of LEAs in an appropriate manner and with reasonable waiting times. Many southern regions (especially Campania and Calabria), on the contrary, are largely defaulting on this aspect: They do not supply all LEAs, sometimes they do not supply them in an appropriate manner, and often they do not provide them in a reasonable time frame. The observation that some regions are largely at fault in guaranteeing LEAs clearly poses a problem of equity in access to care and plausibly in healthcare utilization.

Now it is necessary to draw conclusions about the comprehensiveness of the Italian NHS. Albeit promoting an ample array of procedures, the Italian public health service does not explicitly finance certain types of services. This raises an issue of horizontal equity in both funding and access to care. Add to this the fact that many regions (even though they are required to do so), in fact, are incapable of delivering all LEAs and delivering them in an appropriate and timely manner. We must therefore conclude that the principle of healthcare's comprehensiveness is not fully satisfied.

How the Italian NHS is Funded

The NHS funding process can be broken down into two phases. First, the national government determines the total amount of financial resources to be allocated to the NHS. The budget allocated at the national level is then divided among the individual regions.

The first step in the financing process is the responsibility of the national government, which must decide, each year, how many resources to allocate to the NHS. The budget allocated to the NHS is fed by a mix of direct and indirect taxes; the NHS financing system, as a whole, is to be considered progressive (Hussey and Anderson 2003; Toth 2021a). In principle, the budget for the NHS should be calculated in proportion to LEAs and the population's health needs; thus, the central government is required to provide the regions with the financial resources necessary to ensure LEAs for the entire population. Over the past two decades, however, the amount of the health budget appears to have been determined more pragmatically (Toth 2014b, 2020a). This decision was the result of bargaining both within the government and between the national government and regional presidents.

Since 2001, there has also been an attempt to plan the budget on a 3-year basis: On the basis of negotiations with the regions, the national government has made a habit of indicating how much money it would allocate to the NHS in subsequent years. However, this planning was inevitably subject to revisions, and the government was often forced to reduce the amounts agreed on. These reconsiderations by the national government naturally provoked complaints from regional governments.

The dispute between the state and the regions over the size of the healthcare budget has been going on for a long time; since at least the early 1990s, regions have accused the national government of allocating too few resources to the NHS. It is useful, in this regard, to provide some data. During the decade 2010–2019, public funding of the NHS was on average 110 billion euros (corresponding to roughly 6.6% of the GDP). In 2010, the NHS budget was 105.6 billion euros and 114.5 billion in 2019. This means that, in a decade, public health spending increased by less than 9 billion, growing by 0.9% each year on average, a rate lower than that of the average annual inflation. A sudden acceleration of public spending was recorded in the year 2020 due to the Covid-19 pandemic—that is, the budget allocated to the NHS exceeded 117 billion euros. In the years to come, further substantial increases in public health spending are expected.

The process through which the NHS budget is determined takes on great significance as it touches on the interests of many stakeholders. The stakes are high. The NHS accounts for more than 15% of all public spending in Italy and employs around 650,000 people (ISTAT [Istituto Nazionale di Statistica] 2020), which corresponds to 19% of all civil servants. Healthcare is also, by far, the main sector of regional intervention: If we consider the budgets of regions with ordinary statutes, they allocate over 80% of their budgets to healthcare.

The healthcare sector cannot, however, be considered just a public expenditure item. The health supply chain, which includes not only outpatient and hospital services but also the pharmaceutical sector and the medical device industry, plays a major role in the Italian economy; thus, it is worth around 11% of the GDP (Confindustria 2019). The healthcare sector employs more than 1.5 million workers, which rises to almost 2.4 million if the allied industries are also taken into account.

Therefore, regional governments are not the only ones interested in the adequate funding of the NHS. In addition to citizens, local authorities, and NHS employees, many private stakeholders have an interest at stake (Di Giulio and Toth 2014; Toth 2020a). It should be borne in mind that, in Italy, private healthcare is also closely linked to the fate of the public service. About a third of the NHS budget is used to pay private providers. Family doctors, for example, although employees of the NHS, have a contractual relationship with it and are paid by it. Most private hospital facilities and pharmacies are also contracted with the public service. Also, the amount of pharmaceutical expenditure charged to the public health service—to which the companies producing and distributing drugs are naturally interested—is estimated in proportion to the NHS budget.

In short, many players operating in the healthcare sector have a strong interest in ensuring that the financing of the public healthcare service is adequate (to maintain the quality of healthcare delivery) and possibly increased from 1 year to the next—that is, cuts (or lack of increases) in the NHS budget affect many components of the healthcare sector.

Once the total amount of resources to be allocated to the NHS has been established, the next step is to allocate these resources to the individual regions. As noted above, these regions are responsible for providing services to users. The issue of equity in resource allocation arises here. When it comes to deciding how much money to allocate to the NHS, the regions present a united front against the national government, putting pressure on it to provide as much money as possible. Instead, when it comes to discussing the criteria for distributing the budget, the regions find themselves in competition with one another, and each tries to push through the allocation criteria it deems most advantageous for itself.

For several years now, NHS budget allocation has been based primarily on the number of residents in each region. In addition to the number of residents, the age structure of the regional populations is also taken into account. This means that regions with older populations on average are allocated more resources than regions with younger populations. This constitutes an explicit attempt to achieve vertical equity. Weighting the population only on the basis of age is not sufficient, however; other variables should also be considered, such as the incidence rates of certain diseases, hygienic and environmental conditions, the lifestyles of the population, socioeconomic levels, and any deficits in infrastructure and technology. For this reason, some regions have for some time advocated for the introduction of a "deprivation index," which would take into account not only the health conditions of the population, but also its general socioeconomic conditions. The introduction of such a criterion would greatly enhance vertical equity by allocating funds to regions based on need. To date, however, the regions have failed to agree on how to calculate such an index of deprivation, and such a criterion has not been adopted.

Private Spending

As mentioned, over the decade from 2010 to 2019, Italian public health spending grew by an average of 0.9% per year. Over the same decade, private health spending increased an average of 2.5% annually.

These figures can be interpreted as a transfer of spending from the public to the private sector: Since the state has tightened its purse strings, individual citizens have been forced to compensate by paying more out of their own pockets. In 2010, the public component accounted for 78% of total healthcare spending, with the private component accounting for the remaining 22%. In 2019, the proportion was 74% public spending to 26% private spending (OECD 2020). Over the past decade, a 4% share of total health spending (corresponding to about 6 billion euros) that the state no longer bears has been transferred to individual household budgets (Toth and Lizzi 2019).

In Italy, leaving aside the premiums paid for voluntary private insurance for now, private health expenditure is essentially composed of three items. The first expenditure item is treatments that are not included in the LEAs (e.g., dental care, outpatient physiotherapy, or long-term care). The second item contributing to private spending is copayments charged to patients. A third item contributing to private spending comes from services included in LEAs that Italians nonetheless prefer to purchase from private providers.

With regard to the last category, it should be noted that Italians are accustomed to privately paying (i.e., paying out of their own pockets or being reimbursed by a private insurance company) for many specialist visits and examinations that they would be entitled to receive from the public health service. Several studies (ISTAT 2007; Fabbri and Monfardini 2009; Domenighetti et al. 2010; Glorioso and Subramanian 2014; Toth 2016; Pianori et al. 2020; Intesa Sanpaolo RBM Salute 2021) highlighted how Italians prefer to go private for a number of reasons: (1) Private visits usually have much shorter wait times than public facilities; (2) patients may consider certain private providers to be of higher quality than those guaranteed by the NHS; (3) a private facility may be closer or more convenient than public ones; (4) the booking and payment procedures in private facilities are usually less bureaucratic and more user friendly; (5) for examinations and specialist visits purchased privately, a family doctor's prescription is not required; and (6) patients may want to choose a specific doctor for treatment (this right is not guaranteed in public facilities).

The previously mentioned studies agreed on one important aspect: The medical care and health professionals available in private facilities are not necessarily of higher quality than those provided in NHS facilities. In most cases, the opposite is true. Italians appreciate and choose the private sector above all for the ancillary aspects of care: shorter wait times, easier access, room comfort, and so on.

Italian patients are free to choose among all public facilities and the private facilities that have entered into a special agreement with the NHS. Regarding patient freedom of choice, it should be noted that although Italian healthcare users have the right to choose the outpatient clinics or hospitals where they want to receive treatment, they cannot choose the individual medical practitioner. That is to say, once a user has booked a procedure at a given hospital department, they will be examined by the physicians who are on duty on the day of the appointment. If the patient wants to be sure to see one specialist rather than another, they will have to book a private medical visit. Indeed, all physicians employed by the NHS are also allowed to practice privately outside of their regular working hours (Toth 2014b, 2020b).

Some recent analyses estimated that in Italy, between 40% and 50% of specialist visits and more than 20% of diagnostic examinations are purchased on the private market (Deloitte 2020; Pianori et al. 2020). Italian private health expenditure consists of prescription drug spending (about 26%); dental care (22%); specialist visits (19%); instrumental diagnostic examinations (9%); lenses, glasses, and prostheses (8%); hospital expenses (5%); and other expenses (11%) (RBM-Census 2019).

Private Health Insurance: a Growing Phenomenon

Italy in the last two decades has seen a constant increase in private healthcare spending. According to OECD data (2020), in Italy private health expenditure is for the most part (about 90%) out of pocket and only marginally (just over 10%) intermediated (i.e., patients pay premiums for voluntary private insurance). Although Italians with private health insurance are still a minority—an estimated 23% of the population (Intesa Sanpaolo RBM Salute 2021)—in recent years there has been a sudden increase in private insurance policies. This is a phenomenon that raises an interesting debate. In fact, private health insurance seems to be a silent revolution that significantly affects the relationships between public and private healthcare, on both the financing and delivery fronts (Toth and Lizzi 2019). The expansion of voluntary health insurance poses a threat to the horizontal equity of the entire system, both in financing and in access to care.

It is not easy to briefly present the world of private health insurance in Italy because it presents itself as a decidedly variegated and not fully regulated reality. Italian health insurance encompasses subjects and insurance products that differ from each other in terms of legal nature, size, mode of adhesion, amount of premiums or contributions required, tax benefits, and benefits provided (Gimbe 2019; Toth and Lizzi 2019).

To untangle the jungle of private insurance coverage, it is useful to start from a double distinction. A first distinction is that between complementary and supplementary benefits (Mossialos and Thomson 2002; Hussey and Anderson 2003). In Italy, *supplementary benefits* mean the services and treatments already included in LEAs guaranteed by the public health service. On the other hand, services not included in LEAs are considered *complementary*. A second distinction is that between for-profit insurers (insurance companies) and not-for-profit insurers (mutual aid societies and integrative health funds).

According to data from the Institute for Insurance Supervision (IVASS 2020), in Italy about two-thirds of private healthcare policies are formally issued by not-for-profit insurers, while about one-third are provided by for-profit insurance companies. However, this figure should be viewed with caution: Many small nonprofit organizations prefer to rely on large for-profit companies (this practice is known as "reinsurance"). The private health insurance market thus ends up being dominated by a few large for-profit banking and insurance groups (ANIA 2020).

It is useful to provide some details on how private health insurance is regulated and incentivized in Italy. The Italian state provides tax incentives in favor of the so-called integrative health funds provided that they meet certain conditions.

The matter was regulated by Legislative Decree No. 229 of 1999, known as the Bindi reform (after the presiding minister of health). This reform intended to incentivize and enhance only private policies (collective and nonprofit) that were properly complementary—the integrative health funds. Integrative funds should not overlap with the NHS, but should instead focus on services excluded from LEAs. In anticipation of the recognition of a tax benefit only for funds that are truly complementary to the NHS, Legislative Decree No. 229 provided for the institution of a special register of integrative health funds at the Ministry of Health. The funds enrolled in the register were required to adopt policies of nonselection of risk and were required to use providers accredited by the NHS.

The application decrees issued a few years later (in 2008 and 2009) provided for facilitated tax treatment. This consisted of the deductibility of premiums paid up to a maximum of 3,615 euros per year, but only for funds registered in the ministry's register. To be included in the registry, the funds had to allocate at least 20% of reimbursements to services not covered by the NHS, such as dental care, long-term care, and rehabilitation. The vast majority of Italians who have private health insurance policies are enrolled in integrative health funds recognized by the ministry and therefore receive the tax relief (IVASS 2020).

There is an additional way to enjoy a tax incentive: taking out private insurance through an employer. Starting in 2016, new measures in favor of corporate welfare were introduced. Employees are now allowed to convert performance bonuses into fully tax-free benefits, including premiums paid for the purchase of a private health insurance policy (Toth and Lizzi 2019).

All in all, tax breaks give a big boost to the purchase of private health policies (Dirindin 2018; Gimbe 2019). In fact, the Italian state provides tax relief worth 1.4 billion euros or so against a total intermediated expenditure of 4.3 billion euros (IVASS 2020; Intesa Sanpaolo RBM Salute 2021).

It is not surprising that private health insurance is a growing phenomenon. Until a few years ago, private health insurance concerned only a small minority of the Italian population. Supplementary policyholders were mostly business executives, members of some professional orders, employees of some large companies, members of the historic mutual aid societies, and a few other categories (Toth and Lizzi 2019). In just a few years, the picture has changed radically: It is estimated that Italians with some form of private health insurance today number almost 14 million (Intesa Sanpaolo RBM Salute 2021), compared with the 4.9 million estimated in 2004. The reasons for this growth can partly be found in the financial constraints imposed on the NHS and in the increase in private health expenditure. Having to take on a greater financial burden, many families consider it more convenient to take out a supplementary policy rather than pay for medical treatment in the traditional out-of-pocket mode. Other contributing factors include changes in labor and industrial relations, as well as the effective marketing strategies recently adopted by major insurance companies (Gimbe 2019).

For the past few years, the topic of private health insurance has generated heated debate among experts (Toth and Lizzi 2019). There are essentially two rival coalitions. On the one hand, there are advocates of private healthcare who welcome the strengthening of a "second pillar" in healthcare. This group asks the government to increase fiscal incentives in favor of private health insurance. The opposite side is made up of those who look with concern at the spread of private insurance coverage. They believe that private insurance is crumbling the public, egalitarian, and solidarity-based foundations of the NHS, and that this leads to an unacceptable disparity of treatment between citizens who have some form of private insurance coverage and those who go without it. The clash revolves around the issue of horizontal equity.

Arguments in favor of private health insurance are based on the assumption that insurance coverage is always fairer in general terms than paying for medical care out of pocket on an individual basis; insurance coverage implies a sharing of risk among the insured. A greater diffusion of private insurance coverage would therefore lead to a fairer system than the current one because more families would be protected against the risk of unexpected medical expenses.

These arguments are opposed by those who stand in defense of the public health service (Dirindin 2018; Gimbe 2019). In addition to opposition on the ideal and value level, the issue of public incentives divides the two factions. In fact, a large part of those who proclaim themselves in defense of the NHS do not argue that supplementary coverage should be prohibited. According to NHS defenders, tax breaks should be reserved only for genuinely complementary coverage, not supplementary coverage as well. It should be pointed out that in Italy, private healthcare insurance covers only a small portion of truly complementary services (Intesa Sanpaolo RBM Salute 2021). The majority of insurance reimbursements concern supplementary services, which citizens would be entitled to obtain from the NHS. Therefore, the proposal being put forward is that the financial resources that the state currently commits in tax breaks in favor of private insurance policies and corporate welfare be used differently, to finance the public health service instead (Gimbe 2019). By doing so, it would no longer be just a few privileged people (the 23% of Italians who currently have private insurance) who would benefit from these public resources, but the entire population (Dirindin 2018).

From Paper to Reality: Barriers to Accessing Care

What has been said previously in relation to the healthcare coverage of the entire population and to the provision of LEAs concerns what the NHS should guarantee to patients. However, moving from paper to reality, the picture is different. NHS users encounter various obstacles to accessing many essential services.

Residents in Italy do not have truly comprehensive coverage due to certain limitations of the NHS, which can be traced essentially to four factors: (1) Some services are formally excluded from LEAs; (2) the regions have difficulty providing the full range of LEAs; (3) wait times in public facilities are excessively long; and (4) copayments charged to users can affect the choices of care, especially for the less affluent.

As stated, the first limitation comes from the fact that certain procedures are not included in the LEA list and are therefore not financed by the NHS. For instance, a share of pharmaceutical expenditures, as well as a large portion of dental care and physiotherapy costs, are charged to individual citizens.

A second obstacle to effective access to healthcare services derives from the failures of individual regions to meet their obligations. Many regions do not succeed in providing all LEAs, even though they are required to guarantee them.

Long wait times are another obstacle to accessing care. This is one of the main problems afflicting the Italian NHS, and naturally has the effect of incentivizing the purchase of specialist services from the private sector. In fact, the problem of long wait-lists concerns public facilities almost exclusively; private facilities usually have much shorter response times than public ones. As confirmed by a recent survey (Intesa Sanpaolo RBM Salute 2021), 62% of patients who turned to private providers (thus paying out of pocket) claimed they did so because of the long waiting lists for public facilities.

Finally, a fourth obstacle in accessing care is the copayments charged to patients. Primary care and hospitalizations are free at the time of use. Prescription drugs, inappropriate emergency room visits, specialist visits, and diagnostic tests that do not result in hospitalization may instead be subject to a copayment (called a "ticket") charged to the patient. Copayments vary according to family income and region of residence. People who are affected by certain diseases and those with low income are exempted from paying tickets. On average, every Italian spends around 26 euros annually on copayments for the purchase of medicines and around 22 euros in copayments for specialist outpatient services (Corte dei Conti 2019).

Regional Differences and The North-South Gap

Although the intent of the Italian NHS is to provide uniform service throughout the national territory, in reality the healthcare offered in the various regions is anything but homogeneous. Most of the southern regions offer healthcare services of lower quality than those provided in the central and northern regions. Various indicators and sources can support this statement.

The National Agency for Regional Healthcare Services (AGENAS, Agenzia Nazionale per i Servizi Sanitari Regionali) publishes an annual report, the *National Outcomes Programme*. This report uses dozens of different indicators to provide a comparative assessment of individual regional health services in terms of effectiveness, efficiency, safety, and quality of care provided. On almost all of the indicators considered, the central and northern regions perform systematically better than the southern regions (AGENAS 2020).

In addition to the *National Outcomes Programme* report, other reports assess the quality of healthcare services, ranking the different Italian regions (Osservasalute 2020; Spandonaro, d'Angela, and Polistena 2020; European House—Ambrosetti 2020; Demoskopika 2021; ISTAT 2021). Regardless of the methodology used, all of these rankings agree in identifying a profound north-south divide: the higher-quality healthcare services are provided in the central and northern regions, whereas those provided in the south tend to be of much lower quality. Italians are well aware of this. As shown by a report published a few years ago (Eurispes 2017), only 27% of inhabitants in the southern regions consider themselves satisfied with their regional healthcare service. The level of satisfaction is much higher in the northern regions, where the percentage of satisfied citizens is close to 65%.

Therefore, it is not surprising that residents in southern regions go to regions where they think they can get the best care whenever possible. This is the phenomenon of *interregional healthcare mobility* (Toth 2014a): Each year, hundreds of thousands of patients are admitted to hospitals in regions other than those they reside in. The north-south imbalance is evident here as well. For each patient residing in the center-north admitted to a hospital in the south, more than seven patients make the reverse journey—that is, they travel from the southern regions to be treated in the hospitals of the center-north (Ministero della Salute 2021). Lombardy, Emilia-Romagna, Veneto, and Tuscany are the most attractive regions. Patients tend to flee other regions, especially Calabria and Campania. Considering healthcare mobility, all southern regions show a negative balance, with the sole exception of the small region of Molise (Demoskopika 2021; Gimbe 2020).

Not only the quality of services, but also the health conditions of the population are better in the north-central regions than in the south. Avoidable mortality is more prevalent in the south (18.5 deaths per 10,000 people, standardized rates) than in the north (only 15.9 deaths per 10,000 people) (ISTAT 2021). Life expectancy at birth is higher in central and northern regions than in southern ones (Osservasalute 2020). The infant mortality rate within the first year of life is 2.4 per 1,000 live births in the northern regions and 3.7 in the southern ones (ISTAT 2021). The existence of a deep north-south divide is therefore undeniable.

Inequality in Access to Healthcare and a Safety Net

As argued above, the Italian NHS is unable to "give all to all"; some medical services remain the responsibility of individual citizens. This means that those who have more disposable income can afford healthcare services in addition to those provided by the NHS, shorten their wait times, and have more freedom to choose physicians or medical facilities. The indigent must instead make do with what the public service offers, run the risk of going into debt to pay for healthcare, or, in some cases, renounce care.

In 2020, one in ten Italians said they had forgone necessary visits or diagnostic tests in the past 12 months for reasons related to difficulty of access. The share in the year 2019 was 6.3% (ISTAT 2021). The figure for 2020 is certainly anomalous due to the particular situation related to the Covid-19 pandemic. If we consider the year 2019, the prevailing reasons for forgoing treatment were first cost and second length of wait times. As might be expected, those forgoing care for economic reasons were primarily less-affluent families (Deloitte 2020). Also in this respect, there is a disparity between the north and south of the country: In the year 2019, 5.1% of the population of the northern regions had renounced healthcare for economic reasons, compared to 7.5% in the south (ISTAT 2021).

It has been said before that some categories of individuals, the so-called invisibles (undocumented foreigners, homeless people, etc.), risk being discriminated against and not receiving all the medical care considered essential by the NHS. However, poor and invisible people can rely on a safety net made up of volunteer doctors, charities, the social services of municipalities, and not-for-profit organizations.

Some of these nonprofit entities—including Caritas, Emergency, and MSF (Médecins Sans Frontières)—are large and have a national character; others are smaller local organizations that rely on a few volunteers. This safety net is sparsely distributed throughout the country and varies considerably from one city to another. All larger cities have outpatient clinics managed by volunteer health workers who provide their services at no cost. These clinics mostly provide primary and dental care. ASLs often coordinate and fund programs to protect invisible people. There are also nonprofit organizations such as the Pharmaceutical Bank (Banco Farmaceutico) that distribute free medication to disadvantaged groups, or the National Cancer Association (ANT, Associazione Nazionale Tumori), which provides free home care services to cancer patients.

In short, the not-for-profit sector plays an important complementary role, providing assistance to groups less protected by the public health service. The action of the not-for-profit sector tries to balance some forms of horizontal inequality and, even more, to increase the level of vertical equity, allocating additional resources in favor of the neediest categories of the population.

Conclusions

Here, we underline our arguments in the previous sections, evaluating the extent to which the Italian healthcare system succeeds in guaranteeing equity and quality of healthcare in actual practice. The principle of equity can be applied to different dimensions of the healthcare system, and a crucial distinction is that between vertical and horizontal equity.

Equity in healthcare finance represents one of the founding principles of the Italian NHS. The NHS is in fact funded mostly through general taxation, and the Italian tax system is based on the principle of progressivity. We can therefore conclude that the financing mechanisms of the Italian NHS pursue both vertical and horizontal equity. In practice, however, the overall equity of the financing system is in part weakened by a number of factors, including user charges, a high level of private spending, and the spread of private insurance policies, whose premiums are not calculated according to individual income. In addition, Italy suffers from a long-standing problem of tax evasion.

More than copayments, the elements that most reduce vertical equity in financing stem from the fact that LEAs guaranteed by the NHS exclude certain categories of treatment. Consequently, Italy experiences a high level of private health spending—currently around 40 billion euros per year (around 660 euros per capita). Private spending is largely out of pocket. Italians spend out of their own pockets for both complementary care (treatments that the NHS does not cover) and supplementary services (treatments that citizens are entitled to by the public service). In recent years, there has been impressive growth in private health insurance policies. About one in four Italians currently has a voluntary private insurance policy. Private insurance policies are financially incentivized by the state, and over the last few years they have been included in many national collective bargaining agreements. Tax incentives for voluntary insurance end up favoring specific job categories and employees of certain companies.

Turning to equity in resource allocation, we provided details regarding how the national health budget is distributed among the regions. To date, the Italian national government has assigned per capita quotas to the individual regions that only take limited account of the needs of their populations. More could be done to improve the vertical equity of the allocation mechanisms, taking greater account of the characteristics and health needs of the populations residing in individual regions.

Equity regarding access to care is questionable. Does the NHS in Italy really guarantee "equal access to available care for equal need"? Despite the fact that the NHS strives to guarantee equal opportunities for care for all, we detailed several obstacles to healthcare access. These obstacles are constituted primarily in long wait times and the inability of some regions to fully guarantee LEAs. Profound differences between regions also impact the quality of services offered. Both wait times and regional differences limit horizontal equity in access to care. The spread of voluntary private insurance also affects horizontal equity: Private policyholders have a preferential lane in access to care and can turn more easily to private providers.

For some categories of patients—especially the poor, foreigners, and people with low education levels—access to NHS services can be even more difficult due to language and cultural barriers, bureaucratic procedures, or a lack of awareness of their rights. To support the most disadvantaged, particularly the so-called invisible people, the not-for-profit sector comes to the rescue. Since the declared mission of the not-for-profit sector is to take care of the most disadvantaged people, the presence of a widespread and articulated nonprofit safety net constitutes an element in support of vertical equity.

Finally, concerning equity in healthcare utilization, the Italian NHS certainly applies the principle of vertical equity. In fact, the public health service allocates the majority of its resources to treating a limited number of chronic, serious, and elderly patients. Far fewer resources are allocated to patients in better health. This is true not only in hospital and outpatient settings, but also with reference to territorial care: Chronically ill patients and people in conditions of social distress systematically receive more attention from ASLs and social services. All NHS facilities and staff are required to adhere to the principle of appropriateness of care, which implies that people in different degrees of need are treated in appropriately different ways.

The NHS is also committed to pursuing horizontal equity in care delivery. In practice, however, this objective is not fully realized. First of all, there are marked regional differences. Depending on one's region of residence, the quality of the care provided varies. In addition, the NHS does not provide some types of treatment, and for many nonemergency services, wait times can be long. This means that the more affluent and those with private insurance policies can go private, skipping waiting lists and enjoying greater choice of providers.

Notes

1. In Lombardy, following the 2015 reform, ASLs and AOs no longer exist. In their place, 27 territorial social-health authorities (*Aziende Socio-Sanitarie Territoriali*, ASSTs) and 8 health protection agencies (*Agenzie di tutela della salute*, ATSs) have been established.
2. In most cases, the territory of the ASLs tends to coincide with the provincial territory (Cinelli et al. 2020). In some regions, a single ASL operates that is responsible for the entire regional territory; this is the case in Marche, Molise, Sardinia, and Valle D'Aosta.
3. The STP code guarantees care related to pregnancy and maternity, care of minors, vaccinations, and treatment of infectious diseases. In addition to urgent care, diseases that are not dangerous in the short term, but that could cause greater damage to health or risk of life over time are also treated.

References

AGENAS (Agenzia Nazionale per i Servizi Sanitari Regionali). 2020. *Programma Nazionale Esiti. Edizione 2020*. Rome: Agenzia Nazionale per i Servizi Sanitari Regionali.

ANIA (Associazione Nazionale fra le Imprese Assicuratrici). 2020. *Premi del lavoro diretto italiano 2019. Edizione 2020*. Rome: Associazione Nazionale fra le Imprese Assicuratrici.

Braveman, Paula. 2006. "Health Disparities and Health Equity: Concepts and Measurement." *Annual Review of Public Health* 27(1): 167–194.

Cinelli, Gianmario, Attilio Gugiatti, Francesca Meda, and Francesco Petracca. 2020. "La struttura e le attività del SSN." In *Rapporto OASI 2020*, edited by Cergas-SDA Bocconi, 35–108. Milan: Egea.

Confindustria. 2019. *Patto per la salute. 2019–2021*. Rome: Confindustria.

Corte dei Conti. 2019. *Rapporto 2019 sul coordinamento della finanza pubblica*. Rome: Corte dei Conti.

Culyer, Anthony J. 2001. "Equity: Some Theory and its Policy Implications." *Journal of Medical Ethics* 27 (4): 275–283.

Culyer, Anthony J., and Adam Wagstaff. 1993. "Equity and Equality in Health and Health Care." *Journal of Health Economics* 12(4): 431–457.

Culyer, Anthony J. 2001. "Equity—Some Theory and Its Policy Implications." *Journal of Medical Ethics* 27 (4): 275–283.

Deloitte. 2020. *Outlook Salute Italia 2021. Prospettive e sostenibilità del sistema sanitario*. Rome: Deloitte.

Demoskopika. 2021. *La performance sanitaria. Indice di misurazione e valutazione dei sistemi regionali italiani*. Rome: Demoskopika.

Di Giulio, Marco, and Federico Toth. 2014. "I gruppi di interesse in sanità." *Rivista Italiana di Politiche Pubbliche* 9(3): 377–408.

Dirindin, Nerina. 2018. *È tutta salute. In difesa della sanità pubblica*. Turin: Edizioni Gruppo Abele.

Domenighetti, Gianfranco, Paolo Vineis, Carlo De Pietro, and Angelo Tomada. 2010. "Ability to Pay and Equity in Access to Italian and British National Health Services." *European Journal of Public Health* 20(5): 500–503.

Donatini, Andrea. 2020. "Italy." In *International Health Care System Profiles*, edited by Roosa Tikkanen, Robin Osborn, Elias Mossialos, Ana Djordjevic, and George A. Wharton. Washington, DC: Commonwealth Fund.

Eurispes. 2017. *Rapporto Italia 2017*. Rome: Istituto di Studi Politici Economici e Sociali, Eurispes.

European House—Ambrosetti. 2020. *XV Rapporto Meridiano Sanità. Le coordinate della salute*. Milan: European House, Ambrosetti.

Fabbri, Daniele, and Chiara Monfardini. 2009. "Rationing the Public Provision of Healthcare in the Presence of Private Supplements: Evidence from the Italian NHS." *Journal of Health Economics* 28(2): 290–304.

Gimbe. 2019. *La sanità integrativa*. Bologna: Fondazione Gimbe.

Gimbe. 2020. *La mobilità sanitaria interregionale nel 2018*. Bologna: Fondazione Gimbe.

Glorioso, Valeria, and SV Subramanian. 2014. "Equity in Access to Health Care Services in Italy." *Health Services Research* 49(3): 950–970.

Goddard, Maria, and Peter Smith. 2001. "Equity of Access to Health Care Services: Theory and Evidence from the UK." *Social Science & Medicine* 53(9): 1149–1162.

Hussey, Peter, and Gerard F. Anderson. 2003. "A Comparison of Single—and Multi-payer Health Insurance Systems and Options for Reform." *Health Policy* 66(3): 215–228.

Intesa Sanpaolo RBM Salute. 2021. *IX Rapporto sulla sanità pubblica, privata e intermediata. Annualità 2019–2020*. Venice: Intesa Sanpaolo RBM Salute.

ISTAT (Istituto Nazionale di Statistica). 2007. *Condizioni di salute, fattori di rischio e ricorso ai servizi sanitari*. Rome: Istituto Nazionale di Statistica.

ISTAT (Istituto Nazionale di Statistica). 2020. *Rapporto annuale 2020*. Rome: Istituto Nazionale di Statistica.

ISTAT (Istituto Nazionale di Statistica). 2021. *Rapporto BES 2020. Il benessere equo e sostenibile in Italia*. Rome: Istituto Nazionale di Statistica.

IVASS (Institute for Insurance Supervision). 2020. *Ruolo e prospettive della sanità complementare dopo il Covid-19*. Rome: Istituto per la Vigilanza sulle Assicurazioni.

Lagomarsino, Gina, Alice Garabrant, Atikah Adyas, Richard Muga, and Nathaniel Otoo. 2012. "Moving towards Universal Health Coverage. Health Insurance Reforms in Nine Developing Countries in Africa and Asia." *Lancet* 380: 933–943.

Le Grand, Julian. 1987. "Equity, Health, and Health Care." *Social Justice Research* 1(3): 257–274.

Mapelli, Vittorio. 2012. *Il sistema sanitario italiano*. Bologna: il Mulino.

Ministero della Salute. 2020. *Monitoraggio dei LEA attraverso la cd. Griglia LEA*. Rome: Ministero della Salute, Direzione Generale della Programmazione Sanitaria.

Ministero della Salute. 2021. *Rapporto annuale sull'attività di ricovero ospedaliero. Dato SDO 2019*. Rome: Ministero della Salute, Direzione Generale della programmazione sanitaria.

Mooney, Gavin. 1983. "Equity in Health Care: Confronting the Confusion." *Effective Health Care* 1(4): 179–185.

Mossialos, Elias, and Sarah Thomson. 2002. "Voluntary Health Insurance in the European Union." In *Funding Health Care: Options for Europe*, edited by Elias Mossialos, Anna Dixon, Josep Figueras, and Joe Kutzin, 128–160. Buckingham: Open University Press.

OECD (Organization for Economic Cooperation and Development). 2020. *OECD Health Statistics 2020*. Paris: OECD Publishing.

Osservasalute. 2020. *Rapporto Osservasalute 2019. Stato di salute e qualità dell'assistenza nelle regioni italiane*. Rome: Università Cattolica del Sacro Cuore-Osservatorio Nazionale sulla Salute nelle Regioni Italiane.

Pianori, Davide, Elisa Maietti, Jacopo Lenzi, Mattia Quargnolo, Stefano Guicciardi, Kadjo Y. C. Adja, Maria Pia Fantini, and Federico Toth. 2020. "Sociodemographic and Health Service Organizational Factors Associated with the Choice of the Private versus Public Sector for Specialty Visits: Evidence from a National Survey in Italy." *PLoS ONE* 15(5): e0232827. https://doi.org/10.1371/journal.pone.0232827

RBM-Census. 2019. *IX Rapporto sulla sanità pubblica, privata ed intermediata*. Rome: RBM-Census.

Spandonaro, Federico, Daniela d'Angela, and Barbara Polistena. 2020. *16° Rapporto Sanità-Oltre l'emergenza: Verso una "nuova" vision del nostro SSN*. Rome: CREA, Centro per la Ricerca Economica Applicata in Sanità.

Stuckler, David, Andrea B. Feigl, Sanjay Basu, and Martin McKee. 2010. *The Political Economy of Universal Health Coverage*. Montreux, Switzerland: First Global Symposium on Health Systems Research.

Toth, Federico. 2014a. "How Health Care Regionalization in Italy Is Widening the North-South Gap." *Health Economics Policy and Law* 9(3): 231–249.

Toth, Federico. 2014b. *La sanità in Italia*. Bologna: il Mulino.

Toth, Federico. 2016. "The Italian NHS, the Public/Private Sector Mix and the Disparities in Access to Healthcare." *Global Social Welfare* 3(3): 171–178.

Toth, Federico. 2019. "Prevalence and Generosity of Health Insurance Coverage: A Comparison of EU Member States." *Journal of Comparative Policy Analysis: Research and Practice* 21(5): 518–534.

Toth, Federico. 2020a. "Le Politiche Sanitarie: Un Gioco Strategico." In *Le politiche pubbliche in Italia*, edited by Giliberto Capano and Alessandro Natalini, 147–162. Bologna: il Mulino.

Toth, Federico. 2020b. "Reducing Waiting Times in the Italian NHS: The Case of Emilia-Romagna." *Social Policy & Administration* 54(7): 1110–1122.

Toth, Federico. 2021a. *Comparative Health Systems. A New Framework*. Cambridge: Cambridge University Press.

Toth, Federico. 2021b. "How the Health Services of Emilia-Romagna, Lombardy and Veneto Handled the Covid-19 Emergency." *Contemporary Italian Politics* 13(2): 226–241.

Toth, Federico, and Renata Lizzi. 2019. "Le trasformazioni «silenziose» delle politiche sanitarie in Italia e l'effetto catalizzatore della grande crisi finanziaria." *Stato e Mercato* 39(2): 297–320.

Wagstaff, Adam, and Eddy Van Doorslaer. 2000. "Equity in Health Care Finance and Delivery." In *Handbook of Health Economics*, edited by Anthony J. Culyer and Joseph P. Newhouse, vol. 1, Part B, 1803–1862. Amsterdam: Elsevier.

Whitehead, Margaret. 1992. "The Concepts and Principles of Equity and Health." *International Journal of Health Services* 22(3): 429–445.

WHO (World Health Organization). 2010. *Health Systems Financing: The Path to Universal Coverage*. Geneva: World Health Organization.

9

Healthcare Commodification, Equity, and Quality in Chile and Mexico

Pamela Bernales-Baksai and Ricardo Velázquez Leyer

Introduction

Until the last decades of the 20th century, both Chile and Mexico applied a similar Bismarckian employment-based social insurance path to the organization of their public healthcare systems. That path would begin to diverge in the 1980s. One salient difference in the divergent paths was the way in which public policy established links with private provision. Without completely abandoning Bismarckian logic, an initial wave of neoliberal reforms in Chile created a dual public-private system, characterized by the explicit incorporation of the private sector into healthcare policy and the institutionalized commodification of healthcare provision. After the 1990s, subsequent reforms aimed at ameliorating the effects of commodification processes and expanding protection to certain population groups that had been left especially vulnerable to market forces.

In Mexico, large-scale reforms were not introduced until the early 2000s, when a voluntary health insurance program was created with the aim of expanding public healthcare coverage. The reform reproduced Bismarckian logic, layering an additional public insurance scheme, but without addressing the limitations in the supply of public services, hence preserving the process of implicit commodification that characterizes healthcare provision in this country. Unlike Chile, no links were established between public and private provision. However, given the deficiencies in public supply, large sectors of the population, both before and after the reform, have opted for or been forced to use private services. This need to seek healthcare in the private sector impacts the poor much more than other income groups given their inability to afford private services. This is especially apparent at the secondary

Pamela Bernales-Baksai and Ricardo Velázquez Leyer, *Healthcare Commodification, Equity, and Quality in Chile and Mexico* In: *The Public/Private Sector Mix in Healthcare Delivery*. Edited by: Howard A. Palley, Oxford University Press.
© Oxford University Press 2023. DOI: 10.1093/oso/9780197571101.003.0009

and tertiary levels, as is discussed in this chapter, and signals the failure of markets to guarantee the right to health.

The comparison between Chile and Mexico is interesting because of the different types of healthcare commodification pursued in each case. The concept of commodification in healthcare has been defined as the degree to which its access is dependent on the market position of an individual and the extent to which provision in a given country depends on market arrangements (Bambra 2005). In previous work, it was argued that commodification processes can unfold in explicit or implicit modes, the former referring to the incorporation of market provision as part of the healthcare policy architecture and the latter to the dependence on market provision due to deficiencies in the supply of public services (Bernales-Baksai and Velázquez Leyer 2021). Different commodification modes may have different effects on the equity and quality of healthcare provision.

Healthcare equity has been defined by the World Health Organization (WHO) as the reduction of unnecessary social gaps and the achievement of the optimal healthcare provision for everyone. This definition encompasses equity in the way healthcare resources are allocated, healthcare services are supplied and received, and health services are paid for (WHO 1996). Equity in healthcare represents an imperative to cope with avoidable differences in health outcomes across population groups because of their position, status, and role within society (e.g., gender, ethnic origin, age, employment status, income level) (CSDH [Commission on Social Determinants of Health] 2008) and, therefore, is a core aspect in assessing the impact of the health policy on the path toward universal healthcare.

Equity in healthcare can be horizontal (defined as the absence of differences against similar needs) and vertical (as the upgrade of healthcare provision for greater needs) (Starfield 2001). Horizontal equity can be achieved when all individuals have similar access to and utilization of health services independently of their income, education, gender, or any other sociodemographic condition. Vertical equity requires different treatment for different needs, with greater resources allocated to greater needs.

Healthcare quality is defined by WHO as the degree to which health services for individuals and population groups increases the likelihood of desired health outcomes. It involves effective, safe, and people-centered care and requires timely, equitable, integrated, and efficient health services (WHO 2020b).

The present chapter aims to establish the consequences of current public-private mixes of healthcare provision on healthcare equity and quality outputs. The following section reviews the history of healthcare in both countries, with special mention to the role that private provision has played. The third section compares the policy architectures, focusing on market options and describing the scope of private healthcare services and their interaction with public policy. The fourth section analyzes equity outputs, distinguishing between horizontal and vertical equity, as well as quality outputs. The final section offers the conclusions of the research.

The Development of Healthcare Services

This section offers an overview of the history of healthcare provision in Chile and Mexico. The description of the development of public and private services is distinguished in order to provide the context for the analysis of the current healthcare arrangements and their effects on different population groups. Both countries have historically organized healthcare along Bismarckian principles, but following divergent paths in the configuration of the public-private mix in recent decades: In Chile, private insurance and provision have been incorporated into social security in a process of explicit commodification, while in Mexico private options have remained separated from social security and public services and with low levels of government regulation.

The Chilean Case

In the second decade of the 20th century, Chile was one of the pioneers in Latin America in developing a welfare system (Mesa-Lago 1985). Until the early 1970s, welfare provision, including healthcare, followed a progressive trajectory based on the Bismarckian model, which encompassed different schemes according to occupational categories (Larrañaga 2010).

In 1952, the government created the National Health Service (Sistema Nacional de Salud, SNS), which integrated most of the government's healthcare services into one entity, thus pioneering the regional efforts toward the desegregation of healthcare (Cotlear et al. 2015). In the late 1960s and early 1970s, healthcare became more inclusive and generous: Social insurance coverage increased from 60% in 1960 to above 70% in 1973, and indigents also received assistance coverage (Mesa-Lago 1986). Moreover, the government settled comprehensive health programs, and health outcomes substantially improved (Castillo-Laborde et al. 2019). These efforts, however, were in-sufficient to tackle the fragmentation and stratification that the system had featured since its foundation (Barrientos 2004; Borzutzky 2002; Mesa-Lago 1985, 1994). Furthermore, despite the advances, by the mid-1970s health provision was fragmented into the SNS for blue-collar workers, agricultural workers, and indigents; the National Medical Service of Employees (Servicio Médico Nacional de Empleados, SERMENA) for white-collar workers and civil servants; schemes for army forces and the police; and some smaller schemes for specific occupations. Fragmentation encompassed significant disparities in quality across the schemes (e.g., white-collar workers had more benefits than blue-collar workers), as well as limitations to healthcare faced by more than 20% of the population without coverage (Mesa-Lago 1985). In this scenario, the private sector was limited to a small part of the population who lacked health insurance but had payment capacity and those enrolled in SERMENA who opted for private health facilities (Castillo-Laborde et al. 2019).

In 1973, a military coup abruptly interrupted the expansionist trajectory of the public provision of social welfare. The "assistance State" turned into a "residual State" subsidiary to the market (Larrañaga 2010), and the health system suffered a significant setback. From 1979, the dictatorship introduced reforms that undermined the public sector, favoring a more substantial role by private actors (Cotlear et al. 2015). Law 2.763 of 1979 merged the SNS and SERMENA, creating the National System of Health Services (Sistema Nacional de Servicios de Salud) and established the National Health Fund (Fondo Nacional de Salud, FONASA) to provide financial administration for the system. In 1980, primary healthcare (PHC) decentralized to municipal-ities (MINSAL-Chile 2012; Cid et al. 2014) and the new political constitu-tion defined that the state has the duty of protecting equal and free access to healthcare through either public or private institutions and that each in-dividual has the right to choose the health system in which to participate (Ministerio Secretaría General de la Presidencia 1980).

In 1981, the health system turned into one composed of a public system and a parallel private option administrated by for-profit institutions (ISAPREs), workers' compulsory contributions rose from 4% to 7%, and employers' contributions were eliminated (Castillo-Laborde et al. 2019). On this basis, workers were permitted to channel their payroll contributions to either the public insurance (FONASA) or the private ones (ISAPREs), which is known as "opting out." Furthermore, ISAPREs benefited from special subsidies (Cid et al. 2014) and were allowed to charge additional premiums and cream the population by health risk (Cid et al. 2014; Huber and Stephens 2012; Pribble and Huber 2013). Meanwhile, the public sector kept the responsibility of covering the poor and those with higher health risks (Barrientos and Lloyd-Sherlock 2002), and financial resources fell from 2% to 0.8% of the gross domestic product (GDP) (Cid et al. 2014).

Lack of resources impaired the public sector's ability to provide quality care for the poor and those with higher health risks. In this way, the private sector's ability to set prices higher than the payroll contributions for health plans, and skim the population, caused financial damage to the public sector and gave rise to horizontal inequities that still persist between both types of insurance. This has allowed the private sector to possess more resources to serve the population with fewer health needs, while the opposite has occurred in the public sector.

In addition, since 1985, higher-income beneficiaries of FONASA have been allowed to seek attention beyond public providers (known as the Institutional Attention Modality, MAI) and attend private practices and hospitals (known as the Free Choice Modality, MLE) (Castillo-Laborde et al. 2019). This has further deepened the segmentation of the population and inequities between those with and without the payment capacity to access private care. These new transformations have strengthened the participation of private actors and completed the process of a refoundation of the policy architecture of healthcare. Thus, although the unification of previous schemes into FONASA (i.e., public insurance) ended the historical segmentation by occupational categories, new forms of segmentation arose. On this occasion, primarily between the public and private sectors.

In 1990, the resettlement of democracy did not significantly transform the subsidiary role of the state (Barrientos 2004; Draibe and Riesco 2009; Illanes 2004–2005; Martínez Franzoni 2007), and the policy architecture of healthcare maintained the market-based hallmark. Still, governments started to correct the underfunding of the public health sector, removed subsidies to affiliation at ISAPREs, and strengthened the institutionality to regulating the private sector (Barrientos and Lloyd-Sherlock 2002; Cid et al. 2014).

At the turn of the century, like others in Latin America, the country began to advance a universal model of social policies (Cecchini and Martínez 2011). In 2000, the Ministry of Health explicitly included the reduction of health inequities in the health goals for the decade 2000–2010 (MINSAL-Chile 2002). In this context, the most substantial reform was the Universal Access Plan of Explicit Guarantees in Health (AUGE-GES), approved in 2004, which would have guaranteed the entire population quality and standardized health services and financial protection for a group of health problems (MINSAL-Chile 2012).

Nevertheless, the government´s proposal of reform was amended in parliament, losing part of its redistributive potential. The most striking setback was the replacement of the solidarity single fund[1] by separate public and inter-ISAPREs funds (Cuadrado 2015; Huber and Stephens 2012), meaning the limitation of solidarity to horizontal solidarity and the validation of a dual system with significant horizontal inequity. Also, the increase in the value-added tax and copayments substituted the proposal of financing through alcohol and cigarette taxes, and covered illnesses were cut from 56 to 25 (Pribble and Huber 2013). However, in 2007 they increased back to 56, then in 2010 to 69, and are currently at 85 (MINSAL-Chile 2019). Moreover, the AUGE-GES does not tackle the inequities and the problem of lack of quality of care that persists in the noncovered health area (Frenz et al. 2018). This is reinforced by the significant participation of private actors in both AUGE-GES' provision and the overall system (Bernales-Baksai 2020).

The Mexican Case

In Mexico, the origins of government intervention in healthcare can be traced back to the second half of the 19th century, when the introduction of a program of liberal reforms included the nationalization of the properties of the Catholic Church, among them hospitals and orphanages (Rodríguez de Romo and Rodríguez 1998; López Antuñano 1993). Different government offices were created in the following decades with the aim of organizing and coordinating healthcare, and several public hospitals were built in urban centers. Contributory schemes for certain groups of workers, such as railroad and oil workers and some groups of civil servants, emerged in the first decades of the 20th century.[2] Reforms of the 1930s included the creation of a network of rural medical practices and the establishment of the obligation of medical students to perform a year of social service in rural areas (López Antuñano 1993; Rodríguez 2017; Rodríguez de Romo and Rodríguez 1998). This compulsory social service of all medical students remains an important but frequently overlooked feature of healthcare provision in the country. Yet, all these were isolated measures with a limited scope and without the adoption of a national healthcare policy.

Mexico is not placed among the pioneer countries in Latin America regarding the introduction of welfare programs (Mesa-Lago 1986). The social revolution that began in 1910 can explain the late introduction of national social policies in this country compared to others in the same region; the country was not fully pacified until the 1930s, and political instability and violent conflict impeded policy development in all areas. Hence, it was not until 1943 that a national public healthcare program was introduced, with the creation of the Mexican Social Insurance Institute (IMSS), which offered protection against social risks like illnesses and accidents to workers and their families, hence including healthcare provision. The IMSS acted as both insurer and provider of services with its own resources, funded by tripartite contributions of employers, workers and the state.

Expansion of IMSS would be gradual, prioritizing urban areas, where industrial workers were found—the core group whose benefit was sought as part of the import substitution industrialization strategy. The mode of gradual geographical expansion meant that, even if the legislation mandated social coverage to any person formally employed, during the next decades a large proportion of employees and their families in many parts of the country would still be left unprotected. In addition, because insurance depended on formal employment, large sectors of the population were left without legal coverage, like peasants, domestic workers, and the self-employed (Bonilla-Chacín and Aguilera 2013; Dion 2005).

The Health Secretariat (SSA) was also created in 1943 by fusing two federal government departments that had the aim of overseeing health policy. Besides the responsibility of setting the country's health policy, SSA was given the task of organizing healthcare provision for the population not covered by social insurance. SSA incorporated rural practices and existing hospitals in urban centers, and new hospitals were built but with a high concentration in large cities. SSA services remained with limited access and significant issues with quality of care, no insurance scheme was created, no medical records were kept, and treatment required a copayment at the point of services. The operation of services was decentralized to state governments in the 1980s with the aim of upgrading them, but quality and access problems persisted. Targeted services for poor rural population without social insurance coverage would also be created, notably an IMSS scheme for beneficiaries of antipoverty programs, although also falling short in terms of offering effective protection. Throughout the 20th century, resources devoted to healthcare provision outside social insurance always remained limited, with low levels of access and quality of healthcare for the majority of the population (Bonilla-Chacín and Aguilera 2013; Gómez-Dantes et al. 1997; López Antuñano 1993).[3]

In 1960 the Institute of Social Security and Services for State Workers (ISSSTE) was created to offer protection against social risks for federal civil servants and other public employees. Like IMSS, protection provided health insurance and the provision of healthcare services for covered workers and their families. Many of these categories of workers were already receiving healthcare services under separate insurance schemes, but ISSSTE unified them all. The only groups of public sector employees that would remain with their own social insurance schemes would be the military and workers of the state oil company (PEMEX) (Bonilla-Chacín and Aguilera 2013; Gómez-Dantés et al. 2011; Carrillo Castro 1987). The constitution was reformed in 1982 to establish the right to healthcare protection for all the population, and a new General Health Law (LGS) was passed soon after to secure the compliance of that right, but in practice no policy would be adopted for that aim until 2002, when the System for Health Social Protection (SPSS) was created. A program called Popular Health Insurance (SPS) was introduced as the main instrument of the system to provide health insurance and healthcare to people who lacked social insurance coverage. SPS was a public voluntary health insurance program that required the payment of a premium by families who decided to purchase it, with funding complemented by contributions from the federal government and state governments. Family contributions had a progressive structure, with families of the lowest four income deciles exempt. Insurance covered a basic package of interventions, which was increased throughout the years, but never achieved unlimited coverage equivalent to that provided under social insurance schemes. Services were provided in the medical centers and hospitals administered by state governments. SPS affiliation grew fast, eventually surpassing IMSS insurance, previously the largest public healthcare scheme (CONEVAL 2018; López Arellano and López Moreno 2015; Bonilla-Chacín and Aguilera 2013; Frenk et al. 2006). SPS was replaced by the Institute for Health Welfare (INSABI) in 2020, which targets the same population with no social insurance, utilizing the same infrastructure as SPS, but granting access as a social right, without an insurance logic and eliminating the requirement of the payment of contributions (Reich 2020).

In spite of the expansion of public sector intervention in healthcare, many Mexicans rely on private provision for their healthcare needs. In fact, private healthcare services have grown in parallel to public services since the first half of the 20th century. Private participation may take the form of private outpatient and inpatient services, paid either directly at the point of service by the patient or through the acquisition of private insurance. Unlike Chile, private healthcare has been only marginally incorporated into the country's health-care policy. The LGS established in 1984 that private services formed part of a National Health System, but few links have been built with public serv-ices (González Block et al. 2018; López Arellano and López Moreno 2015; Zurita and Ramírez 2003; Sesma-Vázquez et al. 2005). The sort of implicit commodification observed in Mexico has grave consequences for healthcare quality and equity, as it is mostly the higher-income sector who can afford private services of higher quality through out-of-pocket (OOP) spending. Explicit commodification in Chile generates different, although also unde-sirable, outputs in terms of equity and quality. The dynamics of the public-private mixes of the two case studies is analyzed in the following sections.

Healthcare Policy Architectures and Private Provision

The private sector plays an important role in the provision of healthcare in both Chile and Mexico, although in different ways. The first part of this sec-tion compares the policy architectures and the role assigned to private pro-vision in both countries, grounded on the analytical framework devised by Martínez Franzoni and Sánchez-Ancochea (2016). The second describes the scope of private sector and public-private interactions in each country.

The Comparison of Policy Architectures

The framework proposed by Martínez Franzoni and Sánchez-Ancochea (2016) to analyze social policy architectures and outputs enables the study of the role of the private sector and its impact on the population, consid-ering how it works within the whole policy architecture of healthcare. These authors identified five components or "policy instruments" that make up the architecture of a policy area: eligibility criteria (Under what criteria do people benefit?), funding (Who pays and how?), benefits (Who defines them and how?), delivery (Who does what?), and opt-out options of public pro-vision (How do governments manage market-based alternatives?). The ap-plication of these instruments and their interactions condition the policy outputs in terms of three dimensions: population coverage; generosity of benefits, which encompasses the comprehensiveness and quality of the serv-ices offered; and equity in welfare provision. Table 9.1 compares the health-care policy architectures of Chile and Mexico in 2021.

Table 9.1. Policy architectures of healthcare in Chile and Mexico,[a] 2021

Policy instruments	Chile	Mexico
Eligibility criteria	Contributory scheme: Mandatory insurance for formal salaried workers and self-employed. Contributing workers and their family-dependents are eligible for either the public (FONASA) or private (ISAPREs) insurance. The latter can require the payment of extra premiums. Subsidized scheme: The poor and other vulnerable groups are eligible for enrollment in the public insurance (FONASA) without any payment.	IMSS: Mandatory social insurance for formal private sector workers and their economic dependents. ISSSTE: Mandatory social insurance for civil servants and their economic dependents.[b] INSABI: Social right for citizens not covered by mandatory social insurance. ISSFAM[c]: Social insurance for military personnel and their economic dependents. PEMEX[d] services: Contractual right of workers of state oil company and their economic dependents.
Funding	Subsidies: Free enrollment for FONASA and secondary and tertiary attention at the public network of providers for the poor and other vulnerable groups. Free PHC at the public network of providers for all FONASA holders. Revenue sources: Payroll taxes (monopartite—only workers) directed at either the public or private insurance (opt out). General revenues. Voluntary extra premiums to ISAPREs. Copayments:Pprogressive for secondary/tertiary services in the public network. Unregulated at private providers. Pooling of resources and solidarity: FONASA: General revenues and contributions pooled into a single fund; solidarity in resource allocation. ISAPREs: Multiple funds; no solidarity (individual insurance).	IMSS: Tripartite payroll contributions by employers, employees, and the federal government. ISSSTE: Tripartite payroll contributions by employers (government agency), employees, and the federal government. INSABI: General taxes. ISSFAM: Federal government contributions. PEMEX services: Company budget.
Benefits	Definition of benefits: Ministry of Health. Benefits: FONASA: All services. ISAPREs: Minimum package + other services according to the specific health plan purchased. AUGE-GES services for all.	IMSS: Primary, secondary, and tertiary attention, including medications, without restrictions. ISSSTE: Primary, secondary, and tertiary attention, including medications, without restrictions. INSABI: Prioritization of primary and secondary attention.[e] ISSFAM: Primary, secondary, and tertiary attention, including medications, without restrictions. PEMEX services: Primary, secondary, and tertiary attention, including medications, without restrictions.

Table 9.1. Continued

Policy instruments	Chile	Mexico
Service delivery	Fragmented. Public providers: Mainly population enrolled in FONASA. For-profit private providers: Mainly enrolled in ISAPREs and enrolled at FONASA by the Free Choice Modality.	Fragmented, each scheme delivers services with own infrastructure. IMSS: Decentralized public institute of the federal government, of tripartite administration with representatives of trade unions, employer organizations, and the federal government. ISSSTE: Decentralized public institute of the federal government, administered by a council of representatives from trade unions and the federal government. INSABI: Federal Secretariat of Health. ISSFAM: Decentralized public institute of the federal government, with a board of directors with representatives from the National Defense Secretariat, Marine Secretariat, and the federal government. PEMEX services: Managed by state oil company.
Opt-out options of public provision	A large number of poorly regulated market-based options, including private insurance and providers. Outside market-based options explicitly integrated into the system. Alternatives to opting out from the public sector are institutionalized.	Income tax deductions of spending on private healthcare. Subcontracting of private services by public schemes when public provider deems it necessary to meet demand.

Source: Own elaboration based on Bernales-Baksai and Velázquez Leyer (2021).

[a] For a comprehensive analysis of healthcare architectures and outputs of Chile and Mexico, see Bernales-Baksai and Velázquez Leyer (2021).

[b] Some state governments also operate services for their own civil servants.

[c] Social Security Institute for the Armed Forces, ISSFAM by its acronym in Spanish.

[d] Mexican Petroleum, PEMEX by its acronym in Spanish.

[e] INSABI replaced a program called Popular Health Insurance in 2020. PHI was a voluntary health insurance program financed with contributions from insured families, state governments, and the federal government. The operation of INSABI is still not clear as many rules have not been published yet. For an analysis of this particular scheme, see Reich (2020).

Both countries exhibit a fragmented architecture. This means that there is no unified system that offers similar services for all, but two or more schemes, with differences in eligibility criteria, financing, benefits, and provision. In the two cases, such fragmentation leads to the segmentation of the population, albeit based on different conditions. This means that more advantaged groups are granted more comprehensive benefits and quality healthcare by virtue of either their payment capacity or occupational category, which raises inequities with respect to economically or occupationally disadvantaged groups. In Chile, the fragmented architecture segments the population by income level. Healthcare insurance is mandatory for all workers, with coverage extended to their economic dependents. However, workers are given the option of choosing between public or private insurance, with the latter requiring the payment of extra premiums. In such a way, in practice, only those with higher payment capacity are able to opt for private insurance, despite the important fact that it is financed through social security. In turn, the subsidized scheme only covers those groups that can demonstrate the need for such support because of their low-income levels. In Mexico, the fragmented architecture segments the population by the occupational status of the breadwinner, with coverage also extended to economic dependents. People formally employed in the public or private sector and their families can have access to one of four national contributory social insurance schemes, while the rest of the population (e.g., the self-employed or informal sector workers) are entitled to public services of the recently created INSABI, which replaced Popular Health Insurance (PHI), a voluntary health insurance program for families and individuals without social insurance coverage (Reich 2020). The difference in the eligibility criteria between INSABI and PHI, namely between coverage as a citizen's right of people with no social insurance and as an insurance program for people who did not have social insurance and who chose to join it, did not end the architecture's fragmentation based on formal and informal employment. It also re-created inequalities, with more limited provision levels for outside the social insurance schemes, and generated inefficiencies that obstruct quality improvements in all schemes (González Block et al. 2020).

Besides the different fragmentation and segmentation modes, policy architectures also incorporate private provision through different mechanisms. In Chile, as mentioned, fragmentation is based primarily on the explicit introduction of the private market-based sector as a parallel system to the public one. The private system follows market rules;

therefore, its operation is based on a totally different rationale compared to the public system. In this way, parallel systems coexist with different profiles of holders, independent healthcare centers, and separate resources (Cid et al. 2014; Frenz et al. 2018). Because of the commodification of the private segment, most of such differences are related to the payment capacity and the creaming of the population applied by private insurance (Bernales-Baksai 2020). The commodified private sector captures the better-off and healthiest groups (Frenz et al. 2018; Observatorio Social CASEN 2018; Sojo 2017), offering their insurance plans to those who need them the least, whereas riskier groups are pushed out. This hampers the equalization of resources and care quality regarding the public sector. Also, private providers require copayments that are higher for those enrolled in the public insurance. This allows private providers to raise more resources and offer advantages over the public network. Among these advantages, direct access (i.e., without the need for referrals or waiting lists) to specialty care and more-complex interventions (e.g., surgeries) stands out.

Regarding the public sector, unlike what can be observed in Mexico, the Chilean public system works under a single insurance mechanism, in which all holders have the same benefits and access to the same facilities in the public network of providers (MINSAL-Chile 2012). Besides, all resources are pooled in a single fund, allowing progressivity in revenue collection and redistribution in resource allocation, enabling greater horizontal and vertical equity among those enrolled in the public insurance and a higher overall level of quality of healthcare.

However, the unification of the public sector is undermined by the dynamics of interaction with the private sector. As Table 9.1 indicates, regarding the dimension of outside options, the current architecture provides several institutional mechanisms for opting out of the public sector. The first of these mechanisms is the possibility of channeling compulsory social security contributions to private insurers (ISAPREs). The second mechanism occurs among nonsubsidized holders of the public insurance (i.e., groups B, C, and D of FONASA), who are offered vouchers when they seek to utilize private providers (i.e., the MLE modality). The third mechanism is the purchase of private suppliers by FONASA to face the unavailability of services in the public network of providers, which has steadily increased since 2005 (Goyenechea 2019).

On the other hand, in Mexico private sector participation in the policy architecture seems minimal. There are only two modes in which public policy contemplates private provision. One mode is the tax deduction OOP spending or payment of private insurance premiums. According to the Income Tax Law (Secretaría de Hacienda y Crédito Público [SHCP] 2002), deductions can be done by both individuals and corporations, at 100% from taxable income. This mode in fact represents a public subsidy of private provision (Howard 1999), which occurs in an unregulated manner and without mechanisms for guaranteeing the quality of the private services financed by tax deductions.

The second mode is the option that public social insurance schemes have of subcontracting private providers when the demand for a specific service surpasses available supply in the locality (OECD 2016; ISSSTE 2007; IMSS 1997). IMSS also offers agreements for the reimbursement of contributions by employers who offer private healthcare to their employees as a work benefit (IMSS 1997). No other link is established between private and public provision in this country.

The Scope of Private Services

In spite of the different modes of market incorporation established in the policy architectures, the size and scope of private healthcare sectors is similar in both countries. As shown in Figure 9.1, 50% of current healthcare expenditure in 2018 involved private spending in both countries. Similarly, in both cases a decreasing trend can be observed in the present century. A large proportion of private spending corresponds to OOP spending, which has also decreased in recent decades. Nonetheless, in Mexico that indicator is higher than in Chile (WHO 2020a).

Figure 9.2 compares three indicators of private provision: the percentages of private healthcare facilities and hospital beds and of medical hours or doctors employed in the private sector out of the total numbers in each country. Similar figures are registered for both cases in the first two indicators. Around one-quarter of healthcare facilities and one-fifth of hospital beds belong to the private sector. Regarding the proportion of medical hours or doctors, the indicator is higher in Chile, where more than half of medical hours are in the private sector, while in Mexico about 35% of doctors are employed by private hospitals and practices, with the caveat that in the two countries doctors employed in the private sector might also be employed in public hospitals. This implies that a large amount of resources is channeled

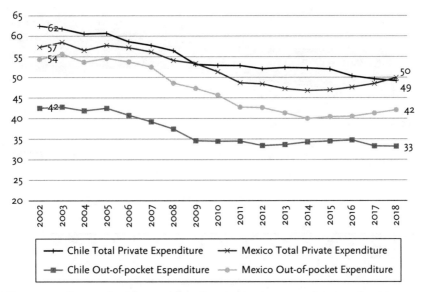

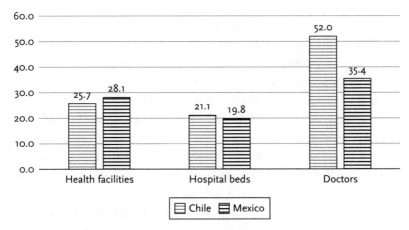

Figure 9.1. Private healthcare expenditure as percentage of current health expenditure, 2002–2018.

Source: WHO (2020a).

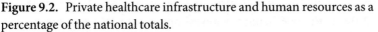

Figure 9.2. Private healthcare infrastructure and human resources as a percentage of the national totals.

Sources: Clínicas de Chile (2018b), DEIS (2021), SS (2021), and González Block et al. (2018).

Notes: In Chile, the column "Doctors" refers to the number of employed hours in the private sector.

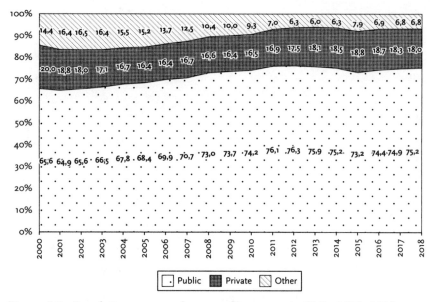

Figure 9.3. Population coverage by type of insurance in Chile, 2000–2018.
Source: Own elaboration from Boletín Estadístico FONASA 2000–2019.

to the private sector, while most of the population seek treatment within the public system, creating significant disparities in terms of quality of care. Thus, while in Chile private insurance holders (i.e., enrolled in the ISAPREs) do not exceed 18% (see Figure 9.3), health facilities, hospital beds, and medical hours in the private sector far exceed that figure.

In Chile, the number of market-based insurance and health providers is high. In 2020, twelve ISAPREs (six open and six for workers of specific companies) managed private insurance in the country (Superintendencia de Salud 2021). By 2018, 18% of the population (3.4 million people) was enrolled at any ISAPRE, which represents a non-negligible part of the population, although it is low compared with the over 75.2% (14.2 million people) covered by public insurance (FONASA) the same year. In fact, the percentage of the population holding private insurance decreased from 19.8% in 2000 to 18.2% in 2018, with 2006 being the lowest point, with 16.4% of population coverage (Superintendencia de Salud 2019).

Nonetheless, the participation of the private sector goes far beyond insurance. By 2014 market-based suppliers delivered about 37% of all health treatment (Cid et al. 2014). In 2018, the association of private providers (Clínicas de Chile) estimated a potential demand of 49.7% of the population (9.3 million people), with the majority (5.8 million people) coming from FONASA and most of the rest from ISAPREs (Clínicas de Chile 2018).

The extent of participation of the private sector is reflected in the large proportion of human resources and medical hours employed by this sector. Thus, 50.4% of physicians and 48% of medical specialists in 2018 exclusively delivered services via private providers (Clínicas de Chile 2018). Likewise, between 2010 and 2019, infrastructure grew faster in the private sector, with a 20.8% increase. Moreover, private beds reached 19% of the country's total beds, while in the same period, beds in the public network increased by 4.5%, reaching 69% (Clínicas de Chile 2018).

As shown above, the significant role of the private sector translates into high levels of private spending on health. Although this spending has progressively declined in recent years, it continues to represent about 40% of the total health expenditure (WHO 2020a). As discussed further in the chapter, since most private expenditure is OOP, this configuration of health spending implies high health-related financial risk.

In turn, despite the governments' efforts to increase spending levels, public spending on health, including payroll contributions, reached 5.4% of GDP in 2017. This proportion is high in Latin America, where average government health expenditure only reached 3.7% of GDP the same year (OECD/WB 2020), but it is below the international recommendation of 6% of GDP (PAHO/WHO 2014; WHO 2010). Such spending levels obstruct improvements in quality and reproduce horizontal inequities and low quality of services, limiting the resources for lower-income groups who do not have the option of seeking private treatment.

In Mexico, coverage levels of public schemes have increased significantly in the last two decades. In 2017, one of the public schemes (INEGI 2021b) insured 83% of the people, and after the latest reform that substituted SPS with INSABI, legally all Mexicans should be covered by the public system. Yet, the scope of private provision is similar to Chile, but with few formal links between public and private services. In Mexico 44% of total consultations and 22% of total hospital discharges correspond to the private sector (González-Block et al. 2018). The reason for such a large scope can be found in the implicit mode in which state action incentivizes private provision, revealed when the specific public-private interactions are analyzed. Implicit commodification in this country has serious implications on equity and quality of healthcare provision; for example, lower-income families are forced to spend a significant proportion of their income on health services, and only to access limited primary care and to buy medicine, as good quality private hospitalization services are out of their reach; demands for improvements of public services are obstructed because middle- and upper-income families are able to opt for private services; with a low degree of regulation, healthcare provision is ultimately left in the hands of market forces (Bernales-Baksai and Velázquez Leyer 2021).

Public-Private Interactions

The dual configuration adopted by the Chilean health system after introducing the private sector implies that far from being isolated from each other, there are multiple and dynamic mechanisms of interaction between the public and private sectors. Three areas can be highlighted where such interactions are especially striking.

The first area of reciprocal impact is insurance, as each sector's different principles and regulations have driven significant segmentation of the insured population. The public insurance gathers groups with lower levels of education and older people (Frenz et al. 2018), females and children (Asociación de Isapres de Chile 2016; Sojo 2017), and groups with lower income (Observatorio Social CASEN 2018). In contrast, ISAPREs have been increasingly gathering the population with less health risk (i.e., males and the middle-aged individuals are progressively overrepresented) (Superintendencia de Salud 2019) and assemble the country's upper and upper-middle classes (Programa de las Naciones Unidas Para el Desarrollo [PNUD] 2017). This marked stratification is based on the lack of regulation that, over the years, has allowed the ISAPREs to cream the population and is supported by the availability of the public insurance to receive those rejected or pushed out (e.g., when they become older or sick) by the ISAPREs (see Cid et al. 2014; Frenz et al. 2018).

Second, the segmentation of the insured population leads to more availability of resources per capita in the private sector vis-à-vis the public sector. ISAPREs attract better-off groups that pay higher payroll taxes and make additional payments to hold better health plans, creating a gap of between 30% (excluding OOP) and 39% (including OOP) of resources compared with FONASA (Frenz et al. 2018). Moreover, the gap is enlarged by the solidarity mechanisms of FONASA, where resource allocation is adjusted to risk calculation (i.e., progressive). In contrast, the individual insurance logic that governs the ISAPREs system excludes any chance of solidarity and, therefore, vertical equity even among holders of private insurance in the same ISAPRE.

Moreover, as examined further here, the accumulation of higher-risk population by the public insurance (first area) along with the higher resource availability in the private sector (second area) lead to the level of health risk not commensurate with the services offered by each sector, thus preventing vertical equity.

Finally, the third area of recurring interaction takes place through healthcare provision. The prominent proportion of private healthcare provision discussed above not only depends on the population that opts out of the public sector, channeling their contributions to the ISAPREs, but also relies on the increasing contracting out of private services with public resources (i.e., the public insurance purchases private attention) (Goyenechea 2019) and the option given to FONASA holders to opt for privately delivered services using vouchers (Bitran 2014; Gómez Bradford et al. 2019). In fact, transfers of public resources to the private sector constantly increased between 2005 and 2018, considering both direct contracting of private services and vouchers delivered to subsidize the demand (see Goyenechea 2019). In turn, purchasing private supply, which is subsidizing the demand instead of the supply side, has become the mechanism increasingly adopted by the public sector to reduce waiting lists and unmet health needs that result from the limitations of resources faced by the public network of providers. By directing these public resources to the private sector instead of strengthening the capacity and quality of the public sector, the quality gaps and inequities, vis-à-vis the private sector, are perpetuated.

In Mexico, as previously stated, few institutionalized links have been built between public and private healthcare services. The subcontracting of private services by public social insurance schemes is not an option offered to patients and is not used extensively, even if unmet demands for services can be high, with budget restrictions affecting the possibility of activation. The use of the mechanism of the reimbursement of social insurance contributions to employers who provide healthcare to their employees has actually been in decline in recent years, amounting to only 1.2% of the total number of insured workers by IMSS in 2014, although it was never extensively used in the first place, having been limited to the banking sector and a few large corporations (González Block 2018; Lara 2018; OECD 2016). Yet, workers who are taken out of the reimbursement scheme lose access to high-quality private services previously offered by their employers, while more pressure is placed on public services as demand increases.

The deductibility of private health spending from income tax represents an important incentive to seek medical attention in the private sector, but it does not establish a direct link between the public and private sectors. Private healthcare services operate in a highly unregulated context, with provision shaped by market rules of supply and demand. Income tax deductions offer an opportunity to obtain healthcare in that market with a public subsidy. On average, taxpayers are able to deduct 30% of spending (Redacción AN 2018). Yet, because of the large size of the informal economy, which in December 2020 accounted for 55% of total employment, that option would exclude many low-income workers who make up the majority of that sector (INEGI 2021d), reproducing horizontal inequities.

Even if the state seems to have neglected private services in the design of its healthcare policy, the private sector still accounts for almost half of total spending and a significant portion of the national infrastructure. A process of implicit commodification unfolds in Mexican healthcare provision, where the existence of a large private sector is explained by the low quality and deficient supply of public services.

Under the current architecture, all Mexicans are formally covered by a public healthcare scheme, either by a social insurance scheme through the employment status of household earners or through INSABI, which is meant to cover all citizens without social insurance. Even before the creation of INSABI in 2020, coverage levels of public schemes were already high: 82% of the population in 2017 (INEGI 2021b). That result was achieved by the creation of SPS in the early 2000s; before the introduction of that voluntary insurance program, only 40% of Mexicans were insured by a public scheme (INEGI 2021b). Nonetheless, in spite of this recent expansion of public healthcare, large numbers of people have continued to seek medical care in the private sector, even if covered by a public scheme.

Due to deficiencies in the supply of public services, many people prefer or are forced to use private services (Bernales-Baksai and Velázquez Leyer 2021). For example, national government surveys of the quality of public services showed that in 2019 only 41% of respondents did not encounter deficiencies with IMSS services and did not have to pay for a private service, percentages that only increased to 42% for ISSSTE and 43% for SPS services, and that practically did not change in the 2015 survey, when they were 39% for IMSS, 40% for ISSSTE, and 43% for SPS. The lowest-rated aspect is the saturation of hospitals and clinics; the weighted average of users that found it to be a problem in 2019 across the three schemes was 83%. This was followed by the lack of medicines, which all public schemes are meant to provide at no cost for the patient, the length of waiting times to be seen, and the insufficiency of doctors, with weighted averages of around 50% of users identifying them as problems in that same year (INEGI 2021a). The 2020 national health and nutrition survey registered that 56% of the total number of people with health problems were treated in the private sector, a proportion that included 45% of IMSS beneficiaries and 57% of ISSSTE beneficiaries with health problems who received care in the private sector. Only 29% of the people surveyed stated that having public insurance was the main reason for selecting their healthcare provider, while 22% declared that the main reason was proximity of the medical unit, 12% that it was the low cost of the services purchased, 11% the time it took to be seen, and 10% that they liked how they were treated (INSP 2021). Regarding the prescriptions given at IMSS medical units and hospitals, 10% of prescriptions are not supplied or are only partially supplied because of lack of medicines, forcing patients to try to purchase them at private pharmacies (Bernales-Baksai and Velázquez Leyer 2021). All these figures reveal the process of implicit commodification that is unfolding in Mexico.

Public/Private Mixes and Healthcare Equity

Because equitable healthcare involves tackling unfair differences among groups of the population, providing everybody similar opportunities to access quality healthcare, we have chosen to focus the analysis on equity outputs, as this reveals the extent of the population coverage and the sufficiency and generosity of health services for all. The next paragraphs offer an analysis of the impact of current public-private arrangements on the equitable provision of healthcare in each country.

The Chilean Case: The Explicit Introduction of the Private Sector

Given the dual structure of the Chilean health system, it is relevant to analyze the inequities that arise from differences in service quality between the public and private sectors. Although evaluating quality is always complex, the examination of available resources can work as a fair proxy. In this area, data show that resource disparities between both sectors may favor inequities. As previously discussed, the public sector insures a population with greater health risks, and therefore with more healthcare requirements, and has fewer per capita resources than the private sector to provide services.

The disparity in resources between FONASA and ISAPREs can imply both horizontal and vertical inequity. Horizontal inequity is apparent as people with similar healthcare needs, but who belong to one or the other insurance, may receive different quality of services. For instance, regarding timely treatment, in the public network waiting lists surpass 1.6 million people, with an average of 400 days waiting for surgeries not included in the AUGE-GES guarantees (Frenz et al. 2018). This is not the case for holders of private insurance, where waiting lists do not exist since anyone who can pay has access to the treatment they require almost immediately.

Moreover, households' OOP spending, which importantly relates to the utilization of private services, exhibited significant increases between 2012 and 2016 (Benítez, Hernando, and Velasco 2018). This is despite the fact that the country´s OOP decreased from 43% (WHO 2020a) to 34% (OECD/WB 2020) of current health expenditure between 2000 and 2020 because of the higher public investment. The increase in households' OOP spending took place across all income quintiles except the first quintile, and among both FONASA and ISAPREs holders, with the exception of those in the subsidized group of FONASA (group A) (Benítez et al. 2018). Thus, those with payment capacity invest in private options to face the barriers to accessing healthcare, as expressed by the growing demand for private services previously discussed. Therefore, horizontal inequities appear as those with the payment capacity have better chances to get quality care.

On the other hand, differences in risk profiles between the public and private sectors imply vertical inequity: The population with higher health risk is concentrated in FONASA, which has fewer resources to respond to these needs. Moreover, as certain socioeconomic and demographic conditions are associated with greater healthcare needs, it is expected that if there is vertical equity, these groups will make greater use of health services. Nonetheless, in the current configuration of the health system in Chile, the reality is ambiguous in this area, and service utilization is not always higher among those groups where it might be predicted. In this regard, we consider five variables that allow us to discriminate among groups with higher healthcare needs: level of income, age, ethnicity, perceived health status, and presence of disability (i.e., the poor, older adults, indigenous population, those with worse self-perception of health, and those with disabilities have more need of healthcare and should have higher levels of service utilization).

Regarding income level, contrary to some arguments found in the literature on higher healthcare needs among the poorest groups, findings from this research show that the richest quintile declared more healthcare needs (21.4%) and higher service utilization (20.1%) vis-à-vis the poorest quintile (17.1% of healthcare needs and 15.6% of service utilization). Consistently, the group affiliated with ISAPREs is the one with the highest service utilization. Among FONASA holders, the population that indicated the need for healthcare and did not receive it reached 6.2% and increased to 6.8% among those subsidized because of their low income (group A), while among those in ISAPREs, the figure decreased to 5.2%.[4] These figures may not be surprising given the fact that ISAPREs assemble the population with the highest income and lower health risks (Cid et al. 2014; Frenz et al. 2018). In fact, the analysis of health insurance[5] showed that 55.8% of those enrolled in ISAPREs belong to the richest quintile and only 5.7% to the lowest income quintile. Meanwhile, the poorest quintile is concentrated in FONASA: 23.5% of its affiliates belong to the first quintile, and only 11.9% to the richest quintile.

Regarding age groups, adults aged 60 and over have more healthcare needs than the population under 60 years old (28.7% vs. 17.2%). Nevertheless, the proportion of people who use health services is similar in both age groups (93% and 94%, respectively).[6] Moreover, the older population is concentrated in FONASA, while ISAPREs favor the enrollment of the younger population.

Regarding ethnicity, the indigenous population perceives fewer healthcare needs and exhibits lower levels of service utilization than the rest of the population (18.1% vs. 19.9% and 16.5% vs. 18.4%, respectively). Nevertheless, these results are contradictory to studies that indicated higher rates of morbidity and mortality in all the indigenous groups in the country, especially in those indicators that trace situations of social injustice such as infant mortality and mortality from tuberculosis (Pedrero and Oyarce 2009).

In terms of perceived health status, those who present a worse self-perception of health use more health services (39.9%) than those with a better self-perception of health (10%). Finally, those with a disability who indicated a health need in the last 3 months use more health services (30.6%) compared with those without disabilities (16.6%).[7,8]

In turn, the analysis of unmet healthcare needs revealed that whereas the percentage of people who did not receive treatment when needed reached 6.2% overall in 2017, only 0.48% were related to healthcare supply. Still, inequities remain by some social conditions that put some groups at a disadvantage. Thus, women, those enrolled in ISAPREs, those in the fourth income quintile, those working as salaried workers, and those living in rural areas are overrepresented among those who did not receive treatment for self-perceived health conditions, compared with men, those enrolled in FONASA, better-off and poorest individuals, self-employed workers, and those living in urban areas[9].

From the perspective of the public-private mix effect, it is striking that the holders of private insurance exhibit higher figures of unmet healthcare needs than those enrolled in FONASA. It implies that there is a group that is opting out of the public sector and still experiencing more barriers to meet their healthcare needs. In the same line, it is significant that the main reason (79.3%) for unmet healthcare needs among those affiliated with ISAPREs was lack of money, while for FONASA holders it was the difficulty of obtaining a medical appointment (48.4%).

Likewise, it was neither the better off nor the poorest who are less likely to receive treatment, but groups that were not poor enough to receive subsidies from the public system or who had sufficient resources to use private services fully. They could, for example, be those who had FONASA but made use of private services through vouchers or those who hired the most exiguous and cheapest health plans offered by the ISAPREs. All of this unveils a system that, although capable of supporting the poorest, continues to produce inequities based on payment capacity.

Other inequities arise from the architecture of the system. As previously discussed, an increasing number of FONASA holders seek treatment from private suppliers (Cid et al. 2014; Clínicas de Chile 2018), either through vouchers and copayments or because of the growing purchase of private services by FONASA. This possibility of opting out of public services raises horizontal inequity among FONASA holders, as only those paying contributions (i.e., groups B, C, and D) and with payment capacity can obtain the vouchers (i.e., the MLE modality of attention) and afford the copayments requested by private providers. Vouchers are perceived as providing access to a better quality of care and pursued by those who can afford the remaining cost of covering the private providers' rates.

A final aspect to consider is that the dual organization of the health system, the coexistence of multiple funds, and particularly the private sector based on individual insurance create financial arrangements that do not leave room for solidarity, which favors progress in achieving greater equity (either vertical or horizontal) except within the public sector, which is also being undermined by the increasing subsidization due to the demand by some for private services.

Table 9.2 below compares the proportions of people who claimed to have had healthcare needs but did not receive care, from either the public or private sector, as described above for the case of Chile. Percentages were calculated from national surveys and considered supply-side related unmet

Table 9.2. Population with supply-side related unmet healthcare needs

Variable	Chile (2017)	Mexico (2020)
Total population with supply-side related unmet needs (self-report)	0.48%	2.1%
Sex	Men = 0.2%*** Women = 0.7%***	Men = 2.2%*** Women = 2.0%***
Position at household	Heads of household = 0.5% Other family members = 0.4%	Heads of household = 2.5%* Other family members = 2.0%*
Health insurance	FONASA = 0.4%** ISAPREs = 0.6%**	Public (compulsory and voluntary insurance) = 0.9%* Private = 0.2%***
Ethnicity	Ethnic groups = 0.5% Nonethnic groups = 0.5%	Ethnic groups = 5.5%* Nonethnic groups = 2.0%*
Income	Quintile 1 = 0.5%** Quintile 2 = 0.5%** Quintile 3 = 0.4%** Quintile 4 = 0.7%** Quintile 5 = 0.3%**	Quintile 1 = 4.7%* Quintile 2 = 1.9%* Quintile 3 = 1.7%* Quintile 4 = 1.5%* Quintile 5 = 0.7%*
Employment status	Self-employed or employer = 0.4%*** Salaried workers = 1.0%***	Self-employed or employer = 3.1%* Salaried workers = 2.4%*
Area of residence	Urban = 0.5%* Rural = 0.7%*	Urban = 1.7%* Rural = 3.2%*

Notes: Out of the total number of people that reported to have had healthcare needs in Chile during the 3 months previous to the survey, 6.2% reported not having received attention for any reason, namely, because they were not able to access care due to either demand-side or supply-side barriers (e.g., had no time to go or could not find a medical unit or hospital to be treated). In Mexico, 24.4% of people with health problems in the previous 3 months did not receive care for any reason. The table shows the proportions of the people with health problems that did not receive care because of problems attributed to the supply-side deficiencies.

*p < .1%, **p < .05%, ***p < .01%.

Sources: Own elaboration from Casen Survey 2017 and INEGI 2021c.

healthcare needs.[10] Thus, the comparison does provide a parameter to evaluate the success of current healthcare arrangements in each country in offering access to all population groups. Indicators showed better results in Chile for all groups. The results for Mexico are discussed in the subsequent section.

The Mexican Case: Effects of Implicit Commodification

There is evidence that the expansion of public healthcare undertaken during this century has yielded some positive results regarding the extent to which households rely on private spending on healthcare. WHO reports increases in general government health spending as a percentage of GDP, from 2% in 2000 to 2.7% in 2018—having peaked at 3.1% in 2013 and 2015—as a percentage of total current spending from 45.2% to 50.1% in the same period (with a peak of 53.2% in 2014), and in terms of per capita spending from 223.1 to 533.7 Purchasing Power Parity (PPP) US Dollars and peaking at 562.7 PPP US dollars in 2015. In 2000, private per capita spending was 20% higher than public spending, while in 2018 it was 0.3% lower, having registered a maximum negative gap of 12% less in 2014. OOP spending, which comprises mostly private spending, declined from 52% to 42% of total current health expenditure between 2000 and 2018 (WHO 2021).

National household surveys registered drops in the number of households that reported spending on private healthcare services, from 67% in 2004 to 54% in 2018 (INEGI 2021c), and in the number of people who declared more frequent use of private services than public services, from 35% in 2004 to 26% in 2017 (INEGI 2021b). On average, in 2018, Mexican households spent 2.6% of their cash income on healthcare, compared to 3.1% in 2008 (INEGI 2021c).

However, in spite of those results, the process of implicit commodification and its consequential horizontal inequities persist. Figure 9.4 compares variations in healthcare spending as a percentage of total cash income for each decile during the current century. Spending trends as a proportion of household income were lower in 2018 than in 2008 for all income deciles, but percentages were also similar across deciles, between 2.2% and 3.1% for all deciles in 2018, with the poorest decile registering the third-highest spending after the 9th and 10th deciles. Moreover, the richest decile was the only one to register a constant decrease in the 3 years (INEGI 2021c).

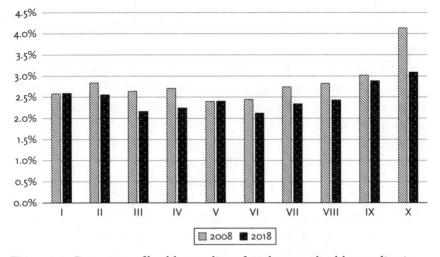

Figure 9.4. Percentage of health spending of total current health spending in Mexico, 2018.
Source: INEGI (2021d).

As mentioned above, even if covered by a public scheme, many people still prefer or have to seek care in the private sector. In addition to the evidence provided in the previous section, the national employment and social security survey of 2017 reported that the proportion of people insured by IMSS who required healthcare but preferred or had to use private services with more frequency was 19%, higher than the indicator of 17% in 2013. In the case of ISSSTE and SPS, during the same period, proportions passed from 18% to 23% and 13% to 16%, respectively. These percentages do not include people who sought care in private pharmacies, which may have a doctor's office attached to them (INEGI 2021b). The percentages registered by the national survey of 2020 were actually higher than these 2017 proportions. The reasons for these trends relate to a deficiency in the supply of public services.

The use of private services displays different shapes and consequences across income groups. The composition of private spending varies by income decile. In 2018, the largest proportions of spending were on medicines with and without prescriptions, which encompassed 29% of total household health spending, and medical services (e.g., payments for private consultations) with 26%. However, for households in the 1st decile almost half of health spending corresponded to medicines, 47% of the total, compared to only 22% for households in the 10th decile. On the other hand, 19%

of spending by households of that 10th decile corresponded to hospitalization services, compared to 13% by the poorest first decile (INEGI 2021c).

Spending on private insurance is heavily concentrated in the wealthiest deciles. It is much lower than in Chile, just 6% of national health spending in 2018. Yet, almost three-quarters of that national total was spent by households in the 10th decile, and if the three top deciles are added, they encompass 89% of the total. Only those three deciles devoted more than 5% of health spending to insurance: 5%, 9%, and 13% for households of the 8th, 9th, and 10th deciles, respectively (INEGI 2021c).

General doctors' offices adjacent to pharmacies of large chains constitute a growing trend across the country; it is estimated that they currently account for 17% of all consultations in the country. While they grant all families, especially lower-income families, access to private provision at a low cost, moral risk is high since there are incentives for them to prescribe as many medications as could be purchased in their employer's establishment. On the other hand, private hospitals, especially those of high quality, are heavily concentrated in urban areas and are mainly accessible by middle- and upper-income families (González-Block et al. 2018). Half of the private hospitals ranked among the best 50 private hospitals in the country in a recent study are found in only two metropolitan areas, Mexico City and Monterrey (Expansión 2021).

Usage and spending indicators showed the inequities and quality problems of healthcare provision in Mexico. Lower-income people are more dependent on public services and are only able to access cheap private provision due to deficiencies in public supply, with a high negative impact on their income since health spending may affect their consumption of other basic products and services. On the other hand, those with a higher income can access private services of higher quality, especially regarding secondary and tertiary care, in some cases through private insurance, which can shield them from catastrophic private expenditures.

The analysis of vertical equity yields important differences in access to services by people from different population groups who require care. In 2018, of people who had a health problem 22%did not receive care, because they either could not access healthcare or chose not to seek care. Older adults and people with disabilities appear to be able to access healthcare to a larger extent than the overall population. Only 16% of adults aged 60 or older who suffered a health problem did not receive healthcare in 2018, less than the unattended proportions of the entire population and of the 23% of the population below that age threshold. In the case of people with disabilities, also 16% of those who had a health issue were not treated, compared to 23% for the population with no disabilities.

When the analysis is restricted to people who did not receive care due to supply-side deficiencies, as shown in Table 9.2 above, 2.1% of people with health problems who sought care in 2018 were not able to access it in either the public or private sector. That percentage includes people who were not able to access public services because of lack of coverage or limitations in the supply of services, because they did not have the financial resources to purchase private services, or a combination of those and various other reasons, and excludes those people who decided not to seek care because they considered that their problem was not serious enough or because they self-medicated at home and other similar reasons (INEGI 2021b, 2021d).

Important inequalities are revealed between income sectors, ethnic groups, and employment categories. In the first quintile, 4.7% of people who sought healthcare were not able to access it, compared with only 0.7% for the fifth-wealthiest quintile, and as can be observed in the table, the proportions of people with unmet healthcare needs decreased as income rose. (INEGI 2021c). Low access rates of two other groups should be highlighted: indigenous people, with 5.5% with health problems not receiving care, and the rural population, with more than 3.2%, compared to 2.0% and 1.7% in the cases of nonindigenous and urban population, respectively (INEGI 2021b, 2021d). According to the national census, in 2020 indigenous people represented 6.1% of the total population, with most inhabiting rural areas, being largely concentrated in southern states and having historically been the most marginalized group in the country (INEGI 2020). Healthcare programs that have targeted poor people in rural areas have existed for many decades, mainly offering primary care with limited resources. Although the voluntary health insurance through PHI did reach coverage of more than 6% of indigenous people, they still suffer from a more serious lack of access to health services than the rest of the population (Leyva-Flores et al. 2013). Finally, another important difference in unmet needs can be observed between the self-employed, who are not entitled to social insurance, 3.1% of whom reported health problems and sought care but did not receive it, and salaried workers, who may be covered by a social insurance scheme, with 2.4% with health problems not able to access healthcare services.

The analysis of horizontal and vertical healthcare equity in Mexico yields mixed results. The expansion of public provision over the two last decades has produced a decrease in private spending and OOP spending. In the 2020s, more people received healthcare from the state, and fewer people depended on market provision than before the expansion in the early 2000s. Nonetheless, results have been far from what is required to face the magnitude of the challenges.

As shown, the analysis of horizontal equity outputs showed that private spending had stronger impact on lower-income families. As previously stated, the proportion that poor households are forced to spend on health might only be sufficient to purchase medicines and primary services, which in fact many of those households are entitled to and should be provided by public schemes. On the contrary, higher-income households are able to access hospitalization services of higher quality than any public program. The market also offers higher protection levels to wealthy groups through private health insurance, an option that is inaccessible to many middle-income and virtually all low-income households (González Block et al. 2018).

Regarding vertical equity, the evidence shows that the public-private mix is able to prioritize care for older adults and people with disabilities. However, low access rates of low-income, indigenous, and the rural population with health problems revealed the failure of the state to provide effective coverage and the inaccessibility of market services for many of them.

Conclusions

Important efforts have been made in both countries to expand healthcare protection in recent decades. In Chile, this has been through the growth of public spending on health, the introduction of the AUGE-GES plan and other reforms aimed at ameliorating the inequalities raised by the dual public-private system, and in Mexico, through the layering of new public programs along social insurance schemes. Positive results can be observed in the two cases, with public coverage spending levels reaching historical records. Yet, commodification processes continue to be reproduced, affecting equity and quality of healthcare services and leaving many people vulnerable to market forces, albeit following different paths that produced distinct public/private mixes in each case.

The explicit process of commodification of the Chilean system encompasses several mechanisms for transitioning from public provision toward the private sector. In this country, the private sector has been formally incorporated into the policy architecture, creating a dual public-private system, where upper-income groups have the possibility of accessing private services subsidized by public resources. In Mexico, the degree of the institutionalization of such private participation is much lower, but the neglect of the private sector in the policy architecture does not mean that it does not play a significant role in healthcare provision. In fact, in this country the role of private healthcare is as large as or even larger than in Chile because deficiencies in the supply of public services implicitly incentivize the use of private services. The two modes of private sector participation have been labeled explicit and implicit commodification (see Bernales-Baksai and Velázquez Leyer 2021). The identification of processes of explicit and implicit commodification shows the variety of the nexus that may develop between the public and private sectors.

The analysis presented in this chapter can show the different instances in which commodification processes may unfold in explicit or implicit modes:

- Private insurance, financed with social insurance resources or indirect public subsidies in the form of tax deductions, or directly purchased by the insured person;
- Private services with public subsidies like vouchers or tax deductions;
- Private services paid by OOP spending with no subsidies; and
- Private services subcontracted by public schemes when supply is deemed insufficient.

The explicit and institutionalized incorporation of these mechanisms that occurs in Chile pushes public resources toward the private sector and empowers private actors to act as veto players and hinder transformations in policy design. Private insurers and suppliers receive public resources from social insurance and general revenues, respectively, but guide their operation by market rules instead of by social welfare principles. The provision of care by the private sector, through insurance by public entities, vouchers that partially cover the treatment cost, or the contracting out of private providers by the government, also means that public resources are pushed toward the private sector. Public resources are transferred to a significant degree to the private sector, instead of improving the actual capacity in the public system, deepening the differences in quality between both sectors and, therefore, healthcare inequities.

In Mexico, institutional links with private services are much weaker. Private provision is promoted through the tax system, which in practice represents a public subsidy not unlike the vouchers offered in Chile, and is enabled by the possibility of contracting them out when public schemes deem their supply to be limited. This is a similar mechanism to the one that operates in Chile as well, but their use and scope is much more limited than in that country. Commodification mostly unfolds by omission, namely, the inability of the state to meet the healthcare demands of the people who have formal public healthcare coverage, under the third mechanism of OOP spending with no government subsidy listed above. Because of the absence of government regulation of private provision, the organization of healthcare in the country is left to a significant extent to the whims of market forces, which result in significant inequities in healthcare delivery as well as different levels of quality of healthcare delivery based on the ability of various groups to access the healthcare market.

The approach of implicit commodification generated in Mexico appears to be even more problematic in terms of securing equitable and adequate healthcare delivery than the process of explicit commodification followed in Chile. Private spending levels are lower in Chile, even if opt-out options are part of the design of healthcare policy, while in Mexico the existence of a large private sector is mostly ignored by public policy. This is not to say that the Chilean system, on the one hand, achieves desirable results; on the contrary, deep inequities are generated and reproduced by the existing public-private mix. The system requires further reforms to address them. In Mexico, on the other hand, what is needed is the formulation and implementation of new institutions to reduce the significant scope of inequities regarding healthcare delivery and different levels of quality of care received by Mexico's population.

Health is a social right that mandates the delivery of public goods in a universal matter. The organization of healthcare cannot be delegated to market forces. The comparison of the Chilean and Mexican cases shows how better institutions in the former and more advanced development of basic healthcare institutions in the latter must be constructed in order to see advances in the equitable provision of healthcare and the provision of quality healthcare services in these two nations.

Acknowledgments

This chapter was prepared with the valuable research assistance of María José Infanzón Valdivieso. Results of the research presented in the chapter was presented at academic events of the International Public Policy Assocation, European Consortium for Political Resarch and the Universidad Iberoamericana of Mexico City.

Notes

1. The single fund supposed solidarity between people enrolled at the public and private insurance.
2. These programs were initially created as private schemes funded by employers and workers but would later be incorporated into public social insurance with state contributions.
3. During the period 1987–1995, only 21% of total health spending was devoted to programs for people with no social insurance coverage. That spending was also highly regressive, because in spite of the creation of targeted programs, the concentration of SSA hospital services in large urban areas meant that it ended up neglecting the poorest regions of the country (Lara et al. 1997)
4. Own calculation using data from CASEN 2017 household survey.
5. Own calculation using data from CASEN 2017 household survey.
6. Own calculation using data from CASEN 2017 household survey.
7. Own calculation using data from CASEN 2017 household survey.
8. A consideration to bear in mind in this analysis is that higher service utilization among older adults, people with a worse perception of health, and those with some disability does not necessarily express vertical equity produced by the characteristics of the health system. The perception of the need for healthcare is higher among these groups than in the general population. Therefore, it is possible that their higher rates of service utilization also respond to more active strategies of healthcare seeking.
9. The analysis also compared position at household and ethnicity, but differences were not statistically significant for these variables.
10. In Chile, the reasons of supply side related unmet healthcare needs include thought about seeking care but had no money; thought about seeking care, but it is difficult to access the healthcare center; and could not get an appointment.

References

Asociación de Isapres de Chile. 2016. *Isapres 1981–2016. 35 años de desarrollo del sistema de salud privado en Chile*. Santiago, Chile: Asociación de Isapres de Chile.

Bambra, Clare. 2005. "Worlds of Welfare and Health Care Discrepancy." *Social Policy and Society* 4(1): 31–41.

Barrientos, Armando. 2004. "Latin America: Towards a Liberal-Informal Welfare Regime." In *Insecurity and Welfare Regimes in Asia, Africa and Latin America: Social Policy in Development Contexts*, edited by Ian Gough, Geoffrey Wood, Armando Barrientos, Philippa Bevan, Peter Davis, and Graham Room, 68–121. Cambridge: Cambridge University Press.

Barrientos, Armando, and Peter Lloyd-Sherlock. 2002. "Health Insurance Reforms in Latin America: Cream Skimming, Equity and Cost-Containment." In *Social Policy Reform and Market Governance in Latin America*, edited by L Haagh and C Helgø, 183–189. London: Springer.

Benítez, Alejandra, Andrés Hernando, and Carolina Velasco. 2018. "Radiografía del gasto de bolsillo en salud en Chile: Análisis del cambio en el gasto entre 2012 y 2016." *Puntos de Referencia* 491. https://www.cepchile.cl/cep/site/docs/20181023/20181023161058/pder491_abenitez.pdf

Bernales-Baksai, Pamela. 2020. "Tackling Segmentation to Advance Universal Health Coverage: Analysis of Policy Architectures of Health Care in Chile and Uruguay." *International Journal for Equity in Health* 19: article 106. https://doi.org/10.1186/s12939-020-01176-6

Bernales-Baksai, Pamela, and Ricardo Velázquez Leyer. 2021. "In Search of the 'Authentic' Universalism in Latin American Healthcare: A Comparison of Policy Architectures and Outputs in Chile and Mexico." *Journal of Comparative Policy Analysis: Research and Practice*. https://doi.org/10.1080/13876988.2021.1908828

Bitran, Ricardo. 2014. *Universal Health Coverage and the Challenge of Informal Employment: Lessons from Developing Countries.* Washington DC: International Bank for Reconstruction and Development/World Bank.

Bonilla-Chacín, M.E., and Nelly Aguilera. 2013. "The Mexican Social Protection in Health." Universal Health Coverage Studies Series (UNICO) No. 1. Washington DC: The World Bank.

Borzutzky, Silvia. 2002. *Vital Connections: Politics, Social Security, and Inequality in Chile.* Notre Dame, USA: University of Notre Dame Press.

Carrillo Castro, Alejandro. 1987. "El ISSSTE: La salud y la seguridad social para los trabajadores al servicio del estado. *Revista de Administración Pública* 69–70: 171–180.

Castillo-Laborde, Carla, Isabel Matute, Claudia González, and Trinidad Covarrubias. 2019. "Historia del sistema de salud chileno." In *Estructura y funcionamiento del sistema de salud chileno*, edited by C. González, C. Castillo-Laborde, and I. Matute, 49–71. Santiago, Chile: CEPS, Fac. de Medicina. CAS-UDD.

Cecchini, Simone, and Rodrigo Martínez. 2011. *Protección social inclusiva en América Latina: Una mirada integral, un enfoque de derechos.* Santiago, Chile: CEPAL, Naciones Unidas.

Cid, Camilo, Ximena Aguilera, Oscar Arteaga, Soledad Barría, Pedro Barría, Carmen Castillo, David Debrott, Marcelo Dutilh, Pedro García, Tomás Jordán, Osvaldo Larrañaga, Fernando Matthews, Mario Parada, Guillermo Paraje, Orielle Solar, and Andras Uthoff. 2014. *Informe final Comisión Asesora Presidencial para el estudio y Propuesta de un Nuevo Régimen Jurídico para el Sistema de Salud Privado.* Santiago, Chile: Comisión Asesora Presidencial para el Estudio y Propuesta de un Nuevo Régimen Jurídico para el Sistema de Salud Privado.

Clínicas de Chile. 2018. *Dimensionamiento del Sector de Salud Privado en Chile. Actualización a cifras año 2018.* Santiago, Chile: Clínicas de Chile AG.

CONEVAL (Consejo Nacional de Evaluación de la Política de Desarrollo Social). 2018. *Sistema de Protección Social en Salud: Seguro Popular y Seguro Médico Siglo XXI.* Consejo Nacional de Evaluación de la Política de Desarrollo Social. https://www.coneval.org.mx/Evaluacion/IEPSM/Documents/Seguro_Popular_Seguro_Medico_Siglo_XXI.pdf

Cotlear, Daniel, Octavio Gómez-Dantés, Felicia Knaul, Rifat Atun, Ivana CHC Barreto, Oscar Cetrángolo, Marcos Cueto, Pedro Francke, Patricia Frenz, and Ramiro Guerrero. 2015. "Overcoming Social Segregation in Health Care in Latin America." *Lancet* 385(9974): 1248–1259.

CSDH (Commission on Social Determinants of Health). 2008. *Closing the Gap in a Generation: Health Equity through Action on the Social Determinants of Health. Final Report of the Commission on Social Determinants of Health.* Geneva: World Health Organization.

Cuadrado, Cristobal. 2015. "Solidaridad: Un análisis del hecho y el valor en el proceso de la reforma del sistema de salud." Magíster, Escuela de Salud Pública, Universidad de Chile.

Dion, Michelle. 2005. "The Political Origins of Social Security in Mexico during the Cárdenas and Ávila Camacho Administrations." *Mexican Studies/Estudios Mexicanos* 21(1): 59–95.

Draibe, S., and Riesco, M., 2009. El estado de bienestar social en América Latina. Una nueva estrategia de desarrollo. Documentos de Trabajo (Fundación Carolina). Madrid: Fundación Carolina.

Expansión. 2021. "Los mejores hospitales privados de México." Blutitute-Fundación Mexicana para la Salud (FUNSALUS). https://expansion.mx/empresas/2021/01/12/ranking-expansion-los-mejores-hospitales-privados-en-mexico

Frenk, Julio, Eduardo González Pier, Octavio Gómez-Dantés, Miguel Lezana, and Felicia Marie Knaul. 2006. "Comprehensive Reform to Improve Health System Performance in Mexico." *Lancet* 368: 1524–1534.

Frenz, Patricia, Izkia Siches, Ximena Aguilera, Oscar Arteaga, Camilo Cid, Roberto Estay, Sylvia Galleguillos, Ricardo Oyarzún, Mario Parada, Andras Uthoff, and Jeanette Vega. 2018. *Propuesta para una reforma integral al financiamiento de la salud en Chile.* Santiago, Chile: Comisión ESP-COLMED, Escuela de Salud Pública Universidad de Chile y Colegio Médico de Chile AG.

Gómez Bradford, María Inés, Anita Quiroga Araya, Isabel Matute Willemsen, Claudia González Wiedmaier, Carla Castillo Laborde, and Rodrigo Fuentes Bravo. 2019. "Prestadores de servicios asistenciales de salud." In *Estructura y funcionamiento del sistema de salud chileno*, edited by C. González, C. Castillo-Laborde, and I. Matute, 91–120. Santiago, Chile: CEPS, Fac. de Medicina. CAS-UDD.

Gómez-Dantes, Octavio, Alejandro Lara, Oswaldo Urdapilleta, and María Lilia Bravo. 1997. "Gasto federal en salud en población no asegurada: México 1980–1995." *Salud Pública de México* 38: 102–109.

González Block, Miguel Ángel, Ricardo Aldape Valdés, Lucero Cahuana Hurtado, Sandra Díaz Portillo, and Emilio Gutiérrez Calderón. 2018. *El subsistema privado de atención de la salud en México. Diagnóstico y retos.* Huixquilucan, Mexico: Universidad Anáhuac.

González Block, and Miguel Ángel. 2018. *El Seguro Social: Evolución histórica, crisis y perspectivas de reforma.* Huixquilucan, Mexico: Universidad Anáhuac.

González Block, Miguel Ángel, Hortensia Reyes Morales, Lucero Cahuana Hurtado, Alejandra Balandrán, and Edna Méndez. 2020. *Mexico. Health System Review.* Health Systems in Transition 22(2). Copenhagen: World Health Organization.

Goyenechea, Matias. 2019. "Estado subsidiario, segmentación y desigualdad en el sistema de salud chileno." *Cuadernos Médico Sociales* 59(2): 7–12.

Howard, C. 1999. *The Hidden Welfare State: Tax Expenditures and Social Policy in the United States*. Princeton, NJ: Princeton University Press.

Huber, Evelyne, and John D. Stephens. 2012. *Democracy and the Left: Social Policy and Inequality in Latin America*. Chicago: University of Chicago Press.

Illanes, María Angélica. 2004–2005. "Política social y modelos de desarrollo: Puntos de saturación histórica: Chile, 1924–2003." *Dimensión Histórica de Chile* (19): 149–204.

IMSS (Mexican Social Insurance Institute). 1997. *Ley del Seguro Social*. Mexico City: Instituto Mexicano del Seguro Social.

INEGI. 2021a. "Encuesta Nacional de Calidad e Impacto Gubernamental." Instituto Nacional de Geografía y Estadística. https://www.inegi.org.mx/programas/encig/2017/

INEGI. 2021b. "Encuesta Nacional de Empleo y Seguridad Social (ENESS)." Instituto Nacional de Geografía y Estadística. https://www.inegi.org.mx/programas/eness/2017/

INEGI. 2021c. "Encuesta Nacional de Ingreso y Gasto de los Hogares." Instituto Nacional de Geografía y Estadística. https://www.inegi.org.mx/programas/enigh/nc/2018/

INEGI. 2021d. "Encuesta Nacional de Ocupación y Empleo (ENOE)." Instituto Nacional de Geografía y Estadística. https://www.inegi.org.mx/programas/enoe/15ymas/

INEGI. 2020. "Censo de Población y Vienda 2020." Instituto Nacional de Geografía y Estadística. https://inegi.org.mx/programas/ccpv/2020/

INSP. 2021. *Encuesta Nacional de Salud y Nutrición 2020 sobre Covid-19. Resultados Nacionales*. Cuernavaca: Instituto Nacional de Salud Pública.

ISSSTE. 2007. *Ley del Instituto de Seguridad Social y Servicios Sociales de los Trabajadores del Estado*. Mexico City: Instituto de Seguridad Social y Servicios Sociales de los Trabajadores del Estado.

Lara, Juan Antonio. 2018. "Patrones pierden interés de proveer servicios médicos particulares." *El Financiero* October 23.

Lara, Alejandro, Octavio Gómez-Dantés, Oswaldo Urdapilleta and María Lilia Bravo. 1997. "Gasto federal en salud en población no asegurada: México 1980-1995". *Salud Pública de México* 39(2): 102–109.

Larrañaga, Osvaldo. 2010. "Las nuevas políticas de protección social en perspectiva histórica." In *Documento de trabajo 2010–4*. Santiago, Chile: Programa de las Naciones Unidas para el Desarrollo (PNUD).

Leyva-Flores, René, César Infante, Juan Pablo Gutiérrez and Frida Quintino-Pérez. 2013. "Inequdidad persistente en salud y acceso a los servicios para los pueblos indígenas de México, 2006–2012. *Salud Pública de México* 55(2): 123–128.

López Antuñano, Franciso. 1993. "Evolución de los servicios de salud de la Secretaría de Salud." *Salud Pública* 35(5): 437–439.

López Arellano, Oliva, and Sergio López Moreno (coords.). 2015. *El derecho a la salud en México*. Mexico City: Universidad Autónoma Metropolitana (UAM).

Martínez Franzoni, Juliana. 2007. "Regímenes del bienestar en América Latina." In *Documentos de Trabajo (Fundación Carolina)*. Madrid: Fundación Carolina; 1–118.

Martínez Franzoni, Juliana, and Diego Sánchez-Ancochea. 2016. *The Quest for Universal Social Policy in the South. Actors, Ideas and Architectures*. Cambridge: Cambridge University Press.

Mesa-Lago, Carmelo. 1985. *El desarrollo de la seguridad social en América Latina*. Santiago, Chile: Comisión Económica para América Latina y el Caribe (CEPAL).

Mesa-Lago, Carmelo. 1986. "Seguridad social y desarrollo en América Latina." *Revista de la CEPAL* 28: 131–146.

Mesa-Lago, Carmelo. 1994. "La reforma de la seguridad social y las pensiones en América Latina. Importancia y evaluación de las alternativas de privatización." In *Serie Reformas de Política Pública.* Santiago, Chile: CEPAL. https://repositorio.cepal.org/bitstream/handle/11362/9550/S9400018_es.pdf?sequence=1&isAllowed=y

Ministerio Secretaría General de la Presidencia. 1980. *Constitución Política de la República de Chile.* Santiago, Chile: Editorial Jurídica de Chile.

Ministerio de Salud de Chile (MINSAL). 2002. "Los objetivos sanitarios para la década 2000-2010." https://www.minsal.cl/portal/url/item/6bdb73323d19be93e04001011f013325.pdf

MINSAL-Chile. 2012. "Sistema de salud en Chile." In *Sistemas de salud en Surámerica. Desafíos para la universalidad, la integralidad y la equidad,* edited by Ernesto Báscolo, Juan Eduardo Guerrero, Juan Garay, Laura Nervi, Ligia Giovanella, Luis Beingolea, and Paulo Buss, 297–347. Rio de Janeiro: UNASUR.

MINSAL-Chile. 2019. *Plan Auge incorpora 5 nuevas patologías y sumará 85 a fin de año.* Santiago, Chile: Ministerio de Salud de Chile.

Observatorio Social CASEN. 2018. *Salud. Síntesis de resultados.* Santiago, Chile: Ministerio de Desarrollo Social.

OECD. 2016. *OECD Reviews of Health Systems: Mexico.* Paris: OECD.

Organisation for Economic Co-operation and Development (OECD)/World Bank (WB). 2020. *Health at a glance: Latin America and the Caribbean 2020.* Paris.

Pan American Health Organization (PAHO)/World Health Organization (WHO). 2014. *Strategy for Universal Access to health.* 53rd Directing Council 66th Session of the Regional Committee of WHO for the Americas. Washington, DC: Pan American Health Organization (PAHO)/World Health Organization (WHO).

Pedrero, Malva Marina, and Ana María Oyarce. 2009. "Una metodología innovadora para la caracterización de la situación de salud de las poblaciones indígenas de Chile: limitaciones y potencialidades." In *Notas de Población.* Santiago, Chile: Comisión Económica para América Latina y el Caribe (CEPAL). https://repositorio.cepal.org/handle/11362/12859

Pribble, Jennifer, and Evelyne Huber. 2013. "Social policy and redistribution: Chile and Uruguay." In *In the resurgence of the Latin American left,* edited by S Levitsky and K Roberts, 117–138. Baltimore: Johns Hopkins University Press.

Programa de las Naciones Unidas para el Desarrollo (PNUD), 2017. Desiguales. Orígenes, cambios y desafíos de la brecha social en Chile. Santiago: PNUD. https://www.undp.org/es/chile/publications/desiguales-or%C3%ADgenes-cambios-y-desaf%C3%ADos-de-la-brecha-social-en-chile

Redacción AN (Aristegui Noticias). 2018. "Gastos médicos solo serán deducibles si el pago se hizo con tarjeta, cheque o transferencia:SAT". February 28. https://aristeguinoticias.com/2802/mexico/gastos-medicos-solo-seran-deducibles-si-el-pago-se-hizo-con-tarjeta-cheque-o-transferencia-sat/

Reich, Michael. 2020. "Restructuring Health Reform, Mexican Style." *Health Systems & Reform* 6(1): 1–11.

Rodríguez, Martha Eugenia. 2017. "La salud durante el cardenismo (1934–1940)." *Gaceta Médica de México* 153: 608–625.

Rodríguez de Romo, Ana Cecilia, and Martha Eugenia Rodríguez. 1998. "Historia de la salud publica de Mexico: Siglos XIX y XX." *História, Ciências, Saúde-Manguinhos* 5(2): 2–19.

Secretaría de Hacienda y Crédito Público (SHCP). 2002. *Ley del Impuesto sobre la Renta.* Mexico, City: Secretaría de Hacienda y Crédito Público.

Sesma-Vázquez, Sergio, Raymundo Pérez-Rico, Tania Martínez-Monroy, and Edith Lemus Carmona. 2005. "Gasto privado en salud por entidad federativa en México." *Salud Pública de México* 47: 27–36.

Sojo, Ana. 2017. *Protección social en América Latina. La desigualdad en el banquillo.* Santiago, Chile: Comisión Económica para América Latina y el Caribe, Naciones Unidas.

Starfield, Barbara. 2001. "Improving equity in health: A research agenda." *International Journal Services* 31(3): 545–566.

Superintendencia de Salud. 2019. *Estudio anual de cartera 2018. Evolución del número de personas beneficiariass del sistema Isapre a diciembre de cada año (2000–2018).* Santiago, Chile: Superintendencia de Salud.

Superintendencia de Salud. 2021. "Directorio de Isapres." Superintendencia de Salud. http://www.supersalud.gob.cl/664/w3-article-2528.html

WHO (World Health Organization). 1996. *Equity in health and health care.* Geneva: World Health Organization.

WHO (World Health Organization). 2010. *The world health report: Health systems financing: the path to universal coverage.* World Health Organization. https://apps.who.int/iris/handle/10665/44371

WHO (World Health Organization). 2020a. "Global Health Expenditure Database." https://apps.who.int/nha/database/Select/Indicators/en

WHO (World Health Organization). 2020b. "Quality Health Services." In *Fact Sheets.* Geneva: World Health Organization.https://www.who.int/news-room/fact-sheets/detail/quality-health-services

Zurita, B., and Ramírez, T. 2003. "Desempeño del sector privado de la salud en México." In *Caleidoscopio de la salud. De la investigación a las políticas y de las políticas a la acción,* edited by J. Frenk, 153–162. Mexico, City: FUNSALUD.

10

Examining Improvements in a Mixed Healthcare System

Equity and Quality of Health Services in Uruguay

Xavier Ballart and Guillermo Fuentes

Introduction

Health reforms developed in the twenty-first century have to cope with health systems that had stratified the population since their foundation (Mesa-Lago 1978; Huber and Stephens 2012). In most Latin American countries, public health services had deteriorated in the 1980s and 1990s, leaving millions of citizens with inadequate quality or with no state-funded care (Barrientos 2004; Filgueira 2007, 2013). However, at the turn of the century, an increased concern with universal health coverage set the way for health reforms, aiming at not only universal access to healthcare but also improved financial protection, equity in the provision of services, and more equal access to quality healthcare across different economic and social groups (WHO [World Health Organization] 2019).

What options do countries have for reforms? European countries developed policies to include all national and foreign residents in one national health system that is financed independently of social security contributions (Béland et al. 2014). This policy was effective at reducing inequity and improving access to quality health services. However, this path is less common in Latin America or Asia, where universal health policies have been based on the idea of adding multiple schemes to reach the whole population, the acceptance of segmentation among population groups, and mixing public and private forms of delivery of health services (Cotlear et al. 2015).

Uruguay is an interesting example of a country following the non-European path with rather good results. It is a good example because it is a good performer in terms of health coverage; it has made a significant effort

Xavier Ballart and Guillermo Fuentes, *Examining Improvements in a Mixed Healthcare System* In: *The Public/Private Sector Mix in Healthcare Delivery*. Edited by: Howard A. Palley, Oxford University Press. © Oxford University Press 2023.
DOI: 10.1093/oso/9780197571101.003.0010

to improve the different dimensions of universalism, and health outcomes are rather good when compared to other countries in the region. It benefits from being a rather small country, with high levels of public governance and economic development. Still, it is an interesting case study as it has high potential to be a useful example for other countries in the region and in other parts of the world.

The analysis was based on a literature review that included official reports from the country and international institutions. We also collected data in order to assess health outcomes in Uruguay 15 years after a significant reform was implemented in 2007. The analysis took into account coverage (population entitled to receive benefits); financial protection (level of state subsidies, level of out-of-pocket spending); equity (evenness of the services received by different social groups); comprehensiveness; and quality of services, according to the conceptualization of universalism by the WHO (2019) and the United Nation's (2019) framework.

Theoretical Framework: Universalism and Political and Social Explanations of Universal Policies

Dimensions of Universalism

Historically, health reform around the world has had to cope with health systems that had stratified the population since the foundation of the systems. In many countries, millions of people were left out of state-funded services. Reforms developed in the twenty-first century followed different paths, but most of them aimed at enhancing access to healthcare and including groups of population that historically remained behind.

In 2012, the United Nations General Assembly adopted a resolution to advance universal health coverage (United Nations 2012). The inclusion of universal health coverage as one of the targets in the post-2015 Sustainable Development Goals (SDGs) reinforced the pursuit of national policies to improve people's access to healthcare. Recently, the 2019 UN Political Declaration of the High-Level Meeting on Universal Health Coverage (United Nations 2019) declared that universal health coverage implies that all people have access to the necessary health services without discrimination, putting a special emphasis on the poor.

In social policy, universalism has often been associated with social programs funded by general revenues that provide benefits to all residents in a country as a right (Béland 2010). However, since universalism in social services can be subject to different interpretations, in this study we distinguish three different dimensions of universalism in healthcare in accordance with the WHO conceptualization of universalism (WHO 2019) and the literature on social policy (Martínez, Franzoni, and Sánchez-Ancochea 2016).

In the first place, there is a horizontal dimension regarding the population covered, which is the number of people who a have access to a certain service. Second, there is the vertical dimension, which is the depth of the system and the extension of the services, treatments, and medicines included in the catalog approved by the government. But there is a third dimension that associates the right to access to the financial protection, disentangling healthcare from capacity to pay.

When universalism is referred to programs aimed at reaching the entire population independently of whether the benefits are sufficient or equal for everyone, this approach does not account for the equity or the quality of services. Equity implies the provision of services according to need and independently of the capacity to pay. Quality implies the right to receive services from similar providers operating with equally trained professionals, with state-of-the-art equipment and infrastructures, whether it is at the hospital or the primary health level.

Paths to Universalism

There are multiple paths to universalism and significant variability among different countries. Policy models where all the citizens are included in the same national health system are more likely to achieve higher levels of equity and quality of services across different population groups (Korpi and Palme 1998). Historically, many countries achieved universal outcomes and high levels of inequity reduction, bringing low-income groups and better-off citizens into the same institutions and programs. This is why it is so relevant for universalism to keep the entire population, or at least the majority, within the same scheme. However, many countries have not followed this policy model when they faced a critical juncture in their reform efforts of one policy domain.

Alternatively, the addition of multiple schemes to reach the whole population may also lead to cover all the population, and, in principle, it should be possible to achieve similar levels of equity and quality for all the citizens. However, this outcome appears to be less likely when the systems continue to segment the population, giving them rights to different service delivery systems (Béland et al. 2014). Often, a significant share of the population continues to rely on private options rather than on services publicly provided, thus limiting financial solidarity. The maintenance of out-of-pocket payments also limits the capacity of important fractions of the population to have access to some services, thus reducing equity. Additionally, the fragmentation of the population and their referral to different providers keeps the system providing uneven quality and the overall degree of universalism at a lower level.

Taking the three dimensions proposed above—coverage of the population, depth and quality of benefits and services received, plus equity across population groups—it makes a lot of sense to consider universalism a question of degree (Martínez, Franzoni, and Sánchez-Ancochea 2016). A universal policy that provides sufficient benefits and quality services to the whole population, reducing inequities, can be considered of a universal character and successful with regard to its main dimensions. On the contrary, a universal policy comprising the coverage of the entire population, where benefits are uneven across social groups and a significant share of the population is exposed to market forces to access benefits that are essential for their welfare, can hardly be considered of a universal character.

Alliances between Social Groups and Electoral Support for Universalist Policies

According to the welfare state literature, in the most advanced countries, the middle classes played a fundamental role for the institutionalization of universal policies and benefits. Esping-Andersen (1990) argued that demands for more generous social benefits required the formation of alliances between the working and the middle classes and the electoral support of the latter.

However, the alliances between the poor and the middle classes do not always take place, and they are less likely in countries with a long trajectory of exclusion of some population groups from social and health policy. In these cases, the government required the electoral support of the middle classes, who either did not trust the state for the provision of public services or considered the fiscal base not broad enough to extend social and health services to the whole population without affecting the quality of the services they received. The principal effect was the maintenance of a two-tiered system that supplies uneven benefits and services to different groups of the population (Ferreira et al. 2013). Additionally, when regulations allowed upper and middle classes to opt for private options, this sector of the population was even less interested in public service and reduced its role as a social group, demanding both the extension and the improvement in the quality of services (Filgueira 2013).

Korpi and Palme (1998) described a similar phenomenon with the "paradox of redistribution." They identified an important risk: Policies that target the poor with the aim to have a higher redistributive effect, in practice, have the opposite result. They argued that the final expenditure could be lower because of the limited political support of programs aimed at a small part of the population vis-à-vis the acceptance of the middle classes to pay for higher taxes when policies have benefits that reach the whole population. More specific to the expansion of public health, Hacker (1998) focused on the path, the political struggle, and the potential vetoes toward a universal healthcare system. Hacker identified three critical issues that could determine the success or failure of health reform. First, the promotion of private health insurance leading to the coverage of a substantial portion of the population, particularly middle classes, can reduce the support of universal public insurance and the delivery of public health services. Second, the building up of the medical private sector prior to expanding access hinders the progress toward universal health insurance because of the segmentation of citizens, the creation of tensions between access and financial protection, and the build-up of resources and political power by opponents to reform. And third, when public health insurance is designed to cover salaried workers, it tends to create a better environment to progressively expand coverage, while, opposite to this, when public health services are residual and cover poor people, the extension of public coverage will face stronger opposition.

Therefore, in this chapter, when reviewing health policy in Uruguay, we focus our attention on the degree of universalism, taking into account depth, equity, and quality of health services, besides population coverage. As Uruguay opted, at the critical junction of the health reform in 2007, for the addition of multiple schemes to reach the whole population, we analyze the extent that the health reform led to cover all the population, reducing inequity and achieving similar levels of quality for all the citizens. Additionally, we discuss the relevance of the middle class for the electoral support of the government in Uruguay and the role played by cross-class alliances between the middle and lower classes to reach universal policies distributing equitable and quality public services. To complete this analysis, we take into account the extent that public services were aimed at a relatively small part of the population, policies promoted private insurance and contributed to build up the economic and political power of opponents to health reforms.

Antecedents and Health Reform

Contextualizing Uruguay

Uruguay is a small country that made the transition to democracy in the midst of a wave that led many Latin American countries to democracy in the 1985–1990 period. Uruguay was governed by the Colorado party most of its 175 years after independence. In 2005, a coalition of center-left political parties (the *Frente Amplio*) won the elections and captured the national government for the first time, with a majority in both chambers of the Parliament.

With less than 3.5 million inhabitants, about 95% of the population lives in urban areas. Most of the population (almost 90%) has a European origin. According to the 2011 census, 7.8% of the population had an African American ascendancy, while only 4.9% were considered descendent from indigenous people (Cabella et al. 2013). Ethnic background appears to be related to health coverage since 46% of African American descendant population received medical care in the public sector in 2015, while this proportion for the non-African American population was 28.2%.[1]

The population is aging by Latin American standards, and it has a low level of births. People 60 or older are more than 18% of the population, life expectancy is 81 for women and 75 for men. Infant mortality is the lowest in the region, along with Chile. There is 100% coverage of skilled attendance at delivery, whether because a doctor, a nurse, or a midwife is present during the labor, and 94% of children are immunized against measles, polio, or other diseases.

According to the Organization for Economic Cooperation and Development (OECD), health expenditures in Uruguay were about 10% of the gross domestic product (GDP) in 2020. Public expenditures represent 70% of the total. About 8% of employed people work in the health sector. Availability of doctors in Uruguay and Chile is higher than in any other Latin American country, about four doctors per 1,000 inhabitants, while Uruguay is the ninth country in the region with respect to the number of nurses (Table 10.1).

Public health services include a primary care network at the local level (some municipal governments provide public primary healthcare services) and a number of regional and national hospitals. The total number of hospitals is over 100, one-half owned by the government, the other half owned mainly by collective medical care institutions (IAMCs for its acronym in Spanish). These are nonprofit, private providers, many of them created at the end of the nineteenth century by European migrants. There is one central university hospital producing significant research in Montevideo. Uruguay has developed an electronic health history system for all the citizens, including health and social data. Having the health history accessible to any authorized doctor is a significant improvement in terms of quality of care. Providers facilitate the access to the health history of patients when there is a change of provider, and health records are accessible to health authorities to use the data to evaluate needs and design health plans. This feature was key for the definition of risk groups and the inclusion of citizens for Covid vaccination.

Table 10.1. Comparative data for Uruguay and other countries in the region

Country	Government Expenditure Health as % of total (2018)	Out of pocket % of current health expenditure (2018)	Life expectancy at birth (years)	Infant mortality rate per 1,000 births (2019)	Vaccination % coverage, 1-year olds BCG vaccine (2019)	Medical doctors per 10,000 people (2019)	Nursing midwife per 10,000 people (2019)
Uruguay	20.77	16.96	77.10	6.07	99	49.40	49.40
Argentina	6.92	27.73	76.58	8.24	93	39.90	25.00
Brazil	6.78	27.54	75.90	12.45	79	23.11	74.01
Chile	15.88	33.24	80.74	5.97	98	51.82	133.20
Colombia	18.14	15.13	79.31	11.84	89	38.44	13.91
Paraguay	11.92	45.33	75.81	16.63	87	13.54	16.60

Source: World Health Data (https://www.who.int/data)

Health Provision in Uruguay before the Reform of 2007

As path dependency is critical for government reforms, in this section, we provide a brief historical account of health provision in Uruguay from the second half of the nineteenth century until 2007, when the government adopted the main health reform.

In 1853, a Spanish Association of Mutual Help was created in Montevideo (Arbulo et al. 2012). This was the first institution that flourished in Uruguay in the form of a mutual aid society. Other community-based clinics and trade union health societies were created at the time. Healthcare associations came to be known as IAMCs. The role that a plethora of small healthcare providers had during the nineteenth and twentieth centuries marked decisively the options the government had when health reform became a central issue in the agenda of the democratic government in 2005.

At the time of the emergence of the first IAMC, some public institutions started to develop based on charity hospitals. In 1889, the government created the first commission to administer charity hospitals scattered over the country. The hospital system evolved to be more dependent on the state with the creation of public hospitals and the Ministry of Health in 1934 (Arbulo et al. 2012). Social security was born in the 1950s when various economic sectors agreed to offer health insurance for workers. Progressively, formal workers were included under the coverage of IAMCs.

In parallel, the Ministry of Health created an administration to manage public hospitals, clinics, and health centers, but it was not until 1987 that the legislation and the management functions were separated with the creation of the State Health Services Administration (ASSE) in Spanish.

As in many other Latin American countries, the health system in Uruguay at the beginning of the twenty-first century could be characterized as composed of many different subsystems with different financing sources, access rules, providers, and benefits attending different groups of the population according to their income level.

By that time, only 25% of the population was included in the social security through IAMCs, but IAMCs covered about 44% of the population. The majority of lower-income citizens received services from ASSE, and the public hospitals, a historical public institution responsible for the administration of the social security contributions (BPS) attended women and their offspring at birth when they did not have social security. The military and the police had their own services, and some municipal governments financed local health clinics, while higher-income people payed for private insurance and private health services.

Uruguay underwent a severe economic and financial crisis at the beginning of the new millennium. GDP declined sharply, unemployment increased, poverty increased up to 15.5% in 2002 (Borgia 2008). The steep economic downturn significantly reduced the capacity of many families to access quality healthcare. It also led many IAMCs to a financial crisis. However, the economy revived, and in 2006 unemployment was below the 2,000 level. This was the landscape in Uruguay at the time of the reform in 2006–2007.

The Reform of 2007

When the coalition of center-left parties captured the government in 2005, they prioritized health reform and income tax reform as their main goals. The two reforms could have been related, particularly if the government had opted for the creation of a national health service financed with taxes independently of social security contributions, but instead, the government opted to separate the two reforms to avoid that a potential crisis in one of the two reforms could influence the other.

The 2007 health reform created three new institutions (Aran and Laca 2011; Arbulo et al. 2012): a National Health Insurance Program, a mixed public-private Comprehensive National Health System (SNIS for its acronym in Spanish), and a new fund, the National Health Fund (FONASA in Spanish) to finance SNIS. The new fund replaced the Social Security Health Insurance Direction that existed before. FONASA was designed to be financed with the contributions of formal employees, their employers, and the state.

Additionally, Uruguay already had an institution that plays an important role for vertical and horizontal equity as it covers highly priced procedures, equipment, and treatments. This National Resource Fund (FNR for its acronym in Spanish) was created in 1981 as a nonstate public entity, which works as a reinsurance of the health providers, providing universal financial coverage. Citizens receive services financed through FNR according to their needs. However, they contribute according to their ability to pay to their provider. Funding of FNR today comes from FONASA and from general revenues of the state.

All the citizens are included in the SNIS, and they are affiliated to one of the two main providers, ASSE and IAMCs. Insured members may opt between the services provided by the IAMCs or the ASSE, while noninsured members receive services from ASSE. Most of the social security members of FONASA chose the services provided by the IAMCs. Opting for ASSE as their provider is less common, but it may happen, either because IAMCs services require the payment of fees at the moment of delivering the service or because only public services by ASSE are available in small towns. In terms of horizontal equity, the principle that people with similar needs receive equal treatment all over the territory is important. The government facilitates access to services through ASSE but cannot guarantee that the levels of quality are exactly the same everywhere.

With the reform, the government introduced more progressivity in revenue collection and increased the contributions by individuals and their employers (Fuentes 2015). Companies contribute with 5% of the salary and workers with between 6% and 3% depending on the salary level and the number of dependents. FONASA includes all the citizens in the contributory scheme (formal workers, dependent family members, and pensioners) and pooled social security resources with general budget transfers.

Another important issue was that the Ministry of Public Health strengthened its authority over IAMCs and ASSE. Both must guarantee a comprehensive benefit plan (PIAS for its acronym in Spanish), which is the publicly guaranteed catalog of services in primary and hospital care (Aran and Laca 2011; Arbulo et al. 2012). Again, the PIAS is important in terms of horizontal equity because, at least in principle, citizens should receive the same health services independently of the provider and the place where they live.

With regard to IAMCs, the ministry sets maximum levels for user fees and authorizes copayments for new services. IAMCs cannot reject the coverage of any social security (FONASA) holder (Arbulo et al. 2012). After the reform, households still must deal with fees at the IAMCs. Fees do not consider payment capacity and differ across providers.

Since the financial position of IAMCs at the beginning of the century was rather weak, some of them reduced fees to attract new clients. However, out-of-pocket payments when receiving the services limit the capacity of middle- to lower-income families to access healthcare through IAMCs.

With regard to the upper-middle and higher income groups, the reform opened the possibility to opt out from the system (Arbulo et al. 2012). Along the same line, the government set a maximum level for contributions above which the social security (FONASA) is supposed to return the surplus. Additionally, the reform included for-profit private insurance as an option for payroll contributions, thus limiting proportionality at the highest income levels.

The government did not regulate for-profit private insurance and payments for non-PIAS services. This type of provision reinforced for-profit insurance and resulted in creaming of the population directly, affecting the horizontal equity of the system. It left the door open to differential access to certain services, equipment or medication, also decreasing the overall re-distributive impact because of the state's financial loss. High premiums for private health plans make them unequally accessible, with the possibility of discriminating against some citizens with higher health needs. For example, people covered by private insurances with cancer have access to certain treatments and medicines, which are not included in the PIAS or financed by the FNR special fund. As they are not affordable for a majority of the population, this kind of provision reinforces inequalities based on payment capacity.

Analysis and Results

Evolution of the Health System since the Reform

After the reform, management of health services in Uruguay has evolved toward a less-hierarchical system. The Ministry of Public Health signs contracts with all the health providers. Contracts describe goals, services, and payments. An external public institution (JUNASA for its acronym in Spanish) controls the execution of the contracts (Aran and Laca 2011). Different parties, including the Ministry of Public Health, the Ministry of Finance, IAMCs, health unions, and various associations of users (ADUSS in Spanish) are also represented in JUNASA.

The Ministry of Public Health negotiates funding with IAMCs, which are financed with per capita payments from the social security according to the risk of the health population they cover, considering gender, age, and the goals set by the health plans. The public provider, ASSE, is funded with a specific budget that is negotiated annually and comes from public budget revenues and with per capita payments from those who choose it as a health provider.

At present, the main provider of social security health services in Uruguay continues to be the IAMCs. These nonprofit associations of health professionals cover nearly 60% of the population, both citizens contributing to the social security and citizens who pay for health insurance out of their pocket. Besides the membership fee, IAMCs charge moderate fees for general or specialized medical attention and medicines, with costs that have been reduced by state regulation; nonetheless, differences between IAMCs persist.

The main provider of public health services continues to be ASSE, covering about 35% of the population and the whole territory. Together with ASSE, the public sector includes the medical services of the University of the Republic in the nation's capital and other specialized institutes for complex diseases. ASSE continues to cover informal workers, unemployed, and, in general, any citizens who are outside of the formal market and their families. This is mainly the part of the population that cannot contribute to the social security and does not have enough resources to pay for private insurance. These citizens continue to be called "subsidized" because their provider of health services is financed with resources coming out of the national budget. In some rural areas, municipal services continue to offer primary health services to the population with less resources, mainly as primary health centers. ASSE remains as the unique provider that covers the entire territory.

The reform did not integrate the military and the police into the general services provided by IAMCs and ASSE. They continue to have their own health plan, covering about 5% of the population. Finally, private insurance covers about 2% of the population. For-profit health companies offer diagnosis and hospital care in private clinics and facilities. All private expenses are financed with out-of-pocket payments. Premiums vary according to the health plans, age, and health status of citizens, and they have the possibility of rejecting applicants with chronic diseases or for other reasons. Although the proportion of people covered by private insurers is quite small, the possibility to select users according to their potential risk undermines the equity of the system.

Immediately after the reform and the creation of the SNIS, many citizens previously uninsured were incorporated to the social security (FONASA). In the following years, while the economy grew and the levels of formal employment improved, the number of citizens not included in the social security decreased. However, in 2016, there was a change of tendency, with the

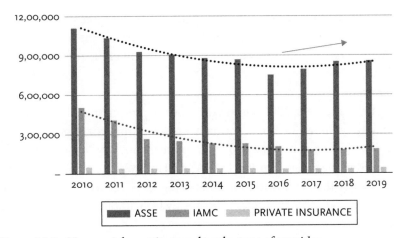

Figure 10.1. Non-social security members by type of provider.
Source: Ministry of Public Health.

economy growing more slowly, unemployment growing, and many citizens returning to ASSE as their health provider. With the COVID crisis, these tendencies are maintained rather than inversed. A significant number of citizens prefer not to contribute to the social security (FONASA), a few pay directly for health services, but non-social security members with private providers remained low in the last 10 years (Figure 10.1).

In principle, thorough the PIAS plan, the government guarantees the same benefits to the entire population (Aran and Laca 2011; Arbulo et al. 2012). However, there are significant performance differences among the five main delivery systems: IAMCs, ASSE, the military, the police, and private insurance. ASSE users have to overcome more barriers to receive services from a more restricted and lower-quality network, which limits their access and their timely, quality healthcare attention. Comparing the two main providers, IAMCs provide higher-quality services in terms of the hospital infrastructure and medical equipment, number of health professionals, and waiting times.

Results

Comparing the situation of universalism in Uruguay before the reform of 2007 and today, we can identify significant changes in the three dimensions of coverage, depth of health services, and financial protection. Changes in the three dimensions have an impact on the overall equity of the system and on the quality of health services experienced by different groups of population.

Coverage

The main challenge in 2006 was to extend health protection to those who did not have any. Today, no one is formally excluded from coverage. In immediate years following the reform of 2007, more than 1.5 million citizens were integrated in the social security (FONASA). However, the population is still segmented by their ability to contribute to the social security, and the population attending ASSE continues to be mostly from lower middle classes and the poor.

At the same time, there was a significant increase in the number of citizens included in social security and attended by IAMCs. The social security progressively included dependents, spouses, minors, pensioners, and different professionals that had their own insurance schemes, but the reform did not advance in the integration of military, police, and municipal workers (Figure 10.2).

The coverage at the IAMCs is today more evenly distributed across different income groups than in 2006 but still higher income groups, working-age population, and males are more represented at the IAMCs than females and younger and older people (Bernales-Baksai 2020).

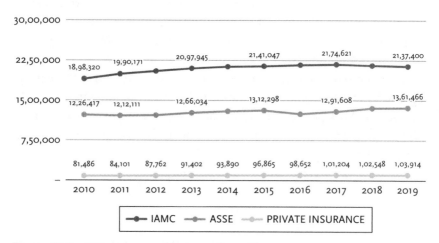

Figure 10.2. Citizens covered by type of provider.
Source: Ministry of Public Health.

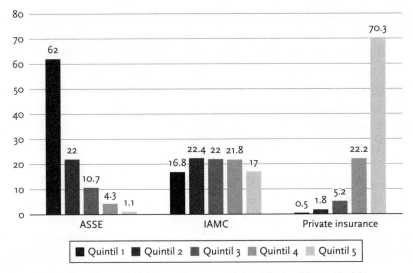

Figure 10.3. Percentage of citizens by type of provider and household income quintiles.

Source: Instituto Nacional Estadística (2019). https://www.ine.gub.uy/

Fourteen years after the creation of SNIS, coverage remains segmented into different providers according to income levels. While more than 60% of the people in the poorest income quintile receive healthcare services from ASSE, the public provider, around 70% of the richest people receive services from a for-profit private insurance scheme. In the middle, IAMCs cover a more diverse group of people in terms of income level (Figure 10.3).

Utilization and Depth of Services

The implementation of health plans like the PIAS and more specific programs set by the Ministry of Health has contributed to guarantee that all citizens have the same right to healthcare. In the last 15 years, there has been less inequality regarding the utilization of services between IAMCs and ASSE beneficiaries, men and women, young and old, and residents in Montevideo and residents in the rest of the country (González and Triunfo 2020).

On the negative side, two main obstacles remain to achieving equality among all the citizens. First, Uruguay continues to have a two-tier system with one type of healthcare for the middle classes and the richer groups of population and another one for the lower middle classes and the poor. Endurance of the distinction between citizens contributing and not contributing to social security and the maintenance of the term "subsidized" for part of the

population stigmatizes ASSE beneficiaries and clearly shows that a significant part of the people does not have an equal right to receive health services
from the same providers. Second, the differences in funding, infrastructure,
and equipment among providers create barriers and logistical difficulties
that are used as a rationing mechanism. Their negative effects are higher for
ASSE beneficiaries than for IAMC beneficiaries. Among ASSE beneficiaries,
citizens who report worse health status and greater healthcare needs and
older than 60 years of age from lower income groups find more administrative obstacles to get the services they need (Balsa et al. 2009). The analysis of the use of medication shows higher degrees of inequity as it is highly
concentrated among higher income groups (González and Triunfo 2020).
Since 2006, the money collected through citizen contributions increased significantly as a direct consequence of the change in the premiums imposed
by the reform. Social security became less dependent on public money, and
the government could reduce the transfers from the public budget to the social security fund. At the same time, the government increased public health
expenditures, reducing the gap in resources per capita between ASSE and
IAMCs from almost 3.5 times to about 1.3 times (Figure 10.4). The fiscal investment in the public health sector raised the availability of resources to finance ASSE, which doubled the budget in 5 years since 2006 (Arbulo et al.

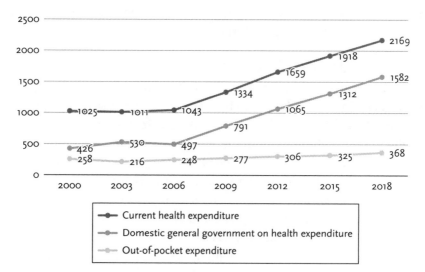

Figure 10.4. Health expenditure per capita.
Source: World Health Data (https://www.who.int/data, at purchasing power parity in dollars).

2012). Overall, the proportion of private health expenditure is now lower than it was in 2006, from about 50% to about 25% (World Health Data, https://www.who.int/data).

Regulations also stabilized and sometimes reduced copayments, tickets, and other fees payable when receiving health services mainly from IAMCs. Overall, there has been a reduction of out-of-pocket spending from 20% in 2006 to 16% in 2020, one of the lowest in the region (Bernales-Baksai 2020).

Additional Protection for Groups with Serious Health Vulnerabilities

An additional financial protection for all the citizens is the possibility to access FNR, the special fund, when they need to be treated with highly specialized equipment or the medication prescribed is extremely expensive. The persistence and enlargement of this institution is a direct attempt to avoid the catastrophic effects of serious diseases on the financial condition of families; therefore, it can be seen as a public tool to increase the vertical equity of the system.

The way COVID-19 was treated is another example of adding resources to the system to respond in a way that reinforces universal coverage according to need under equitable conditions. In terms of outcomes, Uruguay performed particularly well compared to other countries in Latin America. Until the spring of 2020, the country experienced very low community circulation of the virus, with most of the outbreaks occurring in clusters, which it made possible to effectively manage the outbreaks through active search of the cases and their contacts. The government declared a national emergency and created a strategy that was based on increasing the diagnostic testing capacity, the management of suspect cases, and the implementation of telemedicine. In the spring of 2021, the expansion of the Brazilian strain had a significant impact on the number of cases and deaths.

Regarding the vaccination process, the dimensions of the country and the ability to create the necessary infrastructure allowed the country to be one of the best performers at the moment of writing this chapter (Table 10.2).

Political and Social Factors Affecting Health Results

The health system is mixed, and it is based on private and nonprofit provision through IAMCs and on public provision through ASSE. However, health

Table 10.2. Deaths by Covid-19 and vaccinations in selected countries

Country	Cumulative confirmed COVID-19 deaths per million people by April 21, 2021	Share of people who received at least one dose of COVID-19 vaccine by April 21, 2021
Argentina	1.329	12.66
Brazil	1.795	11.72
Chile	1.326	41.06
Colombia	1.368	5.6
Paraguay	780	1.13
Uruguay	599	31.42

Source: www.ourworldindata.org

policy keeps IAMCs, which had played a key role in Uruguay's health history, at the center of the health system.

It can be argued that, at a critical moment, the government rescued IAMCs by helping them to receive new clients and strengthen their financial position (Ballart and Fuentes 2018; Hacker 1998). This explains that private medical services and not-for-profit IAMCs, owned by doctors, clearly aligned with the government policies. Political parties in the opposition could question marginal aspects of the reform but could not oppose a policy that was rather centrist and preserved the private sector initiative in the health sector, limited contributions to maximum levels not to exceed the expected expenditure per citizen, and included the possibility to exit the system and directly opt for private insurance.

The members of the coalition who were more leftist supporting the government and some key stakeholders like unions did not have the power to impose a more radical policy based mainly on public provision, financed with general taxes, and integrating all the citizens in the same national health system to achieve higher levels of equity and quality of services across population groups.

The median voter dominant beliefs were that that Uruguay could not bring low-income groups (the "subsidized") and better-off citizens into the same institutions and programs. The government considered a better option to favor the inclusion of a maximum number of citizens into the formal economy and to extend social security coverage to middle and lower classes. From this perspective, Uruguay was successful at integrating people from a more diverse economic and social origin into the social security, maintaining the participation of higher-income population groups. The Uruguay experience is therefore a good example of incremental progression based on non-disruptive decision-making.

However, the success of the system is dependent on continuous economic growth and the expansion of formal work. The sustainability of the system can be problematic in times of a deep economic recession as it depends on low levels of unemployment and poverty. The change in the trends experienced in 2016 and the recent economic downturn with the Covid-19 epidemic already have sent a warning. Changes could be intensified with the rotation in the national government. In 2019, a center right wing coalition led by the National Party won the elections, putting an end to a number of years with stable policies under the government of Frente Amplio. Promising fiscal adjustments in a context of increasing economic uncertainty, the new government only had 2 weeks in office before the first positive case of Covid-19 was confirmed.

A positive characteristic of the political system of Uruguay is that it is expected that the new government will not unmake the policies that the previous government approved, preserving the health institutions created since 2007. However, the economic context has not been favorable, and it is likely that the general orientation of the government leads to a less interventionist policy and a reduction in the budget allocated to ASSE, the public provider.

As explained before, economic growth has been critical to increase the investment of public resources on the improvement of ASSE and the public provision of health services. However, the dominant idea in Uruguay continues to be that general taxes, paid by middle- and higher-income groups, "subsidize" an important share of the population. The sustainability of this logic could be put into question at any moment by more conservative views, particularly in times of economic recession, putting at risk advances in equity, provision according to need, and quality in the delivery of health services.

Conclusions

The case study about healthcare in Uruguay shows one possible path to improve healthcare universalism. As with any other basic public service, like education or pensions, coverage is not sufficient to guarantee that all the citizens receive services of a similar quality, according to their needs, and independently of their capacity to pay.

Uruguay is a positive example of reinforcing the authority of the state to regulate the health sector (Ballart and Fuentes 2018) when it is composed of a plethora of organizations providing different health schemes based on a public-private mix of health providers. Uruguay shows advances in public sector investment to strengthen the quality of the public sector provider and in the implementation of health plans that progressively extend the catalog of services and treatments to all the citizens. This is an important change in order to reinforce the principle of horizontal equity. Independently of the provider, citizens can expect that they are treated rather similarly if they have a health problem in Uruguay.

The integration of different health schemes within the social security fund increased the financial solidarity among the citizens that are integrated in the economy, although workers with lower wages, who are frequently women, are underrepresented at the IAMCs and for-profit private insurance. Despite this weakness, overall the system has advanced in vertical equity with the creation of FONASA and the maintenance and strengthening of FNR capacities to guarantee that any citizen has access to highly priced procedures and medicines independently of the financial capacity.

The main negative outcome after 15 years of reforms are the differences in timely attention and quality of services across different types of providers that are essentially private (IAMCs) and public (ASSE). Today there is still fragmentation in service provision, which sustains the segmentation to access healthcare and maintains equity gaps in access to quality services because of eligibility criteria. The endurance of fragmentation translates into differences in the sociodemographic profiles of the population covered via social security and via "subsidization," a rather stigmatizing term that is still commonly used.

The case study illustrates the main political and socioeconomic factors as well as institutional constraints affecting healthcare universal reforms in middle-income countries. For many countries in Latin America and Asia, it is unlikely that they will take the route to universal outcomes and increased equity , bringing low-income and better-off citizens into exactly the same institutions and programs. It is more likely that they take the route to add multiple schemes and create compensatory institutions to cover all the population and, at the same time, progress on the goals to reduce inequities and achieve more similar levels of quality in the provision of health services.

This policy option has been effective with respect to improving quality of care in Uruguay, especially between lower-income groups and informal sector workers. They now have better access to some services, and their out-of-pocket expenses have been reduced. According to the Global Burden of Disease published by The Lancet (GBD Universal Health Coverage Collaborators 2020), in 2019 Uruguay occupied position 69 in the world, showing great improvement since previous rounds of this report placed Uruguay in positions above 90.

The key factor is better management and funding of the public sector provider (ASSE) that covers the majority of the poor in Uruguay through an increasing number of clinics and hospitals all over the territory. The network of medical facilities in a rather small country and the absence of large geographic obstacles proved to be critical during the Covid-19 pandemic. Massive testing, keeping track of positive cases, and a rather quick vaccination process, compared with other countries in the region, were key to control the disease and show rather good outcomes.

Uruguay health policy today is very much explained by the historical weight of nonprofit and private health providers. IAMCs played a key role in the delivery of health services to a majority of citizens, including the middle-, middle-upper, and middle-lower classes. The political support of this central part of the population was fundamental to the expansion of universal health services in all its dimensions (Esping-Andersen 1990; Korpi and Palme 1998; Filgueira 2013) and the improvement of the public provider that, in Uruguay, benefited from increasing public budgets for more than a decade. However, this same policy reinforced the private health industry and promoted the private health insurance that was able to keep open the private options (Hacker 1998). This same industry, together with the change of governments, has weakened the positions of those who would like health reforms to continue and progressively turn the public provider into a competitive quality option for any social security member.

Note

1. https://www.gub.uy/presidencia/comunicacion/noticias/46-poblacion-afrodescendie
   nte-recibe-servicios-salud-asse

References

Aran, Daniel, and Hernán Laca. 2011. "Sistema de Salud en Uruguay." *Salud Pública de México* 53(2): 265–274.

Arbulo, Victoria, Juan Pablo Pagano, Gustavo Rak, and Laura Rivas. 2012. *El camino hacia la Cobertura Universal en Uruguay. Evaluación y revisión del financiamiento del Sistema de Salud uruguayo*. Montevideo, Uruguay: Ministerio de Salud Pública (MSP)/ Organización Panamericana de la Salud (OPS) Uruguay.

Ballart, Xavier, and Guillermo Fuentes. 2018. "Gaining Public Control on Health Policy: The Politics of Scaling Up to Universal Health Coverage in Uruguay." *Social Theory and Health* 17(3): 348–366.

Balsa, Ana, Daniel Ferrés, Máximo Rossi, and Patricia Triunfo. 2009. "Inequidades socioeconómicas en el uso de servicios sanitarios del adulto mayor montevideano." *Estudios Económicos* 24(47): 35–88.

Barrientos, Armando. 2004. "Latin America: Towards a Liberal-Informal Welfare Regime." In *Insecurity and Welfare Regimes in Asia, Africa and Latin America: Social Policy in Development Contexts*, edited by Ian Gough, Geog Wood, Armando Barrientos, Philippa Bevan, Peter Davis, and Graham Rooom, 68–121. Cambridge: Cambridge University Press.

Béland, Daniel. 2010. *What Is Social Policy? Understanding the Welfare State*. Cambridge: Polity Press.

Béland, Daniel, Paula Blomqvist, Jorgen Goul Andersen, Joakim Palme, and Alex Waddan. 2014. "The Universal Decline of Universality? Social Policy Change in Canada, Denmark, Sweden and the UK." *Social Policy Administration* 48(7): 739–756.

Bernales-Baksai, Pamela. 2020. "Tackling Segmentation to Advance Universal Health Coverage: Analysis of Policy Architectures of Health Care in Chile and Uruguay." *International Journal for Equity in Health* 19: article 106.

Borgia, Fernando. 2008. "Health in Uruguay: Progress and Challenges in the Right to Health Care Three Years after the First Progressive Government." *Social Medicine* 3(2): 110–125.

Cabella, Wanda, Nathan Mathías, and Mariana Tenenbaum. 2013. *La población Afro-uruguaya en el Censo 2011*. Montevideo, Uruguay: Trilce.

Cotlear, Daniel, Somil Nagpal, Owen Smith, Ajay Tandon, and Rafael Cortez. 2015. *Going Universal: How 24 Developing Countries Are Implementing Universal Health Coverage Reforms from the Bottom Up*. Washington, DC: World Bank.

Esping-Andersen, Gosta. 1990. *The Three Worlds of Welfare Capitalism*. Princeton, NJ: Princeton University Press.

Ferreira, Francisco, Julián Messina, Jamele Rigolini, Luis Felipe López-Calva, María Ana Lugo, and Luis Felipe Vakis. 2013. *La movilidad económica en América Latina*. Washington DC: The World Bank.

Filgueira, Fernando. 2007. *Cohesión, riesgo y arquitectura de protección social en América Latina*. Santiago, Chile: Comisión Económica para América Latina y el Caribe (CEPAL).

Filgueira, Fernando. 2013. "Los regímenes de bienestar en el ocaso de la modernización conservadora: Posibilidades y límites de la ciudadanía social en América Latina." *Revista Uruguaya de Ciencia Política* 22(SPE): 10–27.

Fuentes, Guillermo. 2015. "Actores, intereses y alianzas de cara a la segunda etapa de implementación del SNIS: cambio institucional gradual y posibles escenariosy orientaciones de cambio." In *Economía, política y economía política para el acceso y la cobertura universal de salud en Uruguay* , edited by Fernández Galeano, Miguel, Eduardo Levcovitz, and Daniel Olesker, 197–241. Montevideo, Uruguay: Organización Panamericana de la Salud (OPS).

GBD 2019 Universal Health Coverage Collaborators. 2020. "Measuring Universal Health Coverage Based on an Index of Effective Coverage of Health Services in 204 Countries and Territories, 1990–2019: A Systematic Analysis for the Global Burden of Disease Study 2019." *Lancet* 396: 1250–1284.

González, Cecilia, and Patricia Triunfo. 2020. "Horizontal Inequity in the Use and Access to Health Care in Uruguay." *International Journal for Equity in Health* 19: 127.

Hacker, Jacob. 1998. "The Historical Logic of National Health Insurance: Structure and Sequence in the Development of British, Canadian, and US Medical Policy." *Studies in American Political Development* 12(Spring): 57–130.

Huber, Evelyn, and John Stephens. 2012. *Democracy and the Left: Social Policy and Inequality in Latin America*. Chicago: University of Chicago Press.

Korpi, Walter, and Joakim Palme. 1998. "The Paradox of Redistribution and Strategies of Equality: Welfare State Institutions, Inequality, and Poverty in the Western Countries." *American Sociological Review* 63(5): 661–687.

Martínez Franzoni, Juliana, and Diego Sánchez-Ancochea. 2016. *The Quest for Universal Social Policy in the South. Actors, Ideas and Architectures*. Cambridge: Cambridge University Press.

Mesa-Lago, Carmelo. 1978. *Social Security in Latin America. Pressure Groups, Stratification, and Inequality*. Pittsburgh, PA: University of Pittsburgh Press.

United Nations. 2012. *Global Health and Foreign Policy*, A/67/L.36. General Assembly. Agenda item 123. New York: United Nations, December 6.

United Nations. 2019. *Political Declaration of the High-Level Meeting on Universal Health Coverage. Universal Health Coverage: Moving Together to Build a Healthier World*. New York: United Nations.

World Health Organization (WHO). 2019. "Health Financing for Universal Coverage. What Is Universal Coverage?" https://www.who.int/health_financing/universal_cove rage_definition/en/

11

The Public/Private Sector
Mix in Healthcare

Inequities and Issues of Quality of Care:
The Case of Brazil

Lenaura de Vasconcelos Costa Lobato,
Monica de Castro Maia Senna, and Luciene Burlandy

Introduction

Health services and relations between the public and private sectors in Brazil are conditioned by structural inequities in Brazilian society. Gaping inequalities in income and access to public goods and services feature prominently and persistently in the historical constitution of society itself. These more overall socioeconomic and political inequalities affect conditions of life and health and result in unequal distribution of the risks of falling ill and dying and the possibility of accessing services. Structural inequities affecting conditions of life and work lessen the likelihood that certain segments of the population will face situations of morbidity/mortality and contribute to producing inequities in health service provision and access to and quality of health services.

In the literature, structural inequities and their health impacts have been analyzed on two main approaches: (1) one that favors "health inequalities," that is, that seeks to understand how the epidemiological, nutrition, and morbidity/mortality profile affects the population unevenly, depending on characteristics such as per capita income, place of residence, gender, race, and other factors, and leading to differences in life expectancy and mortality, by sex, level of education, income and socioeconomic position; and (2) another that focuses on inequalities in health service provision and access, which influence the kinds and quality of services offered and how they affect different population groups and the distribution of services in the

Lenaura de Vasconcelos Costa Lobato, Monica de Castro Maia Senna, and Luciene Burlandy, *The Public/Private Sector Mix in Healthcare* In: *The Public/Private Sector Mix in Healthcare Delivery.* Edited by: Howard A. Palley, Oxford University Press. © Oxford University Press 2023. DOI: 10.1093/oso/9780197571101.003.0011 territories (Albert-Ballestar and García-Atlés 2021; Machado and Silva 2019; Viacava et al. 2018).

Structural inequalities also entail power asymmetries that affect health policies themselves and the terms of disputes for public funds that contribute to shaping the configurations of the public/private mix. That is to say, disputes and conflicts over public funds and policies shape the configuration of health systems and consequently their capacity to address structural inequalities and health inequalities. What can be seen in Brazil is a history of intense structural inequality whose impacts on health inequalities are widely acknowledged. Until the 1990s, the characteristics of the health system limited efforts to address these inequalities. The main constraints included the medical-centered care approach, limited coverage, and private sector predominance in service provision, even when funded by the public sector. The creation of a free, universal, public system, the Unified Health System (Sistema Único de Saúde, SUS), in 1998 was designed to break down those constraints. As a result of the democratization process following the military dictatorship, the new system had comprehensive goals, such as supporting the democratization of society by guaranteeing the universal right to health and inverting the logic of medical-centered care by introducing a comprehensive healthcare structure based on promotion, prevention, cure, and rehabilitation.

That system was constructed in parallel with the advance of neoliberal strategies worldwide. In healthcare, these were expressed in recommendations formulated and spread by international organizations that promoted residual policies and favored the private sector (World Bank 1993, 1995). This embodied a conception of equity different from that which informed the SUS: Only the very poorest should be catered for by the state, while those that can pay for services are left to the market (Rizzoto 2015; Travagin 2017). Despite the historical legacy and the constraints on construction of the SUS, its power is to be seen in significant outcomes in health equity. On the other hand, many of its goals have not been achieved, and today its development and very existence are in doubt, given the radical austerity policies introduced recently in Brazil. In healthcare, rather than contributing to equity, the public/private mix has, on the contrary, been one of the factors working against it. This is because, in the case of Brazil, the mix is not cooperative, but essentially conflictive (Lobato, Ribeiro, and Vaitsman 2016).

This chapter examines the public/private mix and its relation to equity in health system configuration and service provision, with special attention to vulnerable groups. The first part describes overall characteristics of Brazil: its historical formation, sociodemographic data, social inequalities, and the background to the health system and the public/private mix in healthcare. Then the public and private systems are described to address the interactions between them in coverage, provision, access, and funding to highlight how these interactions affect equity and quality of health care.

Inequalities and Background to
The Public/Private Mix in Health

Social inequalities in Brazil are among the most extreme in the world. They result from structural factors stemming largely from its colonial slave-owning heritage, the structure of land ownership centered on large estates and the income-concentrating model of economic development in place. Data from the official bureau of statistics, the IBGE, show that in 2019—and thus before the Covid-19 pandemic—the Gini index for Brazil was 0.543, placing it among the 10 most unequal nations in the world. Income appropriated by the wealthiest 10% corresponded to 43% of total per capita household earnings, while the poorest 40% accounted for just 10.2% (IBGE 2020b). A UN report issued in 2019 revealed that the wealthiest 1% of the population received nearly one-third (28.3%) of the country's income—a concentration exceeded only by Qatar (United Nations Development Program [UNDP] 2019).

The economic crisis that began in 2015 and the structural adjustment policies implemented, particularly after the impeachment of President Dilma Roussef in 2016, are now producing impacts in increased poverty. Brazil had recorded historic reductions in extreme poverty (defined as daily income of less than US$1.9), which fell from 28% to 10% between 2003 and 2014. By 2019, that rate had returned to 24.7% (IBGE 2020a). Here, there is a clear race bias: Blacks and mixed race *pardos* represent 56% of the population, but 76.7% of people in extreme poverty, only 22.3% of whom are Whites, who constitute 42.7% of the population. Also contributing to increased poverty are high unemployment, today 14.7%, and the high rate of informal work, which stands at 41.6% overall, but reaches 61% and 56% in Brazil's poorest regions, the North and Northeast (IBGE 2020a).

Social inequalities are expressed in not only income and territories but also race, gender, and sexual orientation, entailing significant disadvantages for Blacks, women, and the lesbian, gay, bisexual, and transgender (LGBT) population. It is these groups that historically have accumulated a series of social deficiencies that are overlaid on one another and structure their relative positions in the social hierarchy. These groups show the highest levels of informal and precarious, unprotected occupation; lower levels of schooling (except for women, who show higher rates of schooling than men); and lack of access to urban infrastructure services and public policies, as well as greater exposure to violence and human rights abuses. The Annual Socioeconomic Report on Women (*Relatório Anual Sócio Econômico da Mulher*, RASEAM) of 2017–2018, the most recent published by the federal government (Brazil 2020), indicated that in 2017 only 28% of women over 16 years old were in formal employment, compared with 40% of their male counterparts. Black women showed the lowest rates of formal occupation, accounting for just over 23% of all women in formal employment. Earnings from work also differed widely and were higher among the White population than among Blacks. In the population over 10 years of age, the mean number of years' schooling is greater among women (9.3 years as against 8.9 years among men), but the mean is much lower among Black women, at 8.6 years' schooling. At all levels of education, however, women earn less than men.

As regards violence, Brazil leads the ranking in number of murders of the LGBT population (Benevides and Nogueira 2020). The *Atlas da Violência 2021* reported that, in 2019, of all homicide victims in Brazil, 77% were from its Black population. The death rate among Black women was 65.8% higher than among non-Black women, demonstrating the enormous vulnerability of this segment of society (Cerqueira 2021).

Added to this situation, there are intense regional and territorial disparities in population size, socioeconomic conditions, and economic dynamism among the different regions of Brazil, which are expressed also in states' and municipalities' differing capacities to provide and manage public policies, which contribute to differentials in access to social policies.

These structural inequalities entail severe inequities in health as regards both the risks of falling ill and dying and the opportunities to access and use health services, which vary by social position. It raises questions about the capability of Brazil's social policies, health policy among them, to alter this dramatic social situation on their own.

Studies indicated that at least until the 1970s, the advances in redistribution and increasing social mobility in Brazil were due much more to policies designed to expand formal employment and increase the real value of the minimum wage than to social policies, as they were in the majority restricted to formal urban workers and the middle class (Viana and Machado 2008). Although Brazil's social protection system began to be built in the early decades of the 20th century, it was directed—as part of national state-building and promotion of Brazil's industrial development policy based on import substitution—only to certain average portions of the urban work-force and established a contractual relationship based on the social security model. Those excluded from the system were left with ad hoc, discontinuous, emergency measures that responded to a rationale that was compensatory, charitable, and stigmatizing.

In this way, it took shape in highly exclusionary form and was strongly segmented and institutionally fragmented. Not even the progressive expan-sion of the system's coverage was able to alter these central characteristics, to which were added—particularly in the long period (1964–1985) of the auto-cratic regime brought in by the military dictatorship—excessive centralism, lack of social participation and preferential treatment for the private sector.

Health policy followed a course dictated by this overall pattern. Before the Unified Health System (SUS) was instituted, the health sector is recognized to have developed with a dual-model system of service provision. Collective health measures intended for the population in general, such as immu-nization and control of epidemics, were the responsibility of institutions connected to the Ministry of Health, while medical care was provided almost exclusively by the social insurance system, which was available only to in-sured workers and their families. This duality reinforced the system's highly segmented and fragmented nature and worsened the inequities in access to healthcare services.

Brazil's health system is also notable for its hybrid nature, expressed by the mix between the public and private sectors, which, over the course of the development of its health policy, has established relations that are complex, overlapping, and at times perverse, resulting in differentiated health service access, funding, and provision. It is argued here that not even introduction of the universal model of healthcare based on recognition of the right to health embodied in the SUS was able to break with what is one of the most salient historical and structural features of the Brazilian system: the strong private sector presence fostered and supported by the state. As argued by Menicucci (2009), the historical legacy from previous policies, associated with a society structurally marked by differentiation, has established patterns that are diffi-cult to reverse, constraining construction of the proposed universal and egal-itarian health system.

The origins of the public/private mix in healthcare date from the process that brought medical care into Brazil's social insurance system in the early decades of the 20th century. Retirement and pension funds (*Caixas de Aposentadoria e Pensões*, CAP) and, soon afterward, retirement and pension institutes (*Institutos de Aposentadoria e Pensões*, IAP)—set up on the social security model and with the prime function of guaranteeing monetary benefits (retirement pensions and other benefits) to the insured—expanded the scope of their activities, coming increasingly even to offer medical care to the insured and their dependents. Provision of these medical services involved primarily (almost exclusively) purchasing private services. Although it was possible for the CAPs to set up their own services, the usual practice was to retain doctors to treat the insured in their private surgeries. The IAPs extended this practice, going on also to purchase hospital services and becoming a major purchaser of private hospital medical services, although strongly guided by the cost-containment logic that prevailed within the IAPs (Oliveira and Teixeira 1989). The schedule of services directly reflected ability to pay and the lobbying power of the various professional categories in their respective institutes, which favored the emergence of a highly segmented system.

From the 1960s onward, the public/private mix in healthcare began to expand and take on new forms, in a situation framed by the rise of the authoritarian regime and expansion of a model of economic development that combined high levels of economic growth with strong income concentration. Unification of the IAPs in 1966 into a single institute, the National Social Insurance Institute (*Instituto Nacional da Previdência Social*, INPS), retained the logic of a social insurance restricted to a small portion of workers, although the numbers of insured grew steadily. During this period, access to social insurance medical care expanded greatly, driven by state action to establish an entrepreneurial medical-industrial and medical care complex (Cordeiro 1980).

At this time, relations between the public and private spheres occurred in three main modalities. The first involved state funding for procurement of hospital medical services, which stimulated supply of private services and medical equipment. Over the following 20 years, the INPS became the major purchaser of private hospital medical services for workers. Unlike the previous period, when these services were purchased through small clinics, hospitals and private surgeries, relations with the private sector came to take place through large private institutions governed by the business rationale.

The second modality involved opening up lines of investment with public funds to build private hospitals, whose services were guaranteed a market by the social insurance system, thus annulling any risk to the private sector. The third modality rested on incentives for firms in any field to offer medical care to their employees by purchasing private services, thus relieving pressure on the public sector and, at the same time, fostering the founding of group medicine companies, medical cooperatives, and the self-managed system (Oliveira and Teixeira 1989; Cordeiro 1980). In this way, a relationship of mutual dependence between public and private sectors was established in health service provision.

That process was assisted by the private sector's enormous capacity to organize as a powerful lobby capable of penetrating the apparatus of the state and allying with the interests of the social insurance technobureaucracy, further reinforcing the system's segmentation. Note here also that the medical profession wielded considerable influence as a significant political actor with veto power over proposals for universal public care.

Not even introduction of the universal public system, the SUS, was able to alter this structural characteristic of the Brazilian health system. Rather, reforms to the system since the late 1980s have ended up introducing new public/private arrangements in both service provision and system management.

The Present Health System and The Public/Private Mix

Brazil is characterized by a universal public system coexisting with a powerful private service system. The public SUS was instituted by the 1988 constitution and was one outcome of the restoration of democracy following the end of the military dictatorship, which lasted from 1964 to 1985. The constitution specified that health was a citizen's right and the state's duty and set down the general outlines of how the public system was to be organized. Public health, drug care, and healthcare at all levels (primary, secondary, and tertiary), as well as health, epidemiological, and environmental surveillance, are all the responsibility of the SUS. Coverage includes the whole population and all its health needs, and access is free of charge. The SUS reaches the whole population in collective health measures (health surveillance, public health campaigns, vaccination, etc.). In medical care, it covers around 71.5% of the population, while 28.5% hold private health insurance. That boundary, however, is not clear cut. As the SUS is universal, joint use is made of services in the two sectors, public and private.

The SUS is unique in all Brazil, and its management is decentralized among the three levels of government (federal, state, and municipal). The public system is funded out of tax revenues (general taxation) by the three levels of government. Total health spending was 9.5% of GDP in 2018, with public expenditures representing 3.96% (less than half of total expenditures). That same year, in Canada and the United Kingdom, also countries with universal systems, public expenditure accounted for 7.3% and 7.86% of GDP, respectively (WHO 2021). Among countries with universal public systems, in Brazil alone public spending is less than private spending, and it also has the lowest capita health expenditure. This is a result of chronic underfunding (Marques 2017; Marques et al. 2016), which, since the tax regime introduced in 2016, has been significantly defunded (i.e., cuts in already insufficient funding) (Funcia 2019). In 2019, public expenditure on health was close to US$70 billion, representing about US$330 per capita/year or less than a dollar a day per capita (Brazil 2021a).

Creation of the SUS did not break with the logic of procuring services from the private sector. Even with significant growth in its own public facilities, the SUS remained highly dependent on private services, particularly at the secondary and tertiary levels of care. Greatest expansion in public services has occurred in primary care, through the Family Health Strategy (*Estratégia de Saúde da Família* ESF), whose goal is to invert the traditional logic of healthcare centered on specialized and hospital services and to make the primary level the gateway to a hierarchical network organized by increasing complexity, as recommended by the SUS (Giovanella and Mendonça 2012). Primary care offers health promotion and disease prevention and control services through health facilities and home care teams that, in addition to doctors, nurses, and health workers, can include dentists and other professions. Despite numerous problems, including the difficulty of retaining personnel in remote areas and lack of materials and equipment, it is primary care that has contributed most to expanding access to health services and improving the quality of healthcare by the lowest-income portions of the population (Oliveira et al. 2017). Coverage by the ESF grew from 48% of the population in 2007 to 64% in 2020. Today, 76.08% of the population is covered by primary care in some form, be it the ESF, primary care clinics, or community health workers (Brazil 2021a). The National Health Survey (*Pesquisa Nacional de Saúde*) (IBGE 2020b) found that 60.0% of households were registered with family health centers in 2019, an increase of 6.7% from 2013, and that coverage was greater in the poorest regions. Among registered households, 38.4% received a monthly visit from a primary care professional in 2019. A number of studies have noted the importance of primary care in reducing regional and territorial service provision inequities, as well as its positive effects on infant mortality and morbidity rates, general morbidity, and life expectancy (Machado and Silva 2019).

The private health sector comprises private health insurers, contracted voluntarily by families and individuals; and group insurance or employer-based insurance (held by companies for their employees). The sector was unregulated until 1998, when a public agency, the National Supplementary Health Agency (*Agência Nacional de Saúde Suplementar*, ANS), connected with the Ministry of Health, was set up for that purpose. The ANS's functions include specifying mandatory minimum coverages (procedures, tests, and treatments); overseeing; and enforcing compliance with contracts with beneficiaries and guaranteeing market competition. The agency has since been captured by market interests, however (Vilarinho 2010), which has undermined its legal functions of safeguarding the system and protecting users, particularly as regards controlling premium prices and adjustments, inspecting services offered, and ensuring insurance companies' transparency and accountability. The agency only regulates prices and adjustments for individual and family contracts, which represent 18.7% of the market. Group and employer-based contracts are negotiated freely with health insurers, resulting in a clear imbalance between the parties and unilateral adjustments. This has meant that the market has practically eliminated new individual and family plans to induce beneficiaries to join group insurance plans (many of which lack any group feature) in order to circumvent price adjustment controls. Even controlled adjustments have been far greater than inflation, which restricts access. The regulation stipulates that premiums are to be adjusted at specific beneficiary ages, the last of which is 59 years. From that age onward, the plans can be adjusted annually, but the premium cannot be altered. This has meant that insurers have applied abusive increases when beneficiaries turn 59 years old, sometimes making it impossible for older adults to continue insurance.

In 2019, there were 59.7 million Brazilians, corresponding to 28.5% of the population, who held some kind of health, medical, or dental insurance—a percentage that had not changed significantly since 2013, when it was 27.9% (PNS 2020b). However, under the influence of the economic crisis, the numbers of those with medical insurance had been falling since 2015, but then increased in late 2020 as a result of Covid-19 (ANS 2021). The number of beneficiaries of exclusively dental plans, on the contrary, has been growing constantly (ANS 2021). This is due to the novelty of dental plans, the high costs of private dental care, and the difficulties in accessing the public system. Dental care was only incorporated to a large extent in the SUS in 2004, under the creation of the Smiling Brazil Program (*Programa Brasil Sorridente*). However, it still presents gaps of assistance.

The private sector has undergone intense change, involving corporate mergers and concentrations, particularly recently since permission was granted for foreign capital participation in healthcare. The number of health insurers declined 30% between 2011 and 2020. There are various modalities of health insurer: medical cooperatives, group medicine companies (similar to managed care organizations), insurers, mixed companies, and services that also offer insurance of their own (large hospitals, i.e.). These modalities are similar in how they operate in relation to care for beneficiaries. Those that differ most are the vertical or mixed companies, which, at the same time, insure and provide services through their own networks, which allows them greater control over service utilization.

There are three modalities of health plan: outpatient, hospital (with or without obstetrics), and dental, which vary by service coverage, accredited facilities and type of accommodation. One modality that, although not regulated, is widespread among the poorer strata of the population comprises extremely inexpensive plans that cover only doctors' appointments. There are no studies of the impact of these plans on access to, and the quality of, healthcare, but they are known for restricted access and a congruence with out-of-pocket expenses on complementary tests and specialist referrals. The ANS's absence from inspection and oversight of these plans aligns with the plans' persistent plans to reduce mandatory coverages to draw in lower-income clients and expand the market. In 2018, the then health minister, a known advocate of the private sector, set up a working group to prepare what he called "accessible plans." The initiative was aborted after numerous criticisms, but the goal of expanding the market by way of cheap plans offering little coverage remains. Even the cheap plans legalized to date generally offer a much smaller service network. The number of accredited hospitals, for instance, can vary by up to 62% between plans offered by the same operator (Instituto Brasileiro de Defesa do Consumidor 2018).

Health plan coverage is potentially inequitable because it is segmented by income, race, schooling, and region. In 2019, of Brazilians with income up to one-quarter of a minimum wage, only 2.2% had some kind of private health insurance, as against 86.8% of those with income of more than five times the minimum wages. Among Whites, 38.8% held private health insurance, as compared with 20.1% of Blacks. The higher the level of education, the greater the likelihood of holding private health insurance coverage, ranging from 16.1% among those who had no schooling or failed to complete lower secondary school to 67.6% among those with higher education (IBGE 2020b).

Also evident are regional disparities in insurance coverage, which remained unaltered in the 2013 and 2019 National Health Surveys. The Southeast, South, and Midwest regions, which are the wealthiest, displayed the highest percentages of private coverage (37.5%, 32.8%, and 28.9%, respectively), and the poorest regions, the North and Northeast, the lowest (14.7% and 16.6%, respectively). By states, percentage private coverage was well above the national mean in São Paulo, the wealthiest state, and the federal capital, Brasilia (38.4% and 37.4%, respectively). At the other extreme are states such as Maranhão (5.0%), Roraima (7.4%), and Acre (8.3%) (IBGE 2020b).

The Mix in Provision and Inequities in Service Access

The Brazilian mix is characterized by duplicate (public and private) coverage (OECD 2004; Santos, Ugá, and Porto 2008) because the private sector covers the same medical services as offered by the public system. The former is distinguished by not only direct payment, but also by offering hotel services, free choice of provider, and/or readier access than in the public system. On the other hand, clinics, outpatient facilities, and hospitals can provide services to both the public sector and private health insurance plans.

From a legal standpoint, the public sector can contract private sector services whenever its available capacity is insufficient and providing preference is given to nonprofit private services. However, that complementarity has been turned into regularity and dependence. Although the public sector is the major purchaser, its dependence weakens the ability to regulate the private sector. The trend in the mix is for the private sector to specialize in provision of higher-complexity and better-paying services. For example, the SUS pays 95% of the total cost of renal replacement therapy procedures but has only 10.3% of hemodialysis machines, compared with 83.3% under contract from the private sector. The SUS also bears the cost of 96% of transplants, which are not fully covered by private plans. High-cost treatments, such as for HIV/AIDS, are entirely provided by the SUS. The contracting of higher-complexity services is not offset by lower-cost, high-demand services, such as diagnostic tests, specialist appointments, and less-complex surgical procedures, which are the greatest bottlenecks in the SUS. Equity is undermined in that restrictions on SUS services push its users toward direct purchase. Those who cannot pay are left to wait in long queues in order to access services, which harms individual health.

Viacava et al. (2018), who examined the trajectory of supply in the system, confirmed that the mix has persisted throughout the 30 years of the SUS's existence. Most hospitals in Brazil are private and serve both the SUS and the private system. Between 2006 and 2017, there were reductions in the percentages of both private hospitals that serve the SUS exclusively and in establishments that take only private patients, indicating an intensifying mix in the system. They reported that "while on the one hand the SUS needs private services to guarantee the right to healthcare, the majority of private establishments also depend on public resources, either because they provide services exclusively to SUS patients or are mixed facilities, particularly in the case of hospitals and SADT [Therapeutic Diagnostic Support Service] units" (Viacava et al. 2018, 1755). While the private sector predominates in hospitals and therapeutic diagnostic support services, primary care facilities are almost all public (99.2% in 2017), pointing to the private sector's preference for more profitable services, which undermines equity in the mix. The National Health Survey (Brazil 2020b) found that the largest proportion in Brazil (46.8%) identified the primary healthcare facility as the establishment that they went to most often when in need of care, especially in the North (55.3%) and Northeast (54.1%), which are the poorest regions. Private clinics and surgeries were indicated by 22.9% and public emergency services by 14.1%.

In the SUS, the hospital bed ratio (beds of its own or contracted from the private sector) is 1.4 per 1,000 population, while in the private sector it is around 2.6. In the SUS, the ratio is relatively balanced across regions, although slightly lower in the poorest (PROADESS 2021), and has changed little in recent years. That is because the number of private beds has declined, and public beds have increased in numbers. The reduction in private beds was greater in for-profit private hospitals (−24.6%) than in philanthropic private hospitals (−1.6%) (FBH 2019), indicating a tendency for that sector to concentrate in more profitable and sustainable areas (Viacava et al. 2018).

The public system is better distributed, care is comprehensive, and services are universally accessible, guaranteeing greater equity than in the private system, as has been abundantly demonstrated in the international literature. In the case of Brazil, the public system has always clearly offered greater equity in service utilization, while facing difficulties in access and at the gateway. In the private sector, inversely, entry is easier, and there is less equity in service utilization because it is determined by ability to pay (Lobato 2000). With the expansion of the SUS, especially in primary care, access improved for the most vulnerable groups, although serious bottlenecks remain and are not being solved by the mix or by the voluntary private sector. These bottlenecks are mainly at the secondary level and in access to medicines, raising out-of-pocket spending by individuals and families.

Considering hospital admissions recorded in 2019 for the prior year, 64.6% were through the SUS, with the poorest regions reporting the highest percentages (77.8% in the Northeast and 76.2% in the North), as against 56.4% in the Southeast, the wealthiest region (IBGE 2020b). Vulnerable groups account for a considerable share: Of these admissions, some 90.0% of patients had income of half a minimum wage or less. People with earnings of more than five times the minimum wage represented only 6.8% of admissions via the SUS for their last prior hospitalization. The SUS is also a substantial presence in rural areas, where there were more admissions via the SUS (85.9%) than in urban areas (61.4%) (IBGE 2020b).

There is also a relationship between income and obtaining prescribed medicines. As regards the previous instance of healthcare received, nearly all respondents (94.9%) earning five times the minimum wage or more managed to obtain medicines, while in the lower-income brackets, the percentage fell to 78.6%. Considering the SUS alone, only 30.5% (6.2 million) of people managed to obtain prescribed medicines, and the percentage was lower in the Northeast (IBGE 2020b). Nonetheless, vulnerable groups are predominant in access to medicines through the SUS: People who are Black, have low income, have little schooling, and the elderly account for the larger percentages of those who receive medicines by this route (IBGE 2020b). Although the SUS maintains an extensive schedule of free medicines, these are not always available, while the private sector offers no medicines, except to hospitalized patients. Spending on medicines accounts for about 30% of families' direct spending on healthcare.

At the time of a health necessity, people faced constraints on access for lack of means to pay, inadequate supply, difficulty in getting to the service or product, or other reasons, all of which factors lead to inequities. The families' characteristics revealed different degrees of restriction. In Brazil, 16.4% of people belonged to families that faced some kind of restriction on their access to medicines and, 26.2%, to health services. Restricted access to medicines was due primarily to lack of money (11.0%), followed by product supply (4.9%). This also occurred with restricted access to health services: The chief reason was lack of money (16.9%), followed by lack of the product or service (8.1%). Although the SUS is important for enabling the most vulnerable groups to access services, restricted access to both medicines and health services affected families with Black people more, the main reason being lack of money. As compared with families in which the person of reference was White, there was a 5.9% difference in restricted access to medicines and 7.15% in access to health services (IBGE 2020b).

Difficulties in access, which can occur in both the private sector and the SUS, require services to be purchased directly and make the system more complex. As direct purchasing is generally limited to doctor's appointments and low-complexity tests, it has to mesh with both the SUS and the private health insurance sector, introducing yet another layer in the mix and further undermining equity. The relationship among the public and private systems and direct purchasing is intense and mediated by health personnel, particularly doctors, who generally work in both public and private sectors. The private health insurance sector restricts utilization by refusing services, even when guaranteed by contract, or by diverting demand for the more expensive procedures toward the SUS, which is common practice as the network largely serves both systems. In Brazil, the intense judicialization of these refusals is camouflaged by the universal nature of the SUS; that is, the SUS can provide care because it is universal. Although there is provision for the SUS to be reimbursed for care provided to patients with private health insurance, the hazy boundary at the front line makes it difficult for such revenues to be returned, and that difficulty is abetted by the poor ability of the regulatory agency to oversee private health insurance plans.

Contraction of the SUS and Incentives for New Kinds of Mix

The lack of adequate financing for service provision in the SUS is today one of the main factors jeopardizing equity. Chronic defunding of the system has prevented the public network from expanding as hoped, forcing the SUS to contract services from the private sector or leading families to purchase health insurance or pay for services directly. Defunding is associated with policies to reduce public spending and, although less extreme under center-left governments, still entailed shortfalls in funding. Prominent among these policies are the Delinking of Federal Revenues (*Desvinculação dos Recursos da União*, DRU), the Fiscal Responsibility Law (*Lei de Responsabilidade Fiscal*), and, more recently, the Expenditure Cap (*Teto de Gastos*). The DRU, introduced in 1991 and extended regularly ever since, allows part (today 30%) of the federal government's tax revenues to be delinked for the government to use at will in nonhealth areas. One of the innovations of the 1988 constitution was to earmark revenues mandatorily for social security (which, in Brazil, includes healthcare, social insurance, and social assistance); the DRU restricted this funding just as the SUS was coming into being. In 2000 the Fiscal Responsibility Law set up mechanisms to control public spending, especially on payroll, restricting the engagement of the civil servants necessary for the SUS to expand and guarantee universal care through its own services (Lobato et al. 2016).

Instability in funding led to the enactment of a specific law in 2000 to guarantee minimum percentage health expenditure at the three levels of government. Governments' inclusion of expenses not specific to healthcare in these percentages made it necessary to regulate what actually are public health measures and services, which happened only in 2014. Although that regulation was important, the percentages applied to healthcare were never much more than the absolute minimums. The federal government's ability to raise revenues is obviously greater, but its percentage contribution to funding the SUS has declined, increasing the share demanded of states and municipalities: In 2019, SUS funding was 42% federal, 26% state, and 32% municipal. Municipalities contributed, on average, 24% of their revenues to the SUS in 2016 and 2017 (Funcia and Bresciani 2019).

In 2016, shortly after the impeachment of the center-left president, Dilma Roussef, and the installation of a conservative government, the Expenditure Cap Law was passed, introducing a new fiscal regime that drastically limited public expenditures, significantly impacting social policy spending. The new regime limits expenditures to their 2017 levels, correcting only for inflation, for a duration of 20 years, until 2036. Although the measure is designed to control public spending, it applies only to primary expenditures, thus excluding public debt maintenance payments—which thus remain limitless.

We know of no other measure as radical to control public expenditures anywhere in the world. Its effects on healthcare and equity have been dramatic because it disregards future needs connected with population aging, alterations in epidemiological profile and health demands, or the incorporation of technology, research and innovation necessary to a public system that covers a population of 210 million. Ortiz and Funcia (2021) noted that expenditures decreased between 2017 and 2019,[1] and that, in practice, the new regime precludes any increase in health expenditures because it permits increases to occur only if offset by reductions in other areas.

This defunding of the SUS has been accompanied by mounting tax benefits granted to the private sector; these grew fivefold between 2003 and 2011 and have been increasing yearly ever since (Mendes and Weiller 2015). The benefits comprise mainly tax waivers on medical expenses and private health insurance premium payments by both individuals and corporations. As these are payments made by the wealthier strata of society, this constitutes a regressive and inequitable distribution of public health funds.

In spite of the funding constraints, another modality of mix—private management of health facilities—has grown in Brazil. Service outsourcing, another result of policies designed to contain public spending and restrict the size of the state, is intended to transfer management of public health facilities to the private sector. This most commonly takes the form of what are known as "social organizations" (*organizações sociais*, OSs). The issue is highly controversial, and no national diagnostic studies have yet been conducted on the subject. Nonetheless, a growing number of studies have noted adverse effects on equity. Management by OSs generally increases access, but as it is based on contracts, the services specified do not guarantee hierarchically organized care, thus opening up cracks in its comprehensiveness (Lobato 2016). OSs must be nonprofit associations, and, accordingly, they benefit from exemption from several taxes. However, several of them are connected with large, private, for-profit corporations and, in fact, constitute a form of transfer of funds to the private sector (Travagin 2017). Morais et al. (2018) saws OSs as representing a growing trend towards " 'active privatization,' where the State stimulates the formation of a domestic market in health, extends the modalities by which public funds are transferred to the private sector and guarantees the legal instruments for operationalizing this new model, in a context in which the logic of the market is becoming the defining factor in the directions taken by national health policy" (Morais et al. 2018, 3).

Final Remarks

The public/private mix in Brazil is simultaneously the result of structural inequalities, accentuated in the context of governments that restrict the public attributions due to alliances with the commercial private sector and, in a two-way street, reinforce and perpetuate existing inequalities.

Analysis of health policy in Brazil indicates the enormous challenges that have to be met in order to reduce health inequalities, in view of the dynamics of the capitalist market, and reveals the key role that policy—including the positions of governments and the macro political disputes being waged—can play in how these inequalities are shaped (Machado and Silva 2019). Although this chapter was not intended to explore the political relations that support the contradictions in the Brazilian mix and its effects on equity, the constraints identified in funding and in regressive policies warrant the conclusion that political choices are placing constraints on implementation of the public system, which has been proven to be more equitable and able to contribute to reducing Brazil's historical, structural inequalities.

In the Brazilian case, extended models of social protection have been retrenched at the same time as they were being implemented. Health policy, the most extensive policy in the Brazilian welfare state was universal, comprehensive, and tax funded, creating a single, powerful, decentralized legal, organizational, and institutional structure, with federative participation and incorporating a political dimension by way of official mechanisms for social participation. However, its universal aspirations are still thwarted by constraints on access and segmented coverage. Duplication in the health system, even after 30 years since the public system was instituted, procurement of private services privileging the highest-cost procedures, transfer of public funds to the private sector (by either exemptions or the simple transfer of public facilities to private management) all indicate the persistence of choices that undermine the endeavor to achieve equity. Brazil's public/private mix is not directed to solving the nation's health problems. The legacy of favoring the private sector to the detriment of collective health needs does not seem to have been surmounted. On the contrary, it seems to have worsened, at the expense of equity and, for many, the quality of healthcare.

Note

1. As in all countries, in Brazil, too, the Covid-19 pandemic pressured public expenditures, and the spending cap was temporarily altered. However, if expenditures specific to the pandemic are excluded, 2020 saw yet another decrease in funding for the SUS (Ortiz and Funcia 2021). The spending cap is once again at the center of the national political debate because the economy minister of the Bolsonaro government, who supports the new fiscal regime, proposed altering it to contemplate the increase in the income transfer program that the government wants to introduce. This benefit is considered fundamental to boosting the popularity of President Jair Bolsonaro, which is at a critical level, threatening his chances of being re-elected in 2022.

References

Albert-Ballestar, Sergi, and Anna García-Altés. 2021. "Measuring Health Inequalities: A Systematic Review of Widely Used Indicators and Topics". *International Journal for Equity in Health* 20(1): 73. https://doi.org/10.1186/s12939-021-01397-3

ANS (Agência Nacional de Saúde Suplementar). 2021. *Boletim COVID 2021*. Rio de Janeiro: Agência Nacional de Saúde Complementar.

Benevides, Bruna Nogueira, and Sayonara Naider Bonfim. 2020. "Dossiê dos assassinatos e da violência contra travestis e transexuais brasileiras em 2019." São Paulo, Brazil: Expressão Popular, ANTRA, IBTE. https://antrabrasil.files.wordpress.com/2020/01/dossic3aa-dos-assassinatos-e-da-violc3aancia-contra-pessoas-trans-em-2019.pdf

Brazil. 2020. "Relatório Anual Socioeconômico da Mulher RASEAM 2017-2018." Brazilia: Ministério da Mulher, da Família e dos Direitos Humanos. https://www.gov.br/mdh/pt-br/navegue-por-temas/politicas-para-mulheres/publicacoes-1/SPMRaseamdigital.pdf

Brzsil. 2021a. "Informação e Gestão da Atenção Básica." Ministério da Saúde. https://egestorab.saude.gov.br/paginas/acessoPublico/relatorios/relHistoricoCoberturaAB.xhtml

Brazil. 2021b. "Sistema de Informações sobre Orçamentos Públicos em Saúde (SIOPS)." Brazilia: Ministério da Economia. https://bit.ly/3E6t1kS

Cerqueira, Daniel, ed. 2021. *Atlas da Violência 2021*. Rio de Janeiro: IPEA.

Cordeiro, Hésio. 1980. *A indústria da saúde no Brasil*. Rio de Janeiro: Graal.

FBH (Federação Brasileira de Hospitais). 2019. *Cenário dos Hospitais no Brasil*. Brazilia: FBH/CNS.

Funcia, Francisco Rózsa. 2019. "Subfinanciamento e orçamento federal do SUS: Referências preliminares para a alocação adicional de recursos." *Ciência & Saúde Coletiva* 24(12): 4405–4415. https://doi.org/10.1590/1413-812320182412.25892019

Funcia, Francisco Rózsa, and Luis Paulo Bresciani. 2019. "A Gestão Recente do Sistema Único de Saúde: Financiamento Restringido." VIII Encontro de Administração Pública da ANPAD–EnAPG. Fortaleza, Brazil, from May 16 to 18 2019. Available from http://www.anpad.org.br/abrir_pdf.php?e=MjYwNzM=

Giovanella, Lígia, and Maria Helena Mendonça. 2012. "Atenção Primária à Saúde." In *Políticas e Sistema de Saúde no Brasil*, edited by Lígia Giovanella, Sarah Escorel, Lenaura de Vasconcelos Costa Lobato, José Carvalho Noronha, and Antonio Ivo de Carvalho, 2nd ed. Rio de Janeiro: Editora Fiocruz; 493–545.

IBGE (Instituto Brasileiro de Geografia e Estatística). 2020b. *Pesquisa Nacional de Saúde 2019: Informações sobre domicílios, acesso e utilização dos serviços de saúde.* Brazilia: IBGE. https://biblioteca.ibge.gov.br/visualizacao/livros/liv101748.pdf

IBGE (Instituto Brasileiro de Geografia e Estatística). 2020. *Síntese de indicadores sociais: uma análise das condições de vida da população brasileira: 2020.* Estudos & pesquisas Informação demográfica e socioeconômica 43. Rio de Janeiro: IBGE. https://biblioteca.ibge.gov.br/visualizacao/livros/liv101760.pdf

Instituto Brasileiro de Defesa do Consumidor. 2018. "Planos de saúde baratos têm rede de atendimento reduzida". https://idec.org.br/pesquisa-do-idec/planos-de-saude-baratos-tem-rede-de-atendimento-reduzida-aponta-pesquisa-do-idec.

Lobato, Lenaura de Vasconcelos Costa. 2000. "Reforma Sanitária e Reorganização do Sistema de Serviços de Saúde: Efeitos sobre a Cobertura e a Utilização de Serviços." PhD thesis. Escola Nacional de Saúde Pública, Fundação Oswaldo Cruz, Rio de Janeiro.

Lobato, Lenaura de V. C., José Mendes Ribeiro, and Jeni Vaitsman. 2016. "Public/Private Mix in the Brazilian Health System and the Quest for Equity." *Global Social Welfare* 3(3): 213–221. https://doi.org/10.1007/s40609-016-0069-x

Machado, Cristiani Vieira, and Gulnar Azevedo e Silva. 2019. "Political Struggles for a Universal Health System in Brazil: Successes and Limits in the Reduction of Inequalities." *Globalization and Health* 15(S1): 77. https://doi.org/10.1186/s12992-019-0523-5

Marques, Rosa Maria. 2017. "Notas exploratórias sobre as razões do subfinanciamento estrutural do SUS." *Planejamento e Políticas Públicas* 49: 35–53.

Marques, Rosa Maria, and Francisco Rózsa Funcia. 2016. "O SUS e seu financiamento." In *Sistema de saúde no Brasil: Organização e financiamento*, edited by Sérgio Francisco Piola, Alejandra Carrillo, and Rosa Maria Marques. Brazilia: Ministério da Saúde; 139–168.

Mendes, Áquilas, and José Alexandre Buso Weiller. 2015. "Renúncia fiscal (gasto tributário) em saúde: Repercussões sobre o financiamento do SUS." *Saúde em Debate* 39(105): 491–505. https://doi.org/10.1590/0103-110420151050002016

Menicucci, Telma Maria Gonçalves. 2009. "O Sistema Único de Saúde, 20 anos: Balanço e perspectivas." *Cadernos de Saúde Pública* 25(7): 1620–1625. https://doi.org/10.1590/S0102-311X2009000700021

Morais, Heloisa Maria Mendonça de, Maria do Socorro Veloso de Albuquerque, Raquel Santos de Oliveira, Ana Karina Interaminense Cazuzu, and Nadine Anita Fonseca da Silva. 2018. "Organizações Sociais da Saúde: Uma expressão fenomênica da privatização da saúde no Brasil." *Cadernos de Saúde Pública* 34 (1): 1–13. https://doi.org/10.1590/0102-311x00194916

Oliveira, Ana Paula Cavalcante de, Mariana Gabriel, Mario Roberto Dal Poz, and Gilles Dussault. 2017. "Desafios para assegurar a disponibilidade e acessibilidade à assistência médica no Sistema Único de Saúde." *Ciência & Saúde Coletiva* 22(4): 1165–1180. https://doi.org/10.1590/1413-81232017224.31382016

Oliveira, Jaime Antônio de Araújo, and Sônia Maria Fleury Teixeira. 1989. *(Im)previdência Social: 60 anos de história da previdência no Brasil*, 2nd ed. Petropolis, Brazil: Vozes.

OECD (Organization for Economic Cooperation and Development). 2004. *Private Health Insurance in OECD Countries*. Paris: OECD.

Ortiz, Marilia, and Francisco Funcia. 2021. "Desfinanciamento federal do SUS e o impacto nas finanças municipais." *Estadão*. August 17 2021. https://politica.estadao.com.br/blogs/gestao-politica-e-sociedade/desfinanciamento-federal-do-sus-e-o-impacto-nas-financas-municipais/

PROADESS (Projeto de Avaliação do Desempenho do Sistema de Saúde). 2021. *Laboratório de Informação em Saúde*. Rio de Janeiro: Fiocruz.

Rizzotto, Maria Lucia Frizon. 2015. "O Banco Mundial e o sistema nacional de saúde no Brasil." In *Demolição de Direitos: Um exame das políticas do Banco Mundial para a educação e a saúde (1980–2013)*, edited by João Márcio Mendes Pereira and Marcela Pronko, 255–274. Available from https://www.epsjv.fiocruz.br/sites/default/files/l240.pdf. Acessed on 10 July 2022.

Santos, Isabela Soares, Maria Alicia Dominguez Ugá, and Silvia Marta Porto. 2008. "O mix público-privado no Sistema de Saúde Brasileiro: Financiamento, oferta e utilização de serviços de saúde." *Ciência & Saúde Coletiva* 13(5): 1431–1440. https://doi.org/10.1590/S1413-81232008000500009

Travagin, Letícia Bona. 2017. "O avanço do capital na saúde: Um olhar crítico às Organizações Sociais de Saúde." *Saúde em Debate* 41(115): 995–1006. https://doi.org/10.1590/0103-1104201711501

United Nations Development Program (UNDP). 2019. *United Nations Development Programme. Human Development Report 2019. Beyond Income, Beyond Averages, Beyond Today: Inequalities in Human Development in the 21st Century*. New York: UNO. http://hdr.undp.org/sites/default/files/hdr2019.pdf

Viacava, Francisco, Ricardo Antunes Dantas de Oliveira, Carolina de Campos Carvalho, Josué Laguardia, and Jaime Gregório Bellido. 2018. "SUS: Oferta, acesso e utilização de serviços de saúde nos últimos 30 anos." *Ciência & Saúde Coletiva* 23(6): 1751–1762. https://doi.org/10.1590/1413-81232018236.06022018

Viana, Ana Luiza D'Ávila, and Cristiani Vieira Machado. 2008. "Proteção social em saúde: Um balanço dos 20 anos do SUS." *Physis: Revista de Saúde Coletiva* 18(4): 645–684. https://doi.org/10.1590/S0103-73312008000400004

Vilarinho, Paulo Ferreira. 2010. "A percepção da captura política da saúde suplementar no Brasil." *Cadernos EBAPE.BR* 8(4): 694–709. https://doi.org/10.1590/S1679-395120 10000400009

WHO (World Health Organization). 2021. "Global Health Observatory Indicator Views. *2021.*" https://apps.who.int/gho/data/node.main.GHEDGGHEDGDPSHA2 011?lang=en

World Bank. 1993. *World Development Report 1993: Investing in Health*. New York: Oxford University Press.

World Bank. 1995. *A organização, prestação e financiamento da saúde no Brasil: Uma agenda para os anos 90*. Washington, DC: World Bank.

12

The Public/Private Sector Mix
in Healthcare in Russia

Some Impacts on Health Equity and Quality of Healthcare Services

Tatiana Chubarova and Natalya Grigorieva

Introduction

The very nature of healthcare makes the role of the state in providing medical treatment important. However, the necessity of securing both improvement of population health status and cost containment has shifted debates in health policy toward increasing the input of other partners, including the involvement of the private sector into the healthcare system to improve quality and efficiency, to provide patient choice, as well as attracting additional resources into the health system (Buso 2004). This approach should also be considered within a broader framework of growing private sector influence on public sector performance, as reflected in quasi markets and recent public management ideology (Sigamani 2015; Lapuente and Van de Walle 2020).

Quality of healthcare is considered a core dimension of a healthcare system and thus is a well-shaped concept developed by such international organizations as the United Nations, WHO (World Health Organization), EU (European Union), and OECD (Organization for Economic Cooperation and Development). According to WHO: "Quality of care is the degree to which health services for individuals and populations increase the likelihood of desired health outcomes and are consistent with evidence-based professional knowledge" (WHO 2018, 15). Health equity is often explained as a concept dealing with inequities that result in "differences in health that are unnecessary, avoidable, unfair and unjust" (Whitehead 1992:430). In practice it means that medical treatment should be provided to all in need regardless

Tatiana Chubarova and Natalya Grigorieva, *The Public/Private Sector Mix in Healthcare in Russia* In: *The Public/Private Sector Mix in Healthcare Delivery*. Edited by: Howard A. Palley, Oxford University Press. © Oxford University Press 2023.
DOI: 10.1093/oso/9780197571101.003.0012

of social and economic characteristics such as income, gender, ethnicity, and geographic location (Chang 2002, Mayberry et al. 2006). Combining quality and equity secures improved outcomes of healthcare systems measured as the betterment of people's health status and increased patient satisfaction.

The Soviet healthcare system (*Semashko* model) was a form of delivery of medical care based on a network of the state-owned health services rendering services to the population (Popovich et al. 2011; Chubarova and Grigorieva 2013). Thus, equity was secured via universal access and free-of-charge (at the point of delivery) medical treatment. Industrial medicine was well developed in the former Soviet Union (USSR, Union of Soviet Socialist Republics), including occupational health services. It is a good example of medical care taking into account the wider social environment—first of all dealing with working conditions and also extending horizontal equity (Chubarova 2001). However, the quality of healthcare was not in line with best international standards, especially in the late USSR, mainly because of the lack of innovative medical equipment and drugs.

Reforms implemented in Russia in the course of a transition from centrally planned to a market-based economy led to serious changes in the healthcare system and involved a gradual increase in the scope and influence of the private sector in terms of both finance and provision of healthcare. Thus, how not to compromise equity and access in changing the landscape of financing and delivery of medical treatment was a problem. In this context the composition of the public/private mix (PPM) is important as a way to get maximum outcome of the limited resources that modern society can allocate to healthcare.

The aim of this chapter is to analyze the PPM in Russian healthcare from the point of view of its influence on healthcare system performance and outcomes for patients. It is based on analysis of literature to include both research articles by Russian and foreign scholars and materials published in the press; official statistical data available as well as results of sociological surveys conducted by either independent research groups (*Levada Center* and *VCIOM*) or commissioned by such official bodies as the Ministry of Health and Federal State statistical agency (*Rosstat*).

The chapter consists of three parts. In the first one, a brief overview of PPM from theoretical and conceptual perspectives is presented as the methodological basis for the study. The second part outlines the main characteristics of the PPM in Russian healthcare along the two main dimensions of health system: organizational and financial. In the third part, the evidence available is used to evaluate the impact of PPM on healthcare system functioning in terms of securing both equity and quality of care.

Public/Private Mix: Methodological Approaches

It is generally accepted that the modern economy is "mixed," and different systems of resource allocation coexist—state, market, and nonprofit sectors. Understanding the real mixed economy involves analysis of not only the scope of each sector, but also complex relationships between them. The question we address is about the limit of interaction, beyond which the basic principles of operation of each sector that differ significantly might be distorted. Healthcare ranks high in these discussions as in modern society the role of the state in financing and provision of healthcare is significant. However, at present, there is consensus that it is precisely a mixed economy that is needed in healthcare (Söderlund, Mendoza-Arana, and Goudge 2003; Phua 2017).

It should be noted that health systems in the modern world are a complex of mixed systems rather than pure models. The scope of private finance and provision is often used as a criterion in elaborating health system classifications.

Changes in healthcare systems are also associated with challenges that they face globally. Population aging; rapid development of health technology innovations, including new drugs and information technology; as well as intensified exchange of information and rising patients' demands and expectations are usually mentioned in research as factors that influence modern developments in healthcare.

According to WHO, PPM may be defined as context-specific approaches to involve all relevant healthcare providers—public and private as well as formal and informal—in the provision of quality-assured healthcare (WHO 2009). Though this definition was elaborated in connection with fighting tuberculosis, it can be applied to the health system as a whole. It stresses the importance of engaging all care providers and enhanced collaboration among them in various settings. WHO also pointed to a significant variety of private providers to include, for example, private clinics operated by formal and informal practitioners; institutions owned by private, voluntary, and corporate sectors (e.g., nongovernmental organizations [NGOs]); faith-based organizations; railway health services; and health insurance organizations.

The mixed economy of welfare in economics and pluralism in politics are basic ideas forming modern attitudes to PPM. *Mixed economy of welfare* assumes that the welfare of citizens is provided by various actors. Thus, it does not matter much what the source of welfare is; rather what matters is that the need is satisfied. Thus, the understanding of the welfare state is expanding, including efforts of all actors rather than government per se.

Pluralism is viewed as a political concept in a democratic society, which in the context of a mixed economy recognizes competing interests when different groups can voice their opinions and ideas. Meeting health needs of citizens in different ways also means recognizing different approaches, values, and norms in addressing health problems. Thus, pluralism means that different approaches exist and should be incorporated into health systems' reaction to any problem. In healthcare systems, it is not only the government that is responsible but also societal-based and/or private actors. The state, NGOs, and the market are involved in the field of healthcare (Marmor and Okma 1998; Moran 2000; Powell 2007). Indeed, "the public's interest and the welfare of individual patients need attention by all parties" (Etheredge Jones 1991, 94).

As a result, government's role in the health system is changing. In the *World Health Report 2000*, it was stressed that governments should fulfill the stewardship function, taking responsibility for the welfare of their populations and securing the benefits the population might obtain from all kinds of healthcare providers, including private ones (WHO 2000; Saltman and Ferroussier-Davis 2000). Fulfillment of this task leads to development of new policy instruments, such as regulation or contracting.

The combination of public and private (PPM) emphasizes the importance of relationships between sectors, engaging all stakeholders, and expanding cooperation between them. The task of fostering relationships between sectors is left to the state. Moreover, the idea of the *enabling state* implies that it should not directly intervene in the decision-making and delivery of public goods and services, but rather create conditions for the development of other sectors through partnerships. This approach is based on the recognition of the existence of common social problems, and partnership is defined as an organizational system for making decisions and their implementation, mobilizing a coalition of interests around a common problem. This perspective maintains that the role of the state is to develop cooperation and ensure dialogue between the parties.

It should be noted that in Russia the term PPM is not used, partly because it is difficult to be translated into Russian. More popular is the idea of public-private partnership (PPP) fixed in legislation. It is understood as a legally binding arrangement between a public partner, on the one hand, and a private partner, on the other hand, based on pooling resources and distribution of risks with the aim of attracting private investment into the economy and thus ensuring the availability and improving quality of goods, works, services, the provision of which falls under the state responsibility. Despite official endorsement, PPPs have not actively developed in Russia and have been limited to certain areas, mainly infrastructure projects. Some authors are skeptical about PPP, understanding it as a means of "hidden privatization" as typically PPP agreements in healthcare include arrangements such as the introduction of separate private wards in public hospitals. Also, local authorities might leave premises that are in poor condition to private providers that proceed to renovate and open private clinics. This, for example, was the case with one of the *MEDSI* (the biggest Russian private healthcare provider) clinics in Moscow in the beginning of 2002.

It is also important to define what exactly "public" and "private" mean in any particular national context. Here it is important to separate economic and legal issues. In economics, usually three sectors are distinguished— public, private, and nonprofit. They have their specific characteristics and features.

Despite the presence of the market paradigm, both researchers and politicians express concerns of possible adverse effects of the profit motive and market behavior of those who provide medical services (Chernichovsky 2000). Because of the very nature of the market economy, private providers in healthcare are inevitably motivated by the aim of making a profit, and as a result their objectives might not coincide with the public goal of providing universal and quality healthcare for the whole population. Such a mismatch of objectives results in particular problems in health systems, such as failure to address public health issues, first of all prevention, lack of integration with government health services, attraction of health professionals out of the public sector, and distortions in provision and spatial distribution of medical facilities and equipment. In any case, often in the private sector access depends on the ability to pay rather than need.

It should be noted that profit motive does not necessarily collide with quality considerations as private providers may also be concerned with quality of healthcare. However, it is still not clear whether quality of medical care in private health services is superior to the public ones as there is conflicting empirical evidence, most studies focusing on hospital care (Kruse et al. 2018).

Among positive aspects, the innovative potential of entrepreneurship, greater responsiveness to needs and desires of patients and doctors, modern approaches to management, and attracting investments should be mentioned. However, commercial healthcare providers are often viewed as not in line with the traditional mission and values of health services, a threat to the autonomy and ideals of medical profession, and as undermining social mechanisms that deliver medical treatment to people who cannot afford to pay. This raises a serious health equity question, namely, if it is fair that people that have money get access to better quality healthcare.

However, government failures also should be discussed, including among other things limited organizational and financial capacity that cause problems with meeting the growing population demand for medical care. For example, lack of public resources allocated to public health services might encourage health personnel to move to the private sector (Reyes-Gonzalez 2015). Thus, by attracting private partners, government aims to release pressures on its budget.

At present, influence of the private sector over the public one in both management and financing issues is strengthening in Russia. In a free market paradigm, government can neither abolish nor ignore the private sector. The best choice would be to regulate the behavior of private providers in order to use their potential and capacity to benefit the public interest. There is a variety of mechanisms that the state can use to regulate the private sector. It is the extent of government capacity to design, implement, and monitor the regulatory system that is likely to determine the success of the interaction between the two sectors. Thus, PPM is not only a conceptual enterprise but also can be considered a mechanism of interaction between the two sectors in question.

In the literature, different approaches to analysis of PPM can be found. For example, Cor van Montfort et al. distinguished four levels in understanding PPM, namely systems, organizations, partnerships, and values (Cor van Montfort et al. 2018). Wendt, Frisina, and Rothgang (2009) generated PPM typology based on three core dimensions of the healthcare system (regulation, financing, and service provision) and three types of actors (state, societal, and private actors). This typology is actively used by researchers, for example, for classifying healthcare systems (Böhm et al. 2012, 2013).

Following it, we suggest that in PPM in healthcare the role of the state and market should be discussed from the three points of view, namely:

- regulation and governance;
- organizational structure of healthcare delivery; and
- financing healthcare from various sources.

It is argued that for an individual patient much depends on who is financing, providing, and regulating healthcare rather than the overall level of health system performance. In this chapter, the focus is on the last two dimensions as they develop in a particular context of Russian society. These two dimensions are selected to analyze areas of potential interaction between public and private sectors. In this sense, legal regulation might be considered as a one-way process.

Also, it is important to understand how PPM might influence health system performance in terms of outcomes for patients. Research indicates that an increase in private sector involvement might affect access to healthcare as influenced by income inequalities even in countries like Canada, with high state involvement in healthcare provision and finance (Marchildon and Allin 2016).

Public/Private Mix in Russian Healthcare: Main Characteristics

Organization and Delivery

Official data on the institutional structure of healthcare in Russia mainly relate to the public sector; information on the private sector is much more limited. Quantitative data come from either Rosstat (the Russian State statistical agency) or reports prepared by various consultant agencies that however are distributed for a fee and are quite expensive. Nevertheless, even the data available indicate the gradual expansion of the private sector in Russian healthcare in terms of number of both health services and health personnel.

With the ending of the Soviet Union, Russia inherited a large hospital network, and the number of hospital beds is still quite high (Table 12.1), though constantly decreasing. For the period 2005–2018, the number of public hospitals decreased from 9,186 to 4,938, or almost by half.

Table 12.1. Number of hospitals and hospital beds in Russia

	2005	2010	2015	2016	2017	2018
Total						
Number of hospitals:	9,479	6,308	5,433	5,357	5,293	5,257
Including nongovernmental	293	224	245	266	294	319
Including private	—	115	180	205	241	259
Number of hospital beds, thousands, total:	1,575.4	1,339.5	1,222.0	1,197.2	1,182.7	1,172.8
Including nongovernmental	32.4	21.7	24.1	23.5	25.4	27.0
Including private	—	4.1	12.8	12.9	15.2	17.3
Per 10,000	110.9	93.8	83.4	81.6	80.5	79.9
Urban						
Number of hospitals	5,820	4,959	4,397	4,351	4,297	4,275
Including nongovernmental	286	216	239	263	288	309
Including private	—	110	176	203	236	252
Number of hospital beds, thousands, total:	1,365.9	1,186.1	1,060.1	1,041.0	1,026.9	1,018.7
Including nongovernmental	32.1	20.2	21.8	22.2	23.0	24.4
Including private	—	3.4	12.1	12.7	14.6	16.5
Per 10,000	130.3	112.5	97.6	95.5	93.9	93.1
Rural						
Number of hospitals	3,659	1,349	1,036	1,006	996	982
Including nongovernmental	7	8	6	3	6	10
Including private	—	5	4	2	5	7
Number of hospital beds, by hundred thousand, total:	209.5	153.4[a]	161.9[a]	156.2[a]	155.8[a]	154.1[a]
Including nongovernmental	0.3	1.6	2.3	1.3	2.4	2.6
Including private	—	0.68	0.6	0.2	0.6	0.8
Per 10,000	55.6	40.9	42.7	41.4	41.5	41.3

Source: Rosstat 2019a.

It should be noted that the logic of reforms changed during post-Soviet years. At the beginning the government just wanted to decrease the number of hospital beds in health services. However, later so-called optimization implied both restructuring and shrinking of the number of health services, with one of the main arguments savings on administrative expenses and rational use of resources. "Efficient use of hospital beds" in practice means mostly a reduction in their total number. But the question remains open if such a re-duction is justified in terms of securing access, taking into account spatial distance factors, as the share of rural population in Russia is high, while pop-ulation density in rural areas is relatively low.

At the beginning of the 2000s serious efforts and money were put into modernization of health systems in regions to both improve technological aspects of healthcare delivery and change patient flow. As a result, many public health services all over the country were able to get new equipment and renovate premises. It should be noted the idea of privatization of public health services has never been discussed in Russia.

As the total number of hospitals decreased, the number of hospitals and hospital beds in the private sector has, on the contrary, increased from 115 in 2010 to 259 in 2018 (Table 12.1). As a result, its share of the total number of hospitals also increased during the period in question, from about 2% to almost 5%, respectively. The number of hospital beds grew even faster—from 4,000 in 2010 to 17,300 in 2018, or more than four times. It should be noted that private hospitals are established predominantly in urban areas.

Between 2010 and 2018, the numbers as well as capacity (visits per shift) of private primary care services mostly organized as *polikliniks* increased from 2,753 to 4,866, or by 30% (Table 12.2). Policlinik is an outpatient health ser-vice that provide both general and specialist examinations, including some

Table 12.2. Primary care services in Russia

	2005	2010	2015	2016	2017	2018
				Public		
Numbers	17,172	12,173	13,985	14,117	14,465	14,424
Capacity (visits per shift, thousands)	3,401.2	3,420.7	3,493	3,500	3,518	3,529
				Nongovernmental		
Numbers	4,043	3,175	4,098	4,494	5,185	5,224
Capacity (visits per shift, thousands)	192.5	226.6	316.6	358.3	390.2	407.0
				Including private		
Numbers	—	2,753	3,749	4,168	4,837	4,866
Capacity (visits per shift, thousands)	—	138.2	252.7	291.5	327.6	348.7

Source: Rosstat 2019a.

Table 12.3. Numbers of healthcare personnel in Russia, selected years

	2005	2010	2015	2016	2017	2018
Total- thousands	**4,357.3**	**4,464.0**	**4,347.2**	**4,328.5**	**4,109.9**	**4,173.1**
Including						
Government	1,837.7	2,059.8	3,550.2	3,588.1	3,374.8	3,423.6
Municipal	2,242.6	2,120.8	343.0	255.2	234.1	205.8
Private	173.1	202.8	367.1	401.3	424.6	460.7
Nongovernmental, including faith organizations	29.5	25.6	23.5	22.8	22.3	21.1
Mixed Russian ownership	56.9	38.5	35.1	30.8	26.3	28.9
Foreign and mixed with Russian participation	17.5	15.7	27.5	29.4	27.8	31.4
Total	**100**	**100**	**100**	**100**	**100**	**100**
Including						
Government	42.2	46.1	81.7	82.9	82.1	82.0
Municipal	51.4	47.5	7.9	5.9	5.7	4.9
Private	4.0	4.5	8.4	9.3	10.3	11.0
Nongovernmental, including faith organizations	0.7	0.6	0.5	0.5	0.5	0.5
Mixed Russian ownership	1.3	0.9	0.8	0.7	0.6	0.7
Foreign and mixed with Russian participation	0.4	0.4	0.6	0.7	0.7	0.8

Source: Rosstat 2019a.

diagnostics procedures under the same roof. Though the number of public primary care services fluctuated slightly, their capacity increased as well.

In the current decade, there is a tendency for the number of doctors and nursing staff to increase (see Table 12.3). The number of personnel working in the private sector is growing in both absolute and relative terms. For the period 2005–2018, it increased from 173,100 to 460,700. Thus, its share in total health employment also increased from 4% to almost 11%.

Rosstat also provides information on average wages of healthcare workers employed in public and private sectors (Table 12.4). Surprisingly, according to official statistics the difference is not as much as one would expect, taking into account the relatively lower wages in public health services. Even more,

Table 12.4. Average nominal wages in health services by form of ownership

	2005	2010	2015	2016	2017	2018
			Rubles			
Average, total	5,906	15,724	**28,179**	**29,742**	**31,980**	**40,027**
Including						
Government	6,603	18,407	28,699	30,266	32528	41,213
Municipal	5,172	12,761	22,616	23,157	24948	30,867
Private	6,844	18,252	26,316	27,118	29385	33,754
Nongovernmental, including faith-based organisations	6,101	13,978	23,347	25,198	26026	29,286
Mixed Russian	7,500	15,523	28,548	27,865	29665	35,203
Foreign and mixed with Russian participation	11,976	34,376	58,983	64,142	71380	74,445
		As share of average wage in health sector				
Average, total	100	100	**100**	**100**	**100**	**100**
Including						
Government	112	117	102	102	101.7	103.0
Municipal	88	81	80	78	78.0	77.1
Private	116	116	93	91	91.9	84.3
Nongovernmental, including faith organizations	103	89	83	85	81.4	73.2
Mixed Russian	127	99	101	94	92.8	87.9
Foreign and mixed with Russian participation	in 2.0 times	in 2.2 times	in 2.1 times	in 2.2 times	In 2.2 times	186.0

Source: Rosstat 2019a.

average wages in the private sector since 2010 have lagged behind those in the public sector. Two reasons might be suggested to explain the situation. First, recently the Russian government undertook massive measures to increase wages in healthcare. Second, it seems that in private health services accounting techniques may be used that appear to lower its wages in order to decrease social security taxes. In actuality, the highest wages are recorded in health services belonging to either foreign or mixed foreign-Russian entities, which are usually more careful with taxation issues. Besides, in the public sector it is a common thing that medical staff perform two functions instead of one; for example, a doctor or a nurse may work two consecutive shifts instead of one. This increases salaries but also means an increase in the workload that is likely to lead to lower quality of healthcare delivery.

Financing

Healthcare in Russia is financed from two sources—public and private. Public sources include compulsory health insurance (CHI) and budget appropriations, while private ones include voluntary private health insurance and out-of-pocket payments (OPPs) (Table 12.5).

In the 1990s Russian GDP dropped dramatically, and resources devoted by the state to public needs had decreased. This was reflected in government health financing, and as a result people had to mobilize private resources. Several important points should be made in connection with this.

The share of public funds devoted to healthcare is quite stable, about 3%–3.5% of GDP, which is very low according to the practice of developed countries.

The share of private finance is high and amounts to about 40% of total current health expenditures in Russia. But what is more important, private expenses mostly consist of OPPs, meaning people pay at the point of receiving medical treatment. The share of OPP amounted to almost 93% of private health expenditures in Russia in 2018. This system of financing is considered by WHO as the most regressive, contributing to horizontal health inequity by putting at a disadvantage those who cannot afford to pay.

Also, voluntary health insurance (VHI) is a controversial issue in Russia. Among the reasons to have VHI in the presence of CHI covering the entire population, experts name low quality of medical care in the underfunded public sector. However, VHI in Russia is rather poorly developed. Typically,

Table 12.5. Health expenditures in Russia, selected years

Indicators	2000	2005	2010	2015	2017	2018
Current health expenditure (CHE) as percentage of GDP	5	5	5	5	5	5
Domestic general government health expenditure as percentage of CHE	59	61	61	59	57	59
Domestic private health expenditure as percentage of CHE	40	39	39	41	43	41
Voluntary health insurance (VHI) as percentage of CHE	3	3	3	2	2	2
Out-of-pocket (OPP) spending as percentage of CHE	30	32	35	39	40	38

Source: WHO, Global health expenditures database.

it is employer based when large mostly foreign companies provide extra healthcare coverage for their employees and sometimes also for members of their families. In some cases, employees might need to contribute. Large corporate clients provide up to 90% of VHI revenues (Kozyrenko and Avdeeva 2019). They provide VHI not only to solve employees' health problems, but also because of broader corporate social responsibility and company image considerations, a social package as part of human resource management.

There are very few individual VHI policies; it is obvious that Russians prefer to contact private clinics directly in case of a particular health problem. Low demand from individual clients is due to low incomes and the high cost of a VHI policy, especially for the elderly. The cost of VHI health insurance for individuals is generally higher than for corporate clients, who have lower expenses due to a higher number of people.

The Russian government does not seem to express a big interest in developing VHI, although it gives some tax incentives for both companies and individuals, for example, exemption of money spent on VHI up to 6% of payroll when calculating a tax on profit.

From January 1, 2015, it became mandatory for labor migrants to buy a VHI policy, which led to a certain growth of the VHI market but caused a decrease in profitability due to frequent visits to health services by migrants with serious illness at an insignificant cost of the policy. As a result, in 2017 many insurance companies increased the cost of a VHI policy for labor migrants by 9% in Moscow and by 7% in other regions. At the same time, corporate VHI programs did not change (Suslyakova 2018).

It should be noted that both public and private health services can provide medical care under VHI. Two basic characteristics of the VHI market should be mentioned. First, VHI is very unevenly distributed geographically, mainly concentrating in Moscow and St. Petersburg. It depends, among other things, on the presence of private medical clinics. In an individual VHI market, almost 66% of contracts and 80% of premiums fall on two cities—Moscow and St. Petersburg. At the end of 2019, the number of contracts by individuals, per 10,000 population, exceeded 1,000 in only 9 regions, while in 11 regions this indicator was less than 100 (DELOVOY PROFIL Group 2021). This can be explained by the low standard of living combined with a high share of rural population and also a small number of health services suitable for VHI programs.

Second, in the VHI market the concentration of providers is very high. Data for the 9 months of 2020 demonstrated that the Top 10 companies accounted for 88.6% of premiums and the Top 20 for 93.4%. *SOGAZ*

JSC remains the leader in terms of premiums, with a 41% market share (DELOVOY PROFIL Group 2021).

At present, VHI contributes to inequality in access to healthcare—not everyone works in large corporations and the contingent covered by them is healthier. There is also an issue of social solidarity—Russian employers keep lobbying lower or even no contributions to CHI, which now amount to 5.1% of payroll, if they pay for VHI.

According to Rosstat, per capita expenditures on medical treatment increased from 764.7 rubles in 2005 to 4,615.4 rubles in 2018. The share of medical treatment in all services for which Russians pay increased from 4.8% to 7% between 2005 and 2018.

The practice of so-called informal payments became widespread in Russia as in other post-Soviet countries in the early 1990s. This included institutional or individual payments to suppliers, in kind or in cash, made outside official channels or paid for services that should be covered by the state. With the reduction of government spending and low wages, paying medical staff directly has become almost a norm. However, the situation changed when state health services were granted the right to charge fees for medical treatment provided in addition to a guaranteed CHI package. Thus, people can now officially pay for medical treatment, with no need for under-the-table informal payments. But the equity issue remains as getting medical care in the instances mentioned above depends on income status.(Chubarova 2019)

Public/Private Mix in Russian Healthcare: Problems and Outcomes

In the PPM in Russian healthcare, the tendency is observed of an increasing role of the private sector, namely:

- a network of private providers in both primary and hospital care is gradually expanding first of all in urban areas (see Table 12.1); and
- the share of private finance in total health expenditures is significant, and OPPs constitute the major share of private health expenditures (see Table 12.5).

The share of "private" in PPM in Russian healthcare is more pronounced in financing than in provision. Public health services can officially offer services for a fee, while private health services can join CHI and receive reimbursement from CHI funds. These parallel developments significantly influence horizontal health equity and quality of healthcare in Russia today.

Starting from 2012, public services can charge fees for certain treatments not included in free government guarantees through CHI, and also one may receive some medical care without a doctor's referral. A patient may also pay for the use of drugs and medical devices as well as medical nutrition that are not included in the standards of medical care. The fee may also be charged when providing medical services not specifically designated, as well as when citizens independently apply for medical treatment. All public health services, especially hospitals, now have special departments dealing with "paying patients," and their websites contain special sections devoted to fee-for-service arrangements.

The main reason for such a development is to improve the financial status of public health services under the conditions of tight public financing. However, there is a big concern—supported by evidence—that health services often make patients pay fees for services that should be provided free of charge (to overcome waiting lists, to visit a certain specialist chosen by the patient). The situation is even more complicated as the paid services are rendered in the same facility, using the same equipment, by the same doctors, etc. as those provided under CHI free of charge. There is a significant distortion of motivation as medical personnel in the public sector is interested in increasing the volume of paid services. Moreover, the expansion of the scope of fee for services is now considered by local health authorities as one of the aims of public health services activities and is used as an important performance indicator. Patients often do not understand why they pay in a public institution; Rosstat survey revealed that about 30.5% of respondents do not know what medical care is free and what is not. The question of fairness arises since citizens who can pay get the opportunity to "jump" the queue, which may not be related to need.

Federal legislation fixes the possibility of obtaining medical treatment under the CHI in health services of any form of ownership. Thus, private health services can join CHI via inclusion into the register of health services operating in CHI as well as having the right to sit in the commission for the development of territorial CHI programs and take part in its activities. The CHI tariffs set in regions within federal regulations are the same for both public and private health services. It should be noted that regional programs of free health care financed from budget appropriations and CHI are adopted annually to fix the level of compensating the cost of medical treatment in health services. Regional tariffs should not be lower than those fixed in the federal program.

Though private health services face difficulties in joining CHI, the latest official data available showed significant growth in the number of private clinics participating in the program of state guarantees for the provision of free medical care to the population funded by CHI. Their number increased from 253 in 2007 to 3,309 in 2020. Thus, the share of private sector clinics operating in the CHI system reached about 36% in 2020 versus 2.2% in 2007. Today, such practice is gradually developing in almost all Russian regions. The range of medical treatment provided by the private sector is expanding from mostly dental and diagnostic services to offices of general practitioners providing primary care, consulting and diagnostic centers, multiprofile clinics, and rehabilitation centers. The composition of private services largely depends on regional needs as private clinics often cover the deficit in certain types of treatment in the public sector.

The hemodialysis procedure is an example of development of PPM. The first private hemodialysis center was opened on the basis of emergency hospital No. 10 in Voronezh region in 2012. According to the latest data available (2018), approximately 45,000 patients receive hemodialysis in Russia; an annual growth rate of 10% and 80% of the need for this procedure is covered by private medical centers. A number of private health services (the most well known and active being Fresenius Medical Care) participate in hemodialysis and peritoneal dialysis projects that develop within the PPP framework (https://medvestnik.ru/content/news/Chastnye-dializnye-centry-obedini lis-v-otdelnuu-associaciu.html).

Initially, private dialysis centers were established in different regions (Nizhny Novgorod, Kazan, Voronezh, Yaroslavl, Lipetsk, Primorsky kray) where there was high unsatisfied demand that the public sector could hardly cope with. It possible to provide services to people in need of chronic life-saving renal replacement therapy and to eliminate waiting lists for receiving hemodialysis. Their services were compensated via CHI. The opportunity to receive guaranteed money from both the CHI and clients' base turned out to be attractive for private hemodialysis centers. Thus, their role became significant, and in some regions they become monopolists.

However, the situation with CHI finance is not that optimistic: The share of private sector in CHI spending is not big, though increasing; in 2007, private clinics received 1.2 billion rubles from CHI, while in 2020 the figure was about 148.5 billion rubles, or 8% of the total CHI expenses. As an illustration, in 2016, the cost of inpatient care provided in private clinics accounted for 1.8% of funds allocated to public health services; outpatient care, including dentistry 4%; and day hospitals 15%.

The private sector claims that one of the main obstacles that prevent it from joining CHI is low CHI tariffs, which are the same for all health services operating in the CHI system regardless of the form of ownership. However, public health services—unlike private ones—receive budget appropriations for equipment and renovation above CHI set levels of compensation. But entering CHI secures the flow of patients who may potentially also use fee-for-service treatments, thus generating additional money for private clinics.

It should be noted that the CHI package is rather comprehensive and covers almost all medical treatments. Initially, some high-tech treatments were provided via special quotas administered by regional and federal health authorities. But at present, they are being gradually included directly into CHI coverage. However, there is still a possibility for a patient to pay to get these treatments in private or public hospitals first of all to avoid waiting lists and administrative bureaucracy.

Thus, in the Russian healthcare system medical treatment can be obtained for a fee in both private and public health services. As a result, competition for patients' money between them is strengthening. This is more prevalent as in recent years state-owned healthcare facilities increased their competitiveness thanks to modern technological equipment and improved customer service supported by state money while the fees they charge are typically less than in the private sector. This is likely to make less-solvent patients seek fee-for-service treatment in public rather than private health services.

It is argued that such a situation in the Russian health system might be referred to as *inverse quasi markets*. Usually in quasi markets the demand is determined by the state money, while in the field of supply, health services of various forms of ownership compete for public money. In Russian inverse health quasi markets, the demand is created by the private (patients') money, and public health services compete formally or informally for private finance with private and nongovernmental providers.

Another issue is increased competition for doctors as an increase in salaries of medical personnel in public health services made it more difficult and more expensive for private clinics to attract and retain good doctors; this is especially relevant to regions with a shortage of qualified medical personnel.

In addition, health insurance companies acting as intermediaries between CHI funds and health services (both public and private) are private entities.

The question arises of a legitimacy of such use of taxpayers' money. Private insurers are interested in profit, which leads to an increase in administrative expenses. The data showed that up to 20% of the CHI funds were spent on intermediaries and an increase in the workflow in this regard. In addition, problems arise in organizing delivery of services with various government agencies. One of the important areas of activities of insurance companies as independent institutions is protection of patients' interests. However, this function could be also be performed by noncommercial or state organizations. Difficulties in debugging the mechanisms of interaction within the CHI system led to the emergence of so-called private insurance brokers, based in health insurance companies, yet another intermediary in the CHI system (Table 12.6).

The Rosstat survey shows that most respondents use public sector facilities, especially in primary care. The share of the private sector is rather substantial in consultants' visits (25%) and diagnostics (19%). In the case of the latter, it is evident that some people use both the public and private sector. The active use of private consultants is explained by recent assignment of a gatekeeping function to primary care physician. Only they can refer patients to certain consultants under CHI.

Table 12.6. Use of health services and payment arrangements in Russian PPM, percentage of respondents

	Primary care	Consultants	Medical tests (diagnostics)
Used public health services, including municipal and those belonging to state departments	95.8	84.4	90.1
Used non-public health services	4	25.4	19.1
Used services of private individual doctors	0.17	1.9	0.5
Other	0.02	0.05	0.05
Received treatment free of charge (CHI)	93	80	87.5
Received treatment for fee, for personal money (OPP or via VHI)	6.1	33.9	23.8
Treatment paid by employers (VHI or individual bills)	0.7	1.3	1.8

Source: Rosstat 2019b.

Among those respondents who paid for diagnostics, 32% mentioned that visiting the public health service was inconvenient (queue, waiting times, etc.), 25.6% indicated that the quality of care in the private sector is better, 22% mentioned the diagnostic procedure was not available in the local public health service, and 13.8% said the visit was suggested by a public doctor. Those who chose to pay for such consultants mentioned first of all quality of care (35.6%), inconvenience of seeing public consultants (26.3%), and absence of a necessary consultant in local public service (19.5%). For 10.5% of respondents, visiting a private consultant was suggested by a public doctor.

All these developments make it quite difficult to evaluate the impact of the composition of PPM on healthcare system functioning. Typically, two problems attract attention in society when the outcome of health system performance is discussed, namely, access and quality of care. The findings of recent research on health expenditure in 13 OECD countries from 1981 to 2007 suggested that the degree to which health services are socialized is regarded as the product of a trade-off between the desire to redistribute income through the fiscal system and the losses some citizens will incur when the public healthcare system expands. Greater income inequality and a higher proportion of an aging population were found to be associated with a smaller share of public health expenditure in total health expenditure (Mou 2013).

The expansion of private finance and provision definitely increased patients' ability to exercise choice in the health system as some people can now seek medical treatment choosing a particular health service or consultants. This also helps to lessen the burden on the public system as some patients now may receive treatment in private health services. Three interesting observations may be made in connection with this.

First, the Levada Center (Analytical Center of Yuri Levada 2016) study showed that the lower the income of the respondents, the more likely they are to apply in case of need to public health services; this option was mentioned by about 80% of respondents from low- and middle-income groups and 66% of respondents from the very affluent group. However, this situation can be looked at from another angle: Wealthy citizens willingly use the free public system.

Second, rich people spent more on healthcare than poor in both absolute and relative terms. The share of expenditures on medical services in total expenditures of the population on services is growing from the first to the top quintile: 1.45% for the 1st quantile, 2.86%- for the 2nd, 3.56%—for the 3rd, 4.50% for the 4th, and 6.92% for the fifths, respectively in 2018. The ratio of the absolute costs of medical treatment between the fifth and the first quantiles was 24.5 times (Rosstat 2019a).

Third, data from the International Social Research Program (ISSP) showed that a significant share of Russian respondents (67.7%) believed that it was unfair that people with higher incomes can afford better health-care than people with lower incomes, while the overwhelming majority of the respondents (93%) thought that the state should be actively involved in healthcare (Kislitsyna 2018). This was confirmed by the 2019 Rosstat survey—93% of respondents considered the increase of fee for services as a negative development damaging health equity and overall quality of health-care for those unable to pay.

It should be stressed that, formally, every Russian citizen is entitled to CHI "on request"; he or she just needs to apply. Thus, the attitude to those covered by CHI is equal in a sense that there is no legally fixed preferences in the federal legislation for providing medical treatment because of income, age, gender, or geography. Rather, there might be some priorities depending on disease; recently, an increased number of measures were introduced by the state to improve services for cancer and cardiology patients. So, both hor-izontal and vertical equity are claimed to be preserved in the public sector. Still, several risks for equity should be highlighted.

Formal entitlements do not often become real ones—the main factors being size of regional resources allocated for healthcare. However, re-gions have some flexibility in health policy within the framework of federal regulations as well as administering many federal arrangements.

In CHI, all citizens are treated equally, but some groups of the population enjoy privileges for drugs and extra healthcare—related services including rehabilitation (staying in a sanatorium), dentures, medical devices—or, for example, free or a 50% discount for drugs and medical devices. The "health" privileged groups include first of all pensioners and the disabled and, in the case of drugs, patients with certain types of disease. Recently it was announced that those suffering stroke and infarction will receive necessary medicine for free.

Some basic preferences are fixed in the federal legislation, but regional authorities can expand the list at their own discretion. In some regions, monthly payment for nutritious food was introduced as measure of social support for the poor. It is given to pregnant and lactating women, as well as children under 3 years of age, subject to doctor's prescription (Moscow, Tyumen, Voronezh, Penza, and Leningrad regions).

Improving medical care for the rural population is one of the most urgent problems of quality and equity in Russian healthcare as about one-third of Russians live in rural areas. However, low access in rural areas is a problem of other large countries as well. In Russia, population density is very low, and the transportation problem is acute.

Data in Tables 12.1–12.4 show that the number of health services and medical personnel in rural areas is much lower than the country averages. The 2019 Rosstat survey (2019b) revealed that seeking medical care was lower in rural areas, but self-medication was more widespread than in the cities. In most rural areas, people can receive medical treatment mostly in feldsher-obstetric points—about 30% use them for primary care, according to the survey data (Rosstat 2019b). (Feldshers are equivalent to physician assistants.) The numbers of feldsher-obstetric points were reduced during modernization reforms, but recently the government policy changed, and they are considered a good solution to provide such primary care in rural settings. Also, medical aviation in emergency cases and mobile health services, such as special medical trains, are considered important in providing access to medical treatment for rural population.

Private medicine is not well developed as it is quite difficult for private providers to operate in the countryside, but 20% of respondents still used private medicine, just a bit less than 26% in urban settings. There were 51% of respondents who received consultant services in other places within the region, 23% of them in the regional center. Thus, people living in rural areas often have to travel elsewhere to receive quality medical care.

To sum, PPM developing in Russian healthcare fee for service is expanding, which might threaten health equity but increase choice and improve the quality of care for those who can pay. The situation is complicated and difficult to analyze as, on one hand, a person might get free treatment at private health services that join CHI, and on the other hand, under certain conditions the person may be asked to pay for public health services.

Recently in Russian healthcare, a number of government initiatives were undertaken aimed to improve both access and quality of care. High-technology treatments should be mentioned as well as construction of pre-natal centers. Modern equipment was purchased and a number of health facilities renovated. Some health status indicators have improved, such as all life expectancy at birth, though some other indicators do not meet developed country standards.

Nevertheless, some discrepancy can be observed between certain positive results, which are fixed in statistics and reports of governmental bodies such as the Ministry of Health and population self-rated health and attitudes to health system. According to sociological surveys, the majority of respondents are not satisfied with their health status and the state of the health system. According to the Levada Center survey conducted for 12 years (2002–2014), the satisfaction rate ranged from 11% of respondents in 2002 to 31% in 2014, with an almost constant number of those who are strongly dissatisfied: 23% in 2002 and 21% in 2012. Probably together with the increasing necessity to pay fees for quality care it is the reason why about 50% of Russians who do not visit health services in case of need prefer self-medication (Rosstat 2019b).

The Rosstat 2019 survey also revealed problems with access connected with the spread of fee for service in Russia. Of respondents, 27.7% had access to fee for services without any or with minor restrictions, while 11.3% of respondents had no access due to lack of funds, for 1.2% more this was due to other reasons, making 12.5% total. However, the majority—59% of respondents—think they would face serious restrictions necessitating cutting expenses for other purposes in case they need to pay for healthcare.

In order to evaluate the outcomes of emerging PPM in Russian healthcare, its financial and institutional implications should be placed into a broader societal context.

In the course of transition in Russia the role of the state in society as well as in healthcare has changed with the emergence of strong individualistic ideology (Chubarova and Grigorieva 2013). In the early 1990s the notion prevailed that the state should withdraw from direct participation in the economy by providing space for private sector and market self-regulation. Such general principles have been automatically transferred to the social sector, including healthcare. In the early years of reform, hopes were high that the market would regulate the relationship between all the actors in the health system, which led to a decreasing role of government in healthcare in post-Soviet Russia.

Among the trends that contributed to financialization of healthcare, the following should be mentioned. First is the changing role of the medical profession, which seems to be adapting quite well to modern market realities; and second is the stress on behavioral factors in understanding determinants of health and evident underestimation of such social factors as income, employment, education, and housing.

Thus, it is suggested that in healthcare financing the role of "individual," rather than just private, financing is growing. As a result, social solidarity is undermined to the extent that the system becomes individualized by greater reliance on fee per service.

The problem of social solidarity is aggravated by high levels of inequality as well as a complicated situation with poverty. The Gini coefficient is 4.1, meaning that Russian society is highly polarized. It is a well-known fact that without redistributive mechanisms high income inequality means also inequality in other areas of social life, including access to healthcare. In such conditions, low levels of state financing results in barriers for people seeking to access health services. Here an important dilemma is whether to support measures to increase people's incomes so they can purchase medical treatment in the market or develop state or other collective forms of financing and provision of healthcare.

Conclusion

We have noted that the national government has made some significant efforts to upgrade medical technology and the availability of critical pharmaceuticals. It has also made significant efforts to upgrade the availability of access to needed healthcare in rural areas.

Nevertheless, limited public resources allocated to healthcare in Russia has not only impeded real access to healthcare for large population groups, but also led to a change in the direction of relevant policies. Government has shifted some responsibilities for healthcare to the individual's responsibility. Therefore, the role of private finance seems to have been gradually institutionalized in the health system. Institutions are likely to continue to develop based on the importance of "individual health financing." In order to deal with the equity and quality issues related to the increasing use of fee for service, some recent development of private hospitals and services, and in order to fulfill universal access to quality healthcare, there needs to be some increase in public resources for underserved areas and for patients whose incomes are not sufficient to meet their healthcare needs. Also, the further development of collective forms of prepayment might help to improve such equity and quality of care.

To conclude, in PPM in Russian healthcare, the "private part," especially in finance, is expanding. The competition between public and private sectors for patients is underway as public health services expand their fee-for-service activities. Still, the relatively large public sector, despite all its problems, provides the possibility for people to obtain a basic level of medical treatment regardless of income status, thus providing a guaranteed minimum level of treatment for individuals with healthcare needs. However, a targeted increase in the financing of the public sector together with building up its administrative capacity is likely to contribute to health equity in forming a better balance between public and private sectors in PPM in Russian healthcare.

References

Analytical Center of Yuri Levada. 2016. *The Confrontation of Logics: The Doctor, the Patient and the Authorities in the Context of Reforming the Healthcare System* [in Russian]. Final report. Moscow, Levada Center.

Bloom, Gerald, and, Hilary Standing. 2001. *Pluralism and Marketisation in the Health Sector: Meeting Health Needs in Contexts of Social Change in Low and Middle-Income Countries.* IDS Working Paper 136. Brighton, UK: Institute of Development Studies.

Böhm, Katharina, Achim Schmid, Ralf Götze, Claudia Landwehr, and Heinz Rothgang.2012. "Classifying OECD Healthcare Systems: A Deductive Approach." TranState Working Papers 165, University of Bremen, Collaborative Research Center 597: Transformations of the State.

Böhm, Katharina, Achim Schmid, Ralf Götze, Claudia Landwehr, and Heinz Rothgang. 2013. "Five Types of OECD Healthcare Systems: Empirical Results of a Deductive Classification." *Health Policy* 113(3): 258–269.

Buso, D. L. 2004. "Public-Private Health Sector Mix—Way Forward. *South African Family Practice* 46(9): 5–8.

Chang, W. 2002. "The Meaning and Goals of Equity in Health." *Journal of Epidemiology Community Health* 56: 488–491.

Chernichovsky, Dov. 2000. *"The Public Private Mix in Modern Health Care System—Concepts, Issues and Policy Options Revisited."* Working Paper no. 7881. NBER, Cambridge MA, USA

Chubarova, Tatiana. 2001. "Occupational Welfare in Russia with Special Reference to Health Care." PhD thesis. University of London, The London School of Economics and Political Science.

Chubarova, Tatiana. 2019. "Inequality of Access to the Health System in Russia: The Case of Out-of-Pocket Payments." In *Social Policy, Poverty, and Inequality in Central and Eastern Europe and the Former Soviet Union Agency and Institutions in Flux*, edited by Sofiya An, Tatiana Chubarova, Bob Deacon, and Paul Stubbs., 87–104. Stuttgart, Germany: Ibidem Press-Verlag.

Chubarova, Tatiana, and Natalya Grigorieva. 2013. "Patterns of Health Care Reforms in Economies Under transition: A Case of Russia." In *Health Reforms in Central and Eastern Europe: options, obstacles, outcome*, edited by James W. Björkman, and Juraj Nemec, 173–192. Hague: Eleven Publishing.

Cor van Montfort, Li Sun, and Ying Zhao. 2018. "Stability by Change—The Changing Public-Private Mix in Social Welfare Provision in China and the Netherlands." *Journal of Chinese Governance* 3(4): 419–437. https://doi.org/10.1080/23812346.2018.1522733

DELOVOY PROFIL Group. 2021. "Analytical Research. VHI Market in Russia: Development Prospects" [in Russian]. https://delprof.ru/upload/iblock/a69/DelProf_Analitika_Rynok-DMS.pdf

Etheredge, Lynn, and Stanley Jones. 1991. "Managing a Pluralist Health System." *Health Affairs* 10(4): 93–105.

Kozyrenko, Elena, and Lilia Avdeeva. 2019. "Current State of Financing Healthcare in Russia" [in Russian]. Astrakhan State Technical University. Series: Economics 1: 153–164.

Kruse, Florien M., Niek W. Stadhouders, Eddy M. Adang, Stef Groenewoud, and Patrick P. T. Jeurissen. 2018. "Do Private Hospitals Outperform Public Hospitals Regarding Efficiency, Accessibility, and Quality of Care in the European Union? A Literature Review." *Health Planning and Management* 33(2): e434–e453. https://doi.org/10.1002/hpm.2502

Kislitsyna, Olga. 2018. "Perception of Injustice of Inequality in Access to Health Care by Russians and Its Determinants" [in Russian]. *Sotsial'ney aspekty zdorov'ya naseleniya.(e-journl).* №3 (61). http://vestnik.mednet.ru/content/view/981/30/lang,ru_ru.cp1251/

Lapuente, Victor, and Steven Van de Walle. 2020. "The Effects of New Public Management on the Quality of Public Services." *Governance* 33(3): 461–475. https://doi.org/10.1111/gove.12502

Marmor, T. R., and K. G. H. Okma.1998. "Cautionary Lessons from the West: What (Not) to Learn from Other Countries' Experience in the Financing and Delivery of Health Care." In *The State of Social Welfare*, International Studies on Social Insurance and Retirement, Employment, Family Policy and Health Care, edited by P. Flora, P. R. de Jong, J. Le Grand, and J.-Y. Kim. Aldershot, UK: Ashgate; 327–350.

Marchildon, Gregory P., and Sara Allin. 2016. "The Public-Private Mix in the Delivery of Health-Care Services: Its Relevance for Lower-Income Canadians." *Global Social Welfare* 3: 161–170. https://doi.org/10.1007/s40609-016-0070-4

Mayberry, Robert M., David A. Nicewander, Huanying Qin, and David J. Ballard. 2006. "Improving Quality and Reducing Inequities: A Challenge in Achieving Best Care." *Proceedings (Baylor University Medical Center)* 19(2): 103–118. https://doi.org/10.1080/08998280.2006.11928138

Moran, Michael. 2000. "Understanding the Welfare State: The Case of Health Care." *British Journal of Politics and International Relations* 2(2): 135–160.

Mou, Haizhen. 2013. "The Political Economy of the Public-Private Mix in Health Expenditure: An Empirical Review of Thirteen OECD Countries." *Health Policy* 113(3): 270–283.

Phua, Kai Hong. 2017. "Universal Health Coverage and Public-Private Participation: Towards a New Balance? *Global Health Journal* 1(2): 3–11. https://doi.org/10.1016/S2414-6447(19)30078-8

Popovich, Larisa, Elena Potapchik, Sergey Shishkin, Erica Richardson, Alexandra Vacroux, and Benoit Mathivet. 2011. "Russian Federation: Health System Review." *Health Systems in Transition* 13(7): 1–190.

Powell, Martin, ed. 2007. *Understanding the Mix Economy of Welfare.* Polity Press; University of Bristol.

Reyes-Gonzalez, Jose Antonio. 2015. *A Critical Assessment of the Mixed Economy of Welfare: Lessons from the UK and Spain*. School of Social Policy and Sociology, University of Nottingham.

Rosstat. 2019a. *Health Care in Russia. Statistics*. Moscow: Rosstat.

Rosstat. 2019b. "Results of the Selective Observation of the Quality and Availability of Services in the Spheres of Education, Health and Social Services, and Promotion of Employment of the Population in 2019." https://rosstat.gov.ru/itog_inspect

Saltman, Richard B., and Odile Ferroussier-Davis. 2000. "The Concept of Stewardship in Health Policy. *Bulletin of World Health Organization* 78: 732–739.

Sigamani, P. 2015. "Delivering Health Services under New Public Management: Is It a Good Model for Emerging Economies?" *Indian Journal of Public Administration* 61(1): 160–168. https://doi.org/10.1177/0019556120150111

Söderlund, Neil, Pedro Mendoza-Arana, and Jane Goudge, eds. 2003. *The New Public/ Private Mix in Health: Exploring the Changing Landscape*. Geneva: Alliance for Health Policy and Systems Research.

Suslyakova, Olga. 2018. "Market Development Prospects for Voluntary Medical Insurance in Russia" [in Russian]. *Nauchno-metodicheskiy elektronnyy zhurnal «Kontsept»* N9 (September): article 1840051.P. e1-e8 http://e-koncept.ru/2018/184051.htm

Wendt, Claus, Lorraine Frisina, and Heinz Rothgang. 2009. "Healthcare System Types: A Conceptual Framework for Comparison." *Social Policy & Administration* 43(1): 70–90.

Whitehead, Margaret. 1992. "The Concepts and Principles of Equity in Health." *International Journal of Health Services* 22: 429–445. (First published with the same title from Copenhagen: World Health Organization Regional Office for Europe, 1990 [EUR/ICP/RPD 414].)

WHO. 2000. *The World Health Report 2000. Health Systems: Improving Performance*. Geneva: World Health Organization.

WHO. 2006. Engaging all health care providers in TB control: guidance on implementing public-private mix approaches. Geneva, World Health Organization, 2006 (WHO/ HTM/TB/2006.360).

WHO. 2018. *Handbook for National Quality Policy and Strategy—A Practical Approach for Developing Policy and Strategy to Improve Quality Of Care*. Geneva: World Health Organization.

13

Taiwan: Achievements and Challenges in a Single-Payer System

Michael K. Gusmano

Introduction

Taiwan has one of the most celebrated healthcare systems in the world. After a decade of planning and incremental reform, it implemented a universal, single-payer healthcare system in 1995. It is a highly equitable system with universal coverage, and healthcare spending is low compared with most advanced healthcare systems in the world. Although many countries have achieved universal coverage, only a few have implemented a single-payer system of the kind that exists in Taiwan. Not surprisingly, advocates for single-payer healthcare systems frequently point to Taiwan as an illustration of why they support this approach.

In this chapter, I discuss the evolution of Taiwan's system and provide an overview of its structure. Next, I discuss its performance, with a particular focus on the degree to which the system has achieved equity in access to healthcare services. Finally, I identify some of the challenges that the system faces, including the perceived inadequacy of the government's health-care spending for achieving a high quality of healthcare services, which has involved the underuse and overuse of healthcare services (National Partnership for Women and Families 2009; Physicians for National Health Program 2017).

Establishing Taiwan's Single-Payer System

After a decade of planning, Taiwan adopted the National Health Insurance Act, which established its single-payer national health insurance system in 1994. It fully implemented the new system by March 1995, less than a year

Michael K. Gusmano, *Taiwan: Achievements and Challenges in a Single-Payer System* In: *The Public/Private Sector Mix in Healthcare Delivery*. Edited by: Howard A. Palley, Oxford University Press. © Oxford University Press 2023. DOI: 10.1093/oso/9780197571101.003.0013 after the law's adoption (, Tsung-Mei Cheng 2020; Hsiao 2019). Before the implementation of national health insurance, Taiwan had multiple public health insurance funds, which only covered 59% of the population. Each of the 10 public insurance schemes in Taiwan covered a particular group, many of which were linked to employment status. This is an approach common to many Bismarkian systems with universal coverage, but in the case of Taiwan, large portions of the public were left out of the system, and some of the funds failed to extend to the dependents of those who qualified. In particular, the fund for employed workers did not cover their family members. Before the adoption of reform, the country had "highly stratified systems" with little or no coverage at all for millions of its poorer citizens (Reinhardt 2008).

Along with limited health insurance coverage, there were complaints that the previous public health insurance funds were inefficient and corrupt, and there was evidence that some providers were filing fraudulent claims (Hsiao 2019). There were also complaints about the adequacy of the healthcare workforce, the hospital infrastructure, and the quality of care (Hsiao 2019). At best, the quality of the healthcare available in Taiwan was "highly variable" and depended on the income of the patient (Reinhardt 2008). As I discuss below, this is a problem that national health insurance helped to minimize, but did not eliminate.

Political Reform and the Health Policy Agenda. By the mid-1980s, political changes in Taiwan, coupled with its growing economy, helped to move health reform onto the policy agenda. For decades following Mao Zedong's victory in the Chinese civil war, Taiwan was governed by an authoritarian one-party system dominated by General Chiang Kai-shek and his Nationalist Party (Fell 2018). In an effort to establish a family dynasty, Chiang Kai-shek was succeeded in office by his son, Chiang Ching-kuo in 1975. Despite continuing the authoritarian system established by his father, Chiang Ching-kuo began a gradual process of liberalization, including the promotion of more native-born Taiwanese to government office and efforts to expand the social welfare system. By 1986, pro-democratic leaders formed Taiwan's first opposition party, the Democratic Progressive Party (DPP). By 1991, lifetime legislators were forced to retire. In 1992, Taiwan held its first full parliamentary election. In 1994, Taiwan-born Lee Teng-hui, who had been selected by Chiang Ching-kuo as his successor, became the first directly elected president.

Although political reform contributed to the eventual adoption of the national health insurance system, the government took steps to improve the healthcare system even before the expansion of formal democratic reforms. Under Chang Kai-shek, the government responded to a combination of political pressure, significant gaps in access to care, and remarkable economic growth, by making improvements to the healthcare system. There was a recognition that the current health system was inadequate and perpetuated inequalities and a growing economic capacity to address it. Starting in the 1950s, the country experienced economic growth that was often referred to as the "Taiwanese miracle." Taiwan began a period of rapid industrialization in the 1950s, stimulated by aid from the US government (BBC News 2019). Thanks to a combination of government policies that promoted manufacturing, currency stabilization that increased the savings rate, and an expansion of education, the gross domestic product (GDP) in Taiwan grew by about 10% each year during the 1960s and 1970s (Olds 2008). The government used some of the country's emerging wealth to address the country's healthcare needs. This included the development of a highly specialized healthcare system (Jan et al. 2017), but it failed to adequately address the need for primary care physicians, something that was not addressed until after the establishment of national health insurance (Wang et al. 2019). Along with the increase in government spending, a number of business groups set up affiliated hospitals. For example, Chang Gung Memorial Hospital was established in 1973 by Wang Yung-ching and Wang Yung-tsai, the founders of Formosa Plastics. This hospital system now operates hospitals in eight locations throughout Taiwan (Rickards 2020).

In 1971, the government established a new Department of Health as a Directorate General in charge of health affairs. This led to an expansion of healthcare resources, particularly in rural areas, in which clinics often had no physicians on staff (Lu and Chiang 2011). These efforts included increasing enrollment in medical schools and the creation of a new hospital construction program (Lu and Chiang 2011). These efforts more than doubled the number of clinicians and increased the number of hospitals and clinics by 57% between 1971 and 1981 (Tables 13.1 and 13.2). This represented a major effort to address the underuse of healthcare services, a component of quality (Figure 13.1).

In 1983, the government worked to address geographic disparities in care through its new "group practice center" program, which established new clinics in underserved areas. To staff these centers, the government subsidized medical schools to send physicians to these centers and allowed physicians working in them to retain 80% of the profits (Lu and Chiang

Table 13.1. Number of registered medical personnel in Taiwan, 1954–2019

Year	Total	Physicians	Doctors of Chinese medicine	Dentists	Pharmacists	Medical radiological techs	Registered & professional nurses	Midwives
1954	10414	3978	1545	709	989	—	1265	1742
1971	18227	6375	1466	910	3304	—	3616	2362
1981	45696	11957	1682	2128	12955	—	13196	2871
1991	96921	21115	2514	5983	18570	1500	41756	1649
2001	165855	30562	3979	8944	24891	3152	85763	518
2010	241156	38887	5354	11656	30001	4913	128955	208
2011	250258	40002	5570	11992	31300	5133	133336	134
2012	258286	40938	5740	12391	32015	5341	137641	120
2013	265759	41965	5977	12794	32668	5507	140915	132
2014	271555	42961	6156	13178	33162	5774	142708	149
2015	280508	44006	6298	13502	33516	5952	148223	150
2016	289174	44849	6441	13912	33908	6164	153509	154
2017	299782	46356	6692	14380	34526	6416	159621	164
2018	312887	47471	6880	14718	34838	6629	167803	179
2019	326691	49542	7096	15126	35316	6840	172966	200

Note: Data do not include Kinmen Country and Lienchiang Country before1993.
Source: Ministry of Health and Welfare

Table 13.2. Number of medical institutions in Taiwan, 1954–2019

End of year	Medical institutions	Hospitals	Hospitals per 10,000 population	Clinics	Clinics per 10,000 population
1954	1,000	—	—	—	—
1971	7,107	—	—	—	—
1981	11,161	—	—	—	—
1991	13,661	821	0.40	12,840	6.25
2001	18,265	637	0.28	17,628	7.87
2010	20,691	508	0.22	20,183	8.71
2011	21,135	507	0.22	20,628	8.88
2012	21,437	502	0.22	20,935	8.98
2013	21,713	495	0.21	21,218	9.08
2014	22,041	497	0.21	21,544	9.19
2015	22,177	494	0.21	21,683	9.23
2016	22,384	490	0.21	21,894	9.30
2017	22,162	483	0.20	22,129	9.39
2018	22,816	483	0.20	22,333	9.47
2019	22,992	480	0.20	22,512	9.54

Note: Data do not include Kinmen County and Lienchiang County before 1993.
Source: Ministry of Health and Welfare.

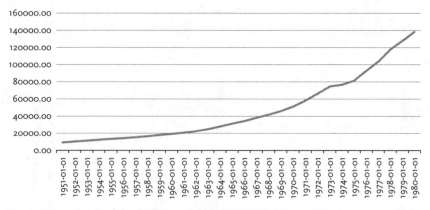

Figure 13.1. Taiwan's real GDP growth in 2017 US$, 1951–1980.

2011). Although this intervention helped to close discrepancies in the geographic access to care, it has not closed this gap. Like other countries that have also adopted incentive programs of this sort (Bärnighausen and Bloom 2009), Taiwan's program has increased the number of physicians practicing in underserved areas (Tikkanen et al. 2020), but challenges remain. Indeed, a study published in 2020 of physician and nurse capacity in Taiwan concluded that there was still a significant gap in medical staff between urban and rural areas, as well as a gap between the mainland and outlying islands (Hu, Chang, and Chung 2020). The authors concluded that these gaps required greater government spending on medical resources (Hu et al. 2020).

One reason the efforts described above fell short was that the expansion of the physician workforce and hospital capacity did not address the significant financial barriers to care faced by a large portion of the country's population. In response, in 1984 the government created a task force to plan for the expansion of the country's social security system, including universal health coverage. The task force was pressured, in these efforts, by the newly established DPP, which made national health insurance an issue about which it criticized the ruling party (Lu and Chiang 2011). Again, these efforts helped, but were insufficient to fully address the problem.

The task force had three goals. The first was to establish universal coverage with equal access to quality healthcare, the second was to improve the efficiency of the system, and the third was to control increases in healthcare spending (Hsiao 2011). To do so, the task force studied health systems in other countries with the hope of adapting practices in other parts of the world to the Taiwanese context (Cheng 2003). To facilitate their work, the task force contacted two prominent health policy scholars in the United States, Dr. William Hsiao from the Harvard University School of Public Health and Dr. Uwe Reinhardt from Princeton University. Reinhardt, a Princeton University economist, recommended that Taiwan's government establish a single-payer system by merging Taiwan's existing public insurance schemes. He argued that the new system should be based on three principles: equity in both access and benefits; effective and egalitarian cost control; and administrative simplicity to help the public understand the system (Cheng 2020). Dr. Hsiao helped the task force organize a 3-day international conference in 1989 with experts from Canada, Germany, Japan, the United Kingdom, and the United States to learn from their experiences. Following the conference, several task force members visited these countries to develop a more in-depth understanding of these systems and how they might be adapted to the Taiwanese context (Hsiao 2011). As Reinhardt noted, the approach led many to call Taiwan's healthcare system "a car made from many parts produced abroad but assembled in Taiwan" (Reinhardt 2008).

Overview of The System

Role of government. The majority of national health insurance systems in the world take the form of "Bismarkian" multipayer systems (Gusmano, Weisz, and Rodwin 2009; Gusmano et al. 2014, 2020). In contrast, Taiwan, like Australia, Canada, and South Korea, relies on a government run "single-payer" health insurance system. In Taiwan, the Ministry of Health and Welfare is responsible for the National Health Insurance (NHI) system and most of the administrative decisions are made by the National Health Insurance Administration (NHIA). Despite important differences among them, all national health insurance systems share certain features in common. Like other systems with universal coverage, the government in Taiwan establishes the benefit package, which is comprehensive and includes inpatient care, outpatient care, prescription drugs, traditional Chinese medicine, dental services, and home nursing care. Payments to hospitals and physicians are established through annual negotiations between the national health insurance fund and providers, and the government establishes an annual budget for the system.

Financing. All countries rely on multiple sources of revenue to pay for healthcare services. The four principal methods of raising funds to pay for health services are (1) general revenue funds through the fiscal tax system; (2) social security/national health insurance (funds from compulsory payroll taxes); (3) private insurance (funds raised through voluntary premiums assessed by private health insurance companies); and (4) out-of-pocket payments from individual patients. National health insurance systems, such as those in Belgium, Canada, France, Germany, Luxemburg, and Japan, tend to be characterized by a dominant share of financing from dedicated payroll taxes. Canada is an exception to this pattern because the dominant share of financing is from general tax revenues (Gusmano et al. 2010).

In Taiwan, the system is financed through a complex combination of payroll taxes, government general revenue, and health insurance premiums. As of 2021, the employee payroll tax rate was 1.4731%, and the employer payroll tax rate was 5.008%. The share of the premium paid by individuals varies considerably and is designed to be redistributive because those with higher incomes pay a larger share of health insurance premiums. For example, self-employed persons pay the entire premium themselves, but the government subsidizes the entire premium for veterans, military personnel, and those in the lowest income brackets (Taiwan Ministry of Health and Welfare 2021). The government has only increased the health insurance premiums twice since 1995, and this has contributed to the system's fiscal challenge. The annual rate of increase in spending on healthcare is 4.83%, but because of a political reluctance to increase premiums and other sources of revenue, the funding for the system has been growing at 4.35% annually. The system has significant reserves, but these are being depleted steadily and placing pressure on the government to look for savings by reducing waste, increasing efficiency, and reducing inflation-adjusted payments to providers (Leong 2018).

The public health insurance system is supplemented by private health insurance for people who can afford it. It is difficult to find estimates of the exact number of people with private health insurance, but reports suggest that the number is growing. There are several for-profit insurance companies that offer plans that cover medical services not already covered by national health insurance. Many of these take the form of disease-specific indemnity plans and are sometimes treated as investments. Private insurance may also be used, as it is in many other countries with universal coverage, to purchase private hospital rooms (Tikkanen et al. 2020).

The system also includes out-of-pocket expenditures on healthcare, but as a percentage of total healthcare spending, it is below the Organization for Economic Cooperation and Development (OECD) average and fell significantly after the implementation of national health insurance in 1995 (Lu 2014). Out-of-pocket spending associated with medical care, dental care, and prescription drugs is about 12% of Taiwan's national health expenditures, compared with an average of about 20% in the OECD. Copayments for outpatient specialist care are modest, but higher if patients do not have a referral from a primary care provider. Taiwan does not use a gatekeeper model, so patients frequently engage in self-referral directly to specialists (Cheng et al. 2019). There are also small copayments for outpatient prescription drugs, but there are limits on how much money people must pay per visit. Copayments for drugs are capped at TWD200 (USD6.6) per outpatient visit regardless of how many prescriptions the patient requires. There is, however, no cap on annual out-of-pocket payments for drugs.

Along with copayments for visits and drugs, there is a coinsurance requirement for inpatient care, so patients are responsible for a percentage of the hospital bill, depending on length of stay and whether they are admitted to an acute (fewer than 30 days) or chronic hospital bed. For patients with an inpatient stay under 30 days, the coinsurance rate is 5% for chronic beds and 10% for acute beds, but there is a cap on coinsurance per hospitalization (TWD38,000 [USD1,254]) and an annual ceiling on coinsurance of TWD64,000 (USD 2,112) for the same condition (Tikkanen et al. 2020).

One study that examined the influence of national health insurance on out-of-pocket spending found that the new system reduced out-of-pocket medical expenditures the most for households with the lowest incomes because it offers a copayment exemption for the lowest-income households (Chu et al. 2005). Similarly, national health insurance helped to address regional inequalities in the financial burden associated with healthcare. The eastern counties of Taiwan, including Taitung, Hualian, and Penghu, are less developed than other parts of the country and have a higher population of indigenous people. The new system adopted several mechanisms designed to increase access to healthcare in these areas. This included offering people living in the mountainous areas in the eastern part of the country and outlying islands an exemption from copayments. The system also provides a higher insurance reimbursement for outpatient physician fees, no limits on the number of insurance-reimbursed visits for patients, and subsidies for transportation costs, including emergency helicopter transportation (Chu et al. 2005). These policies represent important government efforts to enhance vertical equity and provide more healthcare services in areas there were greater needs.

Methods of payment to providers. Taiwan relies, primarily, on fee-for-service payments to physicians in ambulatory care, although it has been experimenting with alternate payment models. Hospital-based physicians are paid salaries with bonuses that are influenced by various measures of productivity. Although overall healthcare spending in Taiwan is quite low by international standards, the government has been worried about the longer-term implications of population aging on healthcare spending. This coupled with limited incentives to guard against the inappropriate overuse of healthcare services led the government to adopt quality and productivity measures and to incorporate these into the physician payment system (S. J. Chang et al. 2011). In 1999, the Department of Health established the Taiwan Joint Commission on Hospital Accreditation (TJCHA) to address hospital efficiency and quality improvement. As they did before adopting national health reform, Taiwan officials examined efforts around the world, including those in the United States and Europe, to develop its own quality metrics and incentive payments (S. J. Chang et al. 2011). In 2000, the country initiated the Taiwan Quality Indicator Project and started collecting data on acute care indicators, psychiatric care indicators, and long-term care indicators (TJCHA 2001).

A few private clinics do not participate in the national health insurance system; nearly all (98%) accept payment from the NHIA to deliver services. There is a single national fee schedule that set by NHIA, but with input from industry stakeholders. The government exerts greater control over this process than in other countries, which rely on corporatists bargaining between the national insurance funds and provider representatives (Anderson et al. 2006; Gusmano et al. 2020). A primary care global budget is divided among and managed by the six NHIA regional offices. To maximize revenue, the clinics within each region compete for patients. As with their French counterparts, Taiwanese physicians have largely resisted efforts to use capitation or value-based payment schemes, and these are accepted by less than 1% of physicians (Gusmano et al. 2020).

To control aggregate hospital expenditures, Taiwan uses a global hospital budget, but within the parameter of the budget, hospitals are paid on a fee-for-service basis with a single national fee schedule. In 2010, Taiwan developed its own version of a diagnosis-related group system (Tw-DRG) for the 50 most common diseases and treatments, so some hospital payments are now based on a case payment scheme, but this represents a small portion of hospital revenue (Yan, Kung, and Chen 2017). Nevertheless, there is some evidence that the implementation of the DRG system reduced the average length of stay in hospitals (Lu and Hsiao 2003). The implementation of DRGs has helped to control spending, but there is more limited evidence on the impact of this system on the quality of care. One study that examined the use of revascularization surgeries for patients with heart disease and knee replacement surgeries found that there was a decline in the intensity of care provided to patients after the implementation of the DRG system, but there were no significant changes in patient outcomes (Wu 2015). This suggests that the implementation of the DRG system may have generated greater value and improved the quality of care.

Organization of care. The delivery system in Taiwan consists of a mix of public and private providers. About one-third of the nation's hospitals are public, and the rest are private, not-for-profit institutions. For-profit hospitals are not allowed to operate in Taiwan. The density of hospitals in Taiwan is 5.7 hospital beds per 1,000 people, which is greater than the OECD average of 4.7 per 1,000 people. The average length of stay in Taiwan is 10 days, which is higher than the OECD average of 7.7 days (OECD Health at a Glance 2019).

With regard to the physician workforce, general practitioners work, primarily, in private clinics, and specialists work in a combination of private clinics and hospital settings. Private clinics are similar to physician offices in the United States, but have a small inpatient capacity for patients who require additional care. This capacity is important for community-based physicians because they do not have hospital admitting privileges (Lu and Hsiao 2003). There are 1.7 practicing physicians per 1,000 people in Taiwan. In contrast to hospital beds, the density of physicians in the country is significantly lower than most of the countries in the OECD, and there are concerns about the adequacy of the healthcare workforce, particularly given the rapid aging of the population (Cheng 2015).

Despite the country's small physician workforce, there is an average number of 12.1 physician visits per person each year, which is comparable to the rate in Japan and significantly higher than the OECD average of 6.8 visits per person (OECD Health at a Glance 2019). The limited number of physicians and high demand for physician visits has led to complaints about the number of hours Taiwanese physicians are forced to work and concerns about physician burnout (Leong 2018). Most physicians in Taiwan work between 80 and 100 hours per week, and they frequently complain about burnout (Leong 2018).

There are also concerns that patients rely too heavily on specialists and engage in "physician-shopping" behaviors (Cheng et al. 2010). The lack of focus on primary care is not new. The shortage of primary care providers preceded the adoption of national health insurance, and efforts to improve the situation, to date, have had limited success. Although family medicine was established as its own specialty in 1988, but by 2015 only 7.8% of the Taiwan's physicians were practicing as family physicians, limiting the system's capacity for care management (Wang et al. 2019). One study examining factors associated with hospitalizations for ambulatory care sensitive conditions found that patients who experienced greater continuity of care were less likely to be hospitalized for these conditions (Cheng et al. 2010). Because the coordination of care in Taiwan is frequently lacking, efforts to improve the continuity of care would serve to improve quality of care (Cheng et al. 2010). To address concerns about the lack of care coordination, Taiwan created the

Family Practice Integrated Care Project in 2003 (Jan et al. 2017). The project creates primary community care networks (PCCNs) made up of primary care physicians from multiple clinics that form a primary care team with an affiliation with at least one community hospital or medical center. To be certified, the physicians in this team are required to take part in a training program that involves administration and education courses (Jan et al. 2017). Before 2009, patient enrollment in the program was voluntary, but the national health insurance administration now enrolls patients with chronic or serious illness that use the healthcare system frequently in order to better coordinate their care and reduce the need for hospitalizations. Patients who are enrolled in this system report high levels of satisfaction and receive more preventive services than other patients in Taiwan. Unfortunately, only about 10% of the population was enrolled in one of these networks as of 2015 (Jan et al. 2017). Nevertheless, for patients enrolled in a PCCN, the outcomes appear to be better. A study published in 2020 found that diabetes care was better among patients enrolled in one of the networks compared with those who were not. Patients in the Family Practice Integrated Care Project were more likely than other patients to complete an annual diabetes examination that included tests for glycated hemoglobin, low-density lipoprotein, urine microalbumin, routine urinalysis, and fundus examination (J. C. J. Chang et al. 2020).

To further strengthen the primary care system, encourage greater care coordination, and reduce wait times for specialists and hospital services, the government set up a referral system in 2016. It is not clear, however, that this system has led to significant changes in physician or patient behavior. One challenge is that the additional costs of self-referring to specialists are relatively low, so most patients do not seek a referral (Leong 2018).

Performance

Access to care. An important dimension of health system performance is the extent to which it provides access to healthcare services. In most countries with universal or near-universal coverage, patients enjoy a relatively equitable distribution of primary care visits across income groups (Van Doorslaer, Masseria, and OECD Health Equity Research Group Members 2004). There is evidence that the introduction of national health insurance in 1995 both increased the use of healthcare services and helped address inequalities in access to ambulatory and hospital care. Among the newly insured, physician visits and hospital stays doubled and reached rates that were comparable to those who had insurance before the reform. Overall, there was a 32.6% increase in physician visits following the implementation of national health insurance, but a 5% decrease in hospitalizations (Gaffney et al. 2021).

But even among countries that provide universal coverage there are differences by socioeconomic status in access to specialty services (Gusmano et al. 2009; Roos and Mustard 1997), and inequalities in access continue to exist in Taiwan as well. For example, a recent study found that residents of Taiwan with incomes below the poverty level have poorer access to trauma care than higher-income residents (L. Kuo et al. 2019). Another study found significant socioeconomic inequalities in 5-year survival among patients with the five most common cancers—liver, colon and rectum, lung, breast, and oral—from 2000–2004 to 2005–2010 (Chien et al. 2018). In addition to studies that have linked poorer access and outcomes to individual-level characteristics, a study by C. Kuo and Chen (2017) found a significant relationship between age-standardized mortality and income of a person's town of residence. According to their analysis, there were almost 30 additional deaths in the lowest income quintile area of Taiwan compared with the highest income area.

Cost. The low cost of Taiwan's healthcare system compared with other advanced healthcare systems around the world is one reason it has been touted as a model for other countries. In 2017, Taiwan's national health expenditures were 6.1% of the country's GDP. This is more than 2% lower than the OECD average (Figure 13.2).

Low spending in Taiwan is also a continual source of concern because critics argue that the system is underfunded, places too much pressure on overworked clinicians, and will be unable to address the needs of the country's aging population without a substantial increase in taxes to fund the system. To illustrate how severely Taiwan has restricted the growth of healthcare spending, one study compared per capita national health expenditures in South Korea, another country in the region with a single-payer national health insurance system, with Taiwan. It found that during this time period, South Korea's health expenditures grew 292% compared with only 83% for Taiwan (Shou-Hsia Cheng et al. 2018). The Cheng et al. study attributed the restriction on spending in Taiwan to the country's global budget cap and, like other observers, expressed concern that these restrictions on spending may be limiting the use of healthcare services.

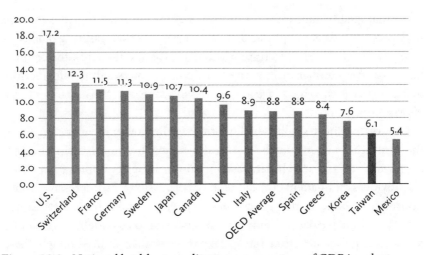

Figure 13.2. National health expenditure as a percentage of GDP in select OECD countries and Taiwan, 2017.
Source: Cheng 2019.

Quality. The focus on quality is a relatively recent phenomenon. For many years, the primary concern of most policymakers, particularly in developed countries, was on overcoming financial barriers to the healthcare system. By the early 1970s, researchers began publishing data that raised serious questions about the quality of medical care and the degree to which clinical decisions are based on evidence. John Wennberg's pioneering research on small-area variations in healthcare delivery, and the subsequent research that it spawned, compared the performance of healthcare systems across small geographic areas (Wennberg and Gittlesohn 1973; Wennberg, Freeman, and Culp 1987). These studies documented extensive variations in rates of hospital admission for certain conditions and rates of surgical procedures between areas that have similar demographic characteristics and similar rates of mortality (Perrin et al. 1990). The findings above suggest that there continues to be unexplained variation in the use of healthcare and in health outcomes within Taiwan (Chien et al. 2018; C. Kuo and Chen 2017; Ling-wei Kuo et al. 2019). One of the concerns with the low level of spending in Taiwan is that it is not sufficient to improve the quality of care available in the system. In 2019, Dr. William Hsiao, who helped the government design the system and has been one of its strongest champions, claimed: "I would like to see the clinical quality of healthcare improved in Taiwan—a real challenge given that quality data are controlled by medical specialty societies that are mostly concerned about physicians' earnings rather than assuring quality of care" (Hsiao et al. 2019). In response to concerns about quality, the country has enacted a number of initiatives, including some small pay-for-performance experiments, but these are limited in scope, and the impact of these efforts is unclear.

One of the most significant investments the government has made in the healthcare system has been in information technology. The national health insurance research database in Taiwan includes information about all providers and patients (Hsiao et al. 2019). Using this impressive health information system, the government generates publicly reported provider performance data on hundreds of quality and cost metrics, including hospital-acquired infection rates (Tikkanen et al. 2020). Although there have been thousands of academic and professional articles published from this database since 2000, the full potential of this database, however, has not yet been tapped (Sung et al. 2020). In addition to privacy protections that limit the availability of the data system, there is about a 2-year lag between when the data are collected and when they are available to researchers (Hsieh et al. 2019). This makes it challenging to generate analysis that is sufficiently timely for policymakers and clinicians. Furthermore, the government offers limited training on how to use the database and does not provide extensive technical support for researchers (Hsieh et al. 2019).

Despite the concerns that quality of healthcare in Taiwan may be uneven and needs to be improved, there is evidence that the expansion of access to care and improvements in quality have generated positive results since the implementation of the national health insurance system. Using broad measures of health status, like life expectancy or mortality rate, to comment on the performance of healthcare systems is problematic because they are not "related directly to the health care system" (Nolte and McKee 2003, 1129) and are influenced by social and economic determinants of health. An alternative is to use concept of mortality amenable to healthcare (amenable mortality), which attempts to capture the consequences of poor access to disease prevention, primary care, as well as specialty services (Nolte and McKee 2012). Of course, few causes of death are entirely amenable, or not amenable to healthcare, and as medical therapies improve, even more deaths may be classified as potentially avoidable. Moreover, the quality of care, including care that is more culturally and linguistically appropriate, not just its volume, may influence this measure.

A cross-national analysis of trends in avoidable mortality in Asia, Europe, and the United States indicated that avoidable deaths have declined much faster over the last three decades than other causes of mortality (Nolte and McKee 2012). This result lends further credence to the validity of avoidable mortality as an indicator for the effectiveness of public health interventions and medical care. More recently, avoidable mortality has been used to evaluate the performance of local healthcare systems in the OECD (Chau et al. 2011).

Examining mortality data from 1981 to 2003, and using the definition of amenable mortality described above, one study found that the adoption of national health insurance in Taiwan led to a significant decline in amenable mortality (Figure 13.3). Specifically, this study found that the adoption of national health insurance led to "a significant acceleration in the rate of decline of causes of death considered to be amenable to health care interventions," but "no clear change in the trend of mortality from conditions not considered to be amenable to health care" (Lee et al. 2010). This is indirect evidence that improvements in access to and quality of healthcare have helped to reduce mortality in Taiwan. If these changes were due to changes in demographics

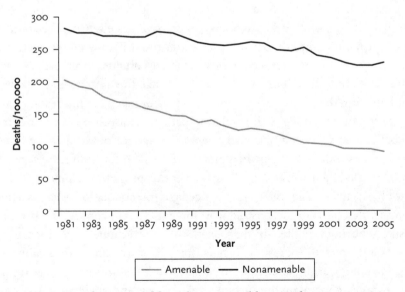

Figure 13.3. Trends in amenable and nonamenable mortality, ages 0–74, in Taiwan, 1981–2005.

Source: Lee et al. 2010.

or broader social conditions only, there would have been a comparable de-crease in mortality not considered to be amenable to healthcare.

Conclusions

During the past quarter century, Taiwan has established one of the most comprehensive healthcare systems in the world. It expanded health insur-ance coverage to more than 99% of its residents. Overall, the implementation of Taiwan's single-payer national health insurance system has been a triumph that has increased access to care and reduced socioeconomic and geographic disparities in access to care. Inequalities in care, particularly among indig-enous populations and those who live in mountainous areas or in outlying islands remain, but in comparison to health systems in the OECD, Taiwan's system is highly equitable. There are currently 16 tribes that are officially rec-ognized by the Taiwan government: Pangcah/Amis, Atayal, Bunun, Paiwan, Pinuyumayan/Puyuma, Rukai/Drekav, Saisiyat, Tao, Thao, Kebalan/Kavalan, Truku, Cou/Tsou, Sakizaya, Seediq, Kanakanayu, and Hla'alua. In addition, there are a number of other tribes that are still seeking official recognition (Teyra 2019).

Despite the clear increase in the use of healthcare services since 1995, through the use of global budgets and aggressive price setting, the country has kept national health expenditures extraordinarily low by international standards. From the perspective of individual patients, healthcare is very affordable. Indeed, critics express concern that the system may insulate patients from the cost of care too much and encourages an unnecessary level of consumption. Along with insulating patients from the cost of care, the global budgeting system has held down the wages of physicians and other clinical personnel at a time when increased demand for healthcare services has increased their workload. Along with concerns that the country has too few physicians to meet the changing needs of the population, there is some concern that parts of the existing workforce may leave clinical practice as a result of burnout. Politically, there seems to be little appetite for increasing taxes for the purpose of raising wages among those working in the healthcare system, but government officials may have to address this in the near future if they hope to maintain the current level of access and quality in the system and to improve access and attention to the healthcare needs of the poorer areas of Taiwan, which include higher levels of the indigenous population.

References

Anderson, Gerard F., Bianca K. Frogner, Roger A. Johns, and Uwe E. Reinhardt. 2006. "Health Care Spending and Use of Information Technology in OECD Countries." *Health Affairs* 25(1): 819–831.

Bärnighausen, Till, and David E. Bloom. 2009. "Financial Incentives for Return of Service in Underserved Areas: A Systematic Review." *BMC Health Services Research* 9(86): 29. https://doi.org/10.1186/1472-6963-9-86

BBC News. 2019. Taiwan profile – Timeline. February. https://www.bbc.com/news/world-asia-16178545 (accessed on June 28, 2022).

Blumenthal, David, and William Hsiao. 2005. "Privatization and Its Discontents—The Evolving Chinese Health Care System." *New England Journal of Medicine* 353(11): 1165–1170.

Cheng, T.M. 2003. Taiwan's new national health insurance program: genesis and experience so far. *Health affairs*, 22(3): 61-76.

Cheng, T.M. 2015. "Universal Health Coverage." *Harvard Public Health Review* 5: 1–12.

Cheng, T.M. 2019. "Health care spending in the US and Taiwan: A response to it's still the prices, stupid, and a tribute to Uwe Reinhardt." *Health Affairs Blog*. February 6. https://www.healthaffairs.org/do/10.1377/forefront.20190206.305164/full/ (accessed on June 28, 2022).

Cheng, T.M. 2020. "The Taiwanese health care system." *International Profiles of Health Care Systems*. New York: The Commonwealth Fund.

Chang, J. C. J., S. J. Hwang, T. J. Chen, Tai Yuan Chiu, Hsiao Yu Yang, Yu Chun Chen, Cheng Kuo Huang, Chyi Feng Jan. 2020. "Team-Based Care Improves Quality of Diabetes Care—Family Practice Integrated Care Project in Taiwan." *BMC Family Practice* 21, 209. https://doi.org/10.1186/s12875-020-01284-w

Chang, S. J., H. C. Hsiao, L. H. Huang, and H. Chang. 2011. "Taiwan Quality Indicator Project and Hospital Productivity Growth." *Omega* 39(1): 14–22. https://doi.org/10.1016/j.omega.2010.01.006Chau, P. H., J. Woo, K. C. Chan, D. Weisz, and M. K. Gusmano. 2011. "Avoidable Mortality Patterns in an Asian World City—Hong Kong." *European Journal of Public Health* 21(2): 215–220.

Cheng, Shou-Hsia, Hyun-HyoJin, Bong-MinYang, and Robert H. Blank. 2018. "Health Expenditure Growth under Single-Payer Systems: Comparing South Korea and Taiwan." *Value in Health Regional Issues* 15: 149–154.

Cheng, Tsung-Mei. 2020. "Taiwan." In *2020 International Profiles*, edited by Rosa Tikkanen, Robin Osborn, Ellias Mossialos, Ana Djordjevic, and George A. Watson. www.commonwealthfund.org.

Cheng SH, and Chiang TL. 1997. "The Effect of Universal Health Insurance on Health Care Utilization in Taiwan. Results from a Natural Experiment." *JAMA* 278(2): 89–93. doi:10.1001/jama.278.2.89.

Chien, Li-Hsin, Tzu-Jui Tsengb, Fang-Yu Tsaic, Jie-Huei Wangc, Chao A. Hsiunga, Tsang-Wu Liuc, and I-Shou Chang. 2018. "Patterns of Age-Specific Socioeconomic Inequalities in Net Survival for Common Cancers in Taiwan, a Country with Universal Health Coverage." *Cancer Epidemiology* 53: 42–48.

Chu, T. B., T. C. Liu, C. S. Chen, Yi-Wen Tsai, and Wen-Ta Chiu. 2005. "Household Out-of-Pocket Medical Expenditures and National Health Insurance in Taiwan: Income and Regional Inequality." *BMC Health Services Research* 5: 60. https://doi.org/10.1186/1472-6963-5-60

Gaffney, Adam, David U. Himmelstein, Steffie Woolhandler, and James G. Kahn. 2021. "Pricing Universal Health Care: How Much Would The Use Of Medical Care Rise?" *Health Affairs* 40(1): 105–112.

Gusmano, M.K., Rodwin, V.G., and Weisz, D. 2010. *Health Care in World Cities: New York, Paris, and London.* Baltimore: Johns Hopkins University Press.

Gusmano, Michael K., Miriam Laugesen, Lawrence D. Brown, and Victor G. Rodwin. 2020. "Getting the Price Right: What Other Countries Do Well." *Health Affairs* 39(11): 1867-1874https://doi.org/10.1377/hlthaff.2019.01804

Gusmano, Michael K., Victor G. Rodwin, and Daniel Weisz. 2014. "Beyond 'US' and 'Them': Access Dimensions of Health System Performance in the US, France, Germany and England." *International Journal of Health Services* 44(3): 553–565.

Gusmano, Michael K., Daniel Weisz, and Victor G. Rodwin. 2009. "Achieving Horizontal Equity: Must We Have a Single Payer Health Care System?" *Journal of Health Politics, Policy and Law* 34(4): 617–633.

Hsieh, Cheng-Yang, Chien-Chou Su, Shih-Chieh Shao, Sheng-Feng Sung, Swu-Jane Lin, Yea-Huei Kao Yang, and Edward Chia-Cheng Lai. 2019. "Taiwan's National Health Insurance Research Database: Past and Future." *Clinical Epidemiology* 11: 349–358.

Hsiao, W.C. 2011. "State-Based Single-Payer Health Care—A Solution for the United States?" *New England Journal of Medicine* 364(13): 1188–1190.

Hsiao, W.C. 2019. "Taiwan's Path to Universal Health Coverage—An Essay by William C Hsiao." *BMJ* 24; 367: l5979. doi:10.1136/bmj.l5979.

Hu, J. L., Chang, M. C., & Chung, H. J. 2020. "Projecting the Target Quantity of Medical Staff in Taiwan's Administrative Regions by the Theory of Carrying Capacity." *International Journal of Environmental Research and Public Health* 17(9): 2998. https://doi.org/10.3390/ijerph17092998

Jan, Chyi-Feng, Shinn-Jang Hwang, Che-Juia Chang, Cheng-Kuo Huang, Hsiao-Yu Yang, and Tai-Yuan Chiu. 2017. "Family Physician System in Taiwan." *Journal of the Chinese Medical Association* 83(2): 117–124. https://doi.org/10.1097/JCMA.0000000000000221

Kuo, Chun-Tung, and Duan-Rung Chen. 2017. "Double Disadvantage: Income Inequality, Spatial Polarization and Mortality Rates in Taiwan." *Journal of Public Health* 40(3): e228. https://doi.org/10.1093/pubmed/fdx179

Kuo, Ling-wei, Chih-Yuan Fu, Chien-An Liao, Chien-Hung Liao, Chi-Hsun Hsieh, Shang-Yu Wang, Shao-Wei Chen, and Chi-Tung Cheng. 2019. "Inequality of Trauma Care under a Single-Payer Universal Coverage System in Taiwan: A Nationwide Cohort Study from the National Health Insurance Research Database." *BMJ Open* 9: e032062. https://doi.org/10.1136/bmjopen-2019-032062

Leong, Siak Hui. 2018. "Health Care for All: The Good & Not-So-Great of Taiwan's Universal Coverage." *News Lens* November 13. https://international.thenewslens.com/article/108032

Lu, Rachel JF, and Chiang TL. 2011. "Evolution of Taiwan's Health Care System." *Health Econ Policy Law* 6(1): 85–107. doi:10.1017/S1744133109990351.

Lu, Jui-fen Rachel. 2014. *Universal Health Coverage Assessment.* Global Network for Health Equity (GNHE), December.

Lu, Jui-fen Rachel, and William Hsiao. 2003. "Does Universal Health Insurance Make Health Care Unaffordable? Lessons from Taiwan." *Health Affairs* 22(7): 77–88.

Nolte, Ellen and C. Martin McKee. Measuring the Health of NationsUpdating an Earlier Analysis." *Health Affairs* 27(1): 58–74.

National Partnership for Women & Families. 2009. "Overuse, Underuse and Misuse of Medical Care. Fact Sheet." National Partnership for Women & Families. http://go.nationalpartnership.org/site/DocServer/Three_Categories_of_Quality.pdf

Nolte, E., and C. M. McKee. 20123. "In Amenable Mortality—Deaths Avoidable through Health Care—Progress in the US Lags that of Three European Countries. *Health Affairs* 31(9): 2114–2122.

Olds, Kelly. 2008. "The Economic History of Taiwan." In *EH.Net Encyclopedia*, edited by Robert Whaples, March 16. http://eh.net/encyclopedia/the-economic-history-of-taiwan/

Physicians for a National Health Program. 2017. "Overuse and Underuse of Medical Care. Right to Healthcare Series." *Lancet Health* January 8. https://pnhp.org/news/overuse-and-underuse-of-health-care/

Reinhardt, Uwe. 2008. "Humbled in Taiwan." *BMJ* 336(7635): 72. https://doi.org/10.1136/bmj.39450.473380.0F

Rickards, Jane. 2020. "Tracking Taiwan's Medical History." *Taiwan Business TOPICS* November 25. https://topics.amcham.com.tw/2020/11/tracking-taiwans-medical-history/

Sung, Sheng-Feng, Cheng-Yang Hsieh, and Ya-Han Hu. 2020. "Two Decades of Research Using Taiwan's National Health Insurance Claims Data: Bibliometric and Text Mining Analysis on PubMed." *Journal of Medical Internet Research* 22(6): e18457.

Taiwan Ministry of Health and Welfare, National Health Insurance Administration. 2021. "How Premiums Are Calculated." https://www.nhi.gov.tw/english/Content_List. aspx?n=B9C9C690524F2543&topn=46FA76EB55BC2CB8

Teyra, Ciwang. 2019. "Who Are the Taiwanese Indigenous Peoples?" https://english. cw.com.tw/article/article.action?id=2495

Tikkanen, Roosa, Robin Osborn, Elias Mossialos, Ana Djordjevic, and George A. Wharton. 2020. "International Health System Profiles: Taiwan." Commonwealth Fund, June 5. ·https://www.commonwealthfund.org/international-health-policy-center/countries/taiwan

TJCHA (Taiwan Joint Commission on Hospital Accreditation). 2001. "The Proceedings of the Second Anniversary of Taiwan Quality Indicators Project (TQIP) Meeting, Taiwan Joint Commission on Hospital Accreditation." Taipei, Taiwan.

Van Doorslaer, Eddy, Cristina Masseria, and the OECD Health Equity Research Group Members. 2004. *Income-Related Inequality in the Use of Medical Care in 21 OECD Countries.* OECD Working Paper. Paris, France: Organisation for Economic Cooperation and Development.

Wang, Y.-J., H.-Y. Liu, T.-J. Chen, S.-J. Hwang, L.-F. Chou, and M.-H. Lin. 2019. "The Provision of Health Care by Family Physicians in Taiwan as Illustrated With Population Pyramids." *INQUIRY: The Journal of Health Care Organization, Provision, and Financing.* 56: 1–10. https://doi.org/10.1177/0046958019834830

Wennberg, J. E., J. L. Freeman, and W. J. Culp. 1987. "Are Hospital Services Rationed in New Haven or Over-Utilised in Boston?" *Lancet* 1(8543): 1185–1189.

Wennberg, J. E., and A. Gittelsohn. 1973. "Small Area Variations in Health Care Delivery." *Science* 182: 1102–1108.

Wu, Jhih-Jhong. 2015. "Implementation and Outcome of Taiwan Diagnosis-Related Group (DRG) Payment System." Master's thesis, Georgia State University. https://scholarworks.gsu.edu/iph_theses/357

Wu, T.Y., Majeed, A., and Kuo, K.N., 2010. "An Overview of the Healthcare System in Taiwan." *London Journal of Primary Care* 3(2): 115–119.

Yan, Y. H., C. M. Kung, and Y. Chen. 2017. "The Exploration of Medical Resources Utilization among Inguinal Hernia Repair in Taiwan Diagnosis-Related Groups." *BMC Health Services Research 17*: article 708. https://doi.org/10.1186/s12913-017-2665-6

Index

For the benefit of digital users, indexed terms that span two pages (e.g., 52–53) may, on occasion, appear on only one of those pages.

Tables, figures, and boxes are indicated by *t*, *f*, and *b* following the page number